AF556717

Recent Advances in the Management of Infertility

NOTICE

Medicine is an ever-changing science. As new research and clinical experience broaden our knowledge, changes in treatment and drug therapy are required. The editors and the publisher of this work have checked with sources believed to be reliable in their efforts to provide information that is complete and generally in accord with the standards accepted at the time of publication. However, in view of the possibility of human error or changes in medical sciences, neither the editors, the publisher, or any other party who has been involved in the preparation or publication of this work warrants that the information contained herein is in every respect accurate or complete. Readers are encouraged to confirm the information contained herein with other sources. For example and in particular, readers are advised to check the product information sheet included in the package of each drug they plan to administer to be certain that the information contained in this book is accurate and that changes have not been made in the recommended dose or in the contraindications for administration. This recommendation is of particular importance in connection with new or infrequently used drugs.

Recent Advances in the Management of Infertility

Editors
Christopher Chen
S.L. Tan
W.C. Cheng

McGRAW-HILL BOOK CO.
Healthcare Group

Singapore Auckland Bogotá Hamburg Lisbon London Mexico Milan
Montreal New Delhi New York Panama Paris San Francisco San Juan
Saō Paulo St. Louis Sydney Tokyo Toronto

Recent Advances in the Management of Infertility

1 2 3 4 5 6 7 8 9 0 CMO PMP 8 9 4 3 2 1 0 9

ISBN 0-07-099144-8

This book was set in Garth Graphic 10/12 pt. by The Fototype Business.

Printed in Singapore

Contents

Contributors

Dr. C. Anandakumar
Department of Obstetrics and Gynaecology, National University of Singapore, National University Hospital, Singapore.

Dr. A. Bongso
Senior Research Fellow, Department of Obstetrics and Gynaecology, National University of Singapore, National University Hospital, Singapore.

Dr. J.K.R. Brodribb
Visiting Obstetrician and Gynaecologist, Queen Alexandra Division, Royal Hobart Hospital, Hobart, Tasmania, Australia.

Dr. C.L.K. Chan
Department of Obstetrics and Gynaecology, National University of Singapore, National University Hospital, Singapore.

Prof. C. Chen
Head and Senior Consultant, Department of Obstetrics and Gynaecology, Kandang Kerbau Maternity Hospital — B Unit; Director, IVF and Gamete Research Centre; Director, National Sperm Bank; Hampshire Road, Republic of Singapore.

Prof. J.F. Correy
Professor of Obstetrics and Gynaecology, University of Tasmania, Hobart, Tasmania, Australia.

Dr. W.C.L. Ford
Senior Research Fellow, University of Bristol, Department of Obstetrics and Gynaecology, Bristol Maternity Hospital, Bristol, UK.

Dr. J.P. Forsey
Clinical Research Fellow, University of Bristol, Department of Obstetrics and Gynaecology, Bristol Maternity Hospital, Bristol, UK.

Dr. R. Fox
Clinical Research Fellow, University of Bristol, Department of Obstetrics and Gynaecology, Bristol Maternity Hospital, Bristol, UK.

Dr. V.H.H. Goh
Department of Obstetrics and Gynaecology, National University of Singapore, National University Hospital, Singapore.

Dr. R.K. Goswamy
Bourn Hall Clinic, Bourn Hall, Bourn, Cambridge, UK.

Dr. P.C. Ho
Reader, Department of Obstetrics and Gynaecology, University of Hongkong.

Dr. M.C. Hsu
Department of Obstetrics and Gynecology, College of Medicine and the Hospital, National Taiwan University, Taipei, Taiwan.

Dr. M.G.R. Hull
Reader and Consultant, University of Bristol, Department of Obstetrics and Gynaecology, Bristol Maternity Hospital, Bristol, UK.

Dr. I. Johnston
Chairman, Reproductive Biology Unit, The Royal Women's Hospital, Melbourne, Australia.

Dr. M.S.W. Kwan
Executive Director, Family Planning Association of Hong Kong.

Prof. T.T.Y. Lee
Department of Obstetrics and Gynecology, College of Medicine and the Hospital, National Taiwan University, Taipei, Taiwan.

Dr. S.C. Ng
Senior Lecturer, Department of Obstetrics and Gynaecology, National University of Singapore, National University Hospital, Singapore.

Dr. J. Parsons
Assisted Conception Unit, King's College Hospital, London, UK.

Prof. S.S. Ratnam
Professor, Department of Obstetrics and Gynaecology, National University of Singapore, National University Hospital, Singapore.

Dr. H. Sathananthan
Lincoln Institute, La Trobe University, Carlton, Victoria, Australia.

Prof. R.W. Shaw
Professor of Obstetrics and Gynaecology, Royal Free Hospital, Pond Street, London, UK.

Dr. C. Sutton
Consultant Gynaecologist, Royal Surrey County Hospital and St. Luke's Hospital, Guildford, Surrey, UK.

Dr. S.L. Tan
Department of Obstetrics and Gynaecology, Kandang Kerbau Maternity Hospital — B Unit; Hampshire Road, Republic of Singapore.

Dr. P.J. Taylor
Bourn Hall Clinic, Bourn Hall, Bourn, Cambridge, UK.

Dr. P.W. Thong
Department of Obstetrics and Gynaecology, Kandang Kerbau Maternity Hospital — B Unit; Hampshire Road, Republic of Singapore.

Dr. P.G. Wardle
Lecturer, University of Bristol, Department of Obstetrics and Gynaecology, Bristol Maternity Hospital, Bristol, UK.

Dr. P.C. Wong
Department of Obstetrics and Gynaecology, National University of Singapore, National University Hospital, Singapore.

Dr. Y.C. Wong
Department of Obstetrics and Gynaecology, National University of Singapore, National University Hospital, Singapore.

Dr. M. Wren
Assisted Conception Unit, King's College Hospital, London, UK.

Dr. Y.S. Yang
Department of Obstetrics and Gynecology, College of Medicine and the Hospital, National Taiwan University, Taipei, Taiwan.

Preface

The field of Infertility or Reproductive Medicine is widely recognised as a subspecialty within the discipline of Obstetrics and Gynaecology. It has made enormous progress over recent years and will undoubtedly continue to do so with the development of the newer reproductive technologies.

In an endeavour to focus on the latest advances in this field, an international symposium on the "Recent Advances in the Management of Infertility" was organised in Singapore in 1988. Leading infertility specialists from various parts of the world came together and imparted the "state-of-the-art" in their respective areas of interest.

This book is the culmination of their efforts. The topics covered are far-ranging and comprehensive. Changing trends in the management of the infertile couple and idiopathic infertility are discussed in the earlier sections of the book. Difficult problems of ovulation and their treatment, including the use of LHRH agonists are then dealt with. This is followed by a discussion on the latest in the management of hyperprolactinaemia and endometriosis. The newer reproductive technologies in assisted conception are given full treatment, including ultrasonography in IVF, GIFT, laboratory IVF, cyropreservation of embryos and eggs, and the microfertilisation of eggs. Sperm dysfunction, antisperm antibodies, immunological infertility, and AID are also given detailed consideration. Finally, the roles of hysteroscopy and lasers are discussed.

It is hoped that this book may serve the needs of many medical practitioners in keeping abreast with the latest in infertility and its management. It is also anticipated that infertility specialists, generalists, and postgraduates in Obstetrics and Gynaecology may find this book of special interest and benefit.

Professor Christopher Chen
Chief Editor

Singapore, 1989

1
Changing trends in the management of the infertile couple

J.F. Correy and J.K.R. Brodribb

Introduction

Prior to 1960, all patients with infertility had ovulation assessed by a basal body temperature (BBT) chart, a biphasic change indicating ovulation, a curettage or endometrial biopsy in the luteal phase of the cycle to demonstrate the appropriate histological transformation associated with ovulation and also the use of cervical mucus changes and vaginal exfoliative cytology. All these methods were used as there was no readily available hormone assay. Tubal function was assessed by hysterosalpingography (HSG) and in some cases practitioners were still using Rubin's test to demonstrate tubal patency.

Irradiation of the pituitary or ovary for ovulation induction was no longer acceptable. Diethylstilbestrol was given to "shock" the pituitary to release luteinizing factors or cortisone if there was evidence of androgen excess (Jeffcoate, 1962). Ovulation induction became a reality following Gemzell's work with human pituitary gonadotrophins (HPG) (Gemzell, 1958) and the use of clomiphene citrate (CC) by Greenblatt in 1961 (Greenblatt, 1961). It was several years before these drugs were to become available in Australia and the steroid assays, essential if the drugs were to be used, were able to be performed. It was not until 1966 that these modalities of treatment could be offered in Tasmania. That year also saw the commencement of laparoscopy in Australia.

Before the advent of gonadotrophins and CC, there was virtually no advance in infertility except perhaps in procedures to establish patency in blocked tubes. Pregnancies occurred after these procedures, as they did after HSG, Rubin's test, or spontaneously after the patient had seen the practitioner. With the experience gained in the in vitro fertilisation (IVF) programmes in patients with clinically diseased and even blocked tubes, it is considered that the operative procedures may not have been as effective as previously thought. From 1983, when the IVF programme in Tasmania was started, 409 patients had 925 cycles of treatment, and 104 clinical pregnancies were achieved. There were, however, 105 spontaneous pregnancies, 54 prior to a treatment cycle and 51 after at least one failed treatment cycle. Approximately 60 per cent of these pregnancies occurred in patients with clinically diseased, and in a few instances, blocked tubes (Correy, 1988).

While there is no doubt that pregnancies do occur in relation to therapies, eg. Danocrine and surgical procedures in endometriosis, CC in ovulatory defects, AIH in mucus/semen problems, and surgical procedures in tubal disease, can it be assumed that such treatments and procedures are indeed as effective as we believe (Collins, 1983)? There have not been adequate controlled, randomised (and, if appropriate, double blind) trials in these conditions. Patients seek attention after a period of infertility and are investigated and treated. In 1971, Schokman and his colleagues (Schokman et al, 1971) pointed out the difficulties of assessing the efficacy of CC. In their series of 71 patients they considered suitable for CC (31 secondary amenorrhea and 40 oligomenorrhea with anovulation), 29 became pregnant on placebo tablets or during investigation.

The authors do not consider the modalities of treatment ineffective but consider that one should not be overconfident in the efficacy of various methods of treatment (Collins, 1983) until such can be shown in a controlled manner.

One problem any practitioner will have in determining pregnancy rates in various conditions, presumably causing infertility, is that patients default at various stages of investigation or treatment. Thus, one can give only the minimum pregnancy rates. Another difficulty in comparing pregnancy rates at various centres is in the criteria for treatment, and particularly the duration of infertility. Our policy, and we believe the policy in reputable centres, is not to investigate or treat infertility until 12 months have elapsed, unless there are pre-existing reasons for the infertility.

Materials and methods

The senior author (J.F.C.), with help from several colleagues, has conducted a Tasmania-wide service in infertility since 1966 in clinics in Hobart and Launceston. Initially, all patients, excluding those with tubal disease, were referred to the clinic, but as more specific modalities of treatment and a wider range of investigations became available to general gynaecologists, the pattern of referral has altered (Brodribb, 1986). Consequently, a larger proportion of referred patients are those who have not conceived after CC or bromocriptine, or after failed insemination with partner's semen (AIH), or after more intensive investigation by the gynaecologists. Furthermore, there has also been an awareness by general gynaecologists in recent years that patients regularly menstruating may not be ovulating or may have ovulatory defects and increasing numbers of patients in this category have also been referred (Brodribb, 1986).

Computer forms for all patients who have become pregnant, moved interstate, transferred to the IVF clinic, signified they wished no further treatment, or have not attended for at least 12 months, have been completed and analysed. All patients currently being treated have been excluded from this study. Every patient's file was reviewed by the senior author (J.F.C.).

The menstrual status has been clinically grouped into the following categories: (a) primary amenorrhea, (b) secondary amenorrhea, (c) oligomenorrhea, (d) regular menses with no greater than six days variation in the cycle, (e) regular or irregular cycles with durations of greater than 35 days but not amounting to oligomenorrhea, and (f) frequent periods.

Although provision is made on the computer form for causes of anovulation or ovulatory defects, because the survey spans 22 years and diagnostic criteria have changed, no attempt has been made to categorise the causes in this manner.

The total number of new patients since 1966, excluding those currently being treated, was 1370. One hundred and sixty five were seen again after a pregnancy had been achieved, making the total number of infertility treatments 1535. One hundred and sixty patients were transferred to the IVF programme and will not be discussed further in this paper.

Only certain aspects of infertility, mainly illustrating trends, will be highlighted in this paper

Results

General features

During the period 1966 to 1987, 1535 patients were seen at the clinics with a complaint of infertility. Of these, 64.2 per cent were primary, and 35.8 per cent secondary infertility. The average ages were 26.6 years and 28.8 years (Table 1-1). Thirty-six patients did not have a designated date of first attendance. There were other patients seen at these clinics with gynaecological cndocrine disorders in whom infertility was not a factor, and for the purpose of this review have not been included.

When related to parity, 64.2 per cent were nulliparous and 33.8 per cent had one or two previous children. However, there were 30 patients who had previously had three or more children, but of these almost all had no children by the current relationship.

Infertility factors

Ovulatory disorders were the most common problems (69.5 per cent overall: 71.2 per cent for primary and 66.4 per cent for secondary infertility). Semen problems were the next most common, 28.5 per cent, while tubal factors accounted for 18.2 per cent of the patients. Mucus problems were found in 12.4 per cent; endometriosis in 5.2 per cent, and unexplained infertility in 1.1 per cent. The combined factors present were ovulatory/tubal factors 10.4 per cent, ovulatory/semen factors 19.4 per cent, and tubal/semen problems 3.8 per cent (Tables 1-2 and 1-3).

Non-attendance at the clinic

For the purpose of assessing the effectiveness of counselling by the staff, particularly the nursing staff, an attempt was made to identify those patients who failed to attend for further investigations, as against patients who elected to cease active investigation, moved interstate, or who were transferred to the IVF programme.

The distribution of infertility factors in the defaulters was similar to the general clinic population, with the exception of patients with tubal factors, in whom the default rate was lower. There was a marked reduction in the percentage of defaulters in the period 1982 to 1987 (Table 1-4).

Pregnancy rates

Overall clinic population

The total pregnancy rate, spontaneous pregnancy rate and the pregnancy rate as a result of specific therapy are shown in Table 1-5. There were a further 25 ongoing pregnancies achieved in 1987 which have not been included in the detailed analysis in this survey.

There is a significant spontaneous pregnancy rate (b of each category) in each of the infertility categories. Even in documented tubal disease, which included complete tubal occlusion at times, there is a spontaneous pregnancy rate from 13.0 per cent to 25.0 per cent.

The defaulters have not been excluded from these results and therefore the figures presented are a minimum pregnancy rate.

Early pregnancy outcome

This has been determined for only three main groups (Table 1-6), ie. ovulatory dysfunction, tubal disease and abnormal semen profiles. There were 81 patients in whom the outcome was not known.

The overall pregnancy rate was 51.7 per cent; ovulatory disorders 57.7 per cent; tubal disease 35 per cent and for semen abnormalities 40 per cent.

The spontaneous abortion rate of 14.7 per cent is higher than that for the community as a whole (9.0 per cent) (Correy, 1987). The overall multiple pregnancy rate was 4.4 per cent, with a rate of 4.2 per cent for those with ovulatory disorders.

Overall, in this clinic population, the ectopic pregnancy rate was 2.2 per cent for pregnancy > 20 weeks, whereas the ectopic pregnancy rate for Tasmania in 1986 was 1.1 per cent for pregnancies of greater than 20 weeks gestation. As expected, the highest ectopic pregnancy rate (8 per cent) occurred in patients with tubal disease.

Patients who had both laparoscopy and HSG

There were four groups comprising 227 patients who had both a laparoscopy and HSG performed. These groups were designated as both normal (group A): normal laparoscopy/abnormal HSG (group B); abnormal laparoscopy/normal HSG (group C) and both abnormal (group D) (Table 1-7).

The pregnancy rate of 45.2 per cent in patients with no abnormality (group A) was 7 per cent lower than that for total patients. The pregnancy rate for patients with demonstrated abnormalities in either the HSG or laparoscopy or both (groups B, C and D) was 40 per cent, which is only 11 per cent less than the pregnancy rate for the total series.

Menstrual status at first visit

The pregnancy rates are tabulated in Table 1-8. Forty-six per cent of the clinic population had regular menses (Category 4); 16 per cent had oligomenorrhea (Category 3); 17.8 per cent had secondary amenorrhea (Category 2), and 11 per cent had long cycles (Category 5). In Categories 3 and 5, ovulatory dysfunction was the major problem (86.6 per cent and 76.1 per cent with tubal and semen defects being of a similar incidence in these two categories. In those with regular menses, only 53.3 per cent had ovulatory defects, with a greater proportion having tubal disease (26 per cent, and semen abnormalities (31.9 per cent).

The pregnancy rates in those patients with ovulatory dysfunction in Categories 2, 3 and 5 were similar and significantly higher (> 12 per cent) than those in the regular menses category. It would appear that this difference is due to the higher proportion of patients in this category having tubal disease and semen abnormalities.

When the ovulatory disorders were associated with either tubal or semen abnormalities, the pregnancy rates were significantly lower (Table 1-5). However, some caution is needed in the interpretation of these subgroups, as the numbers involved are small.

Discussion

There have been difficulties in the collation of data over a 22-year period. This is so because the changes in diagnostic tests, operative procedures and the understanding of the infertility disease processes, combined with the advent of newer modes of therapy, have made the concept of uniformity in investigative and therapeutic processes impossible. As such, we accept it is not possible to apply the rigorous controls that are now becoming widely accepted by clinicians as necessary to interpret the success or otherwise of the various treatment modalities (Lillford, 1987; Olive, 1986).

However, it is possible to analyse the broad experience over 22 years. We have included in our total patient population those patients who defaulted (and hence would tend to reduce the pregnancy rates) as well as other patients who, for one reason or another (poor attendance etc.), we would ideally prefer to exclude as they do not reflect the results of sustained investigation and treatment.

As shown by our results, it is disappointing that for the clinic population, in certain respects such as total pregnancy rates, there has been no change over 22 years (Table 1-5, line c of "overall"). In other areas such as in the defaulting population (Table 1-4), there appears to be a reduction in defaulters occurring toward the latter part of the period of investigation. Finally, we have demonstrated that the continuation of certain procedures, eg., HSG, would not appear to be justified for routine investigation of tubal function, a conclusion others have commented on in recent times (Randolph, 1986; WHO Taskforce, 1986).

In assessing couples with infertility, reliance is placed on published series indicating the relative proportions that each factor contributes towards the overall problem of infertility. This has guided us in a sequence of investigations to allow a maximal detection rate. However, it is necessary that local figures are assessed so as to avoid unnecessary investigations on couples.

Such an example comes from our state where Correy and Schokman (1977) demonstrated, when investigating anovulatory and secondary amenorrheic patients, four of 58 HSG's were abnormal but that with ovulation induction three of these patients became pregnant. Only one of 60 patients who had a laparoscopy had a potentially treatable tubal condition, the implication being that assessment of tubal function was not an essential early investigation in such patients as had been suggested in the past. As well, it only confirms the opinion of others that, although there may appear to be significant tubal disease including bilateral occlusion, pregnancy occurring spontaneously cannot be discounted (Gomel, 1981; Correy, 1988).

In this discussion we will highlight a number of areas that appear to be important to our practice and indicate changing trends in the management of some aspects of infertility. We will not include the more sophisticated and specific regimens of treatment with human menopausal gonadotrophins, follicle stimulating hormone, GnRH infusion or analogues etc., but will refer to these only in the suggested protocols of management.

Infertility factors

It is apparent that in our clinic population there is a very high incidence of ovulatory dysfunction, 69.5 percent overall, and this is so for both primary and secondary infertility. Overall, in both primary and secondary infertility, there is no significant difference in the proportion of other factors, including combined etiological factors. On the basis of previously published data, our expectation would have been for a lower incidence of ovulatory disorders (Hull, 1985; Thomas, 1980; Cox, 1975). Hull et al. reported 21 per cent as having ovulatory failure, Thomas and Forrest in Melbourne reported 50.2 per cent while our incidence is 69.5 per cent. This lends further support to the assertion that it is important to assess the local population in order to understand where the required attention is needed.

The incidence of 20 per cent tubal factors is higher than the 6.5 per cent to 14 per cent reported in other series (Hull, 1985; Thomas, 1980; Cox, 1975). There is a slightly higher incidence of tubal factors in our primary infertility population, 22.9 per cent in primary infertility compared to 20.4 per cent in secondary infertility. Thomas and Forrest in Melbourne also reported a slightly higher incidence in primary infertility, 7.8 per cent as compared to 4.5 per cent.

Semen abnormalities accounted for 28.5 per cent of the overall factors in this series. This compares with 21 per cent (Hull, 1985), 6.2 per cent (Thomas, 1980), and 19.7 per cent (Cox, 1975). Since 1986 we have as a routine investigated male and female partners for antisperm antibody status using the immunobead test. Of a total of 191 men, 11 (5.8 per cent) had significant sperm head attachment of IgG (> 50 per cent). This is similar to reported figures by Harding et al. (1987). The antibody status was also determined in the serum of 183 women and, of these, 3.8 per cent had sperm head attachment of IgG in significant levels (> 50 per cent). Immunological factors would appear to play an important part in infertility, but at this time the status of immunological aspects of infertility, while being intensively investigated, has yet to be fully clarified, particularly in relation to therapeutic procedures, one of which (steroid therapy) is not without significant risks.

The whole subject of antisperm antibodies is unclear because (a) antibodies may occur in the serum of children, (b) they may transiently appear in both males and females, (c) pregnancies may occur in the presence of immobilising antibodies, (d) in vitro fertilisation occurs but pregnancies in patients with immobilising antibodies, particularly in the female, are rare, (e) the post coital test may still be reasonable, and (f) inconsistency in detection of antibodies in various laboratories (Bronson, 1985). At this stage the authors consider that AIH is not helpful in the presence of significant antibodies in the female.

Trends in infertility factors in the clinic population

In Table 1-3 there is a summary of infertility factors given as a percentage of the annual number of patients attending the clinic. It can be seen that overall numbers of patients attending the clinic had progressively increased but there appears to be a reduction in this trend in the last two years. This is probably due to the ready availability of CC to general gynaecologists and the aforementioned changing pattern of referral.

Over the 22 years there has been a gradual reduction in the proportion of ovulatory disorders. This can be explained in several ways. Firstly, the treatment of ovulatory disorders by general gynaecologists with CC. Secondly, the clinic was set up to manage ovulatory disorders, hence it is not surprising that 85 per cent of patients were initially in this category. However, as the clinic developed there were, and are, referrals for other reasons with a consequent dilution effect. Diagnostic methods for ovulation and its disorders have improved, so that we no longer rely on vaginal cytology, cervical mucus and BBT charts to determine ovulation. Basal body temperature charts have been shown to be a poor predictor of ovulatory events (Lenton, 1977; Schokman, 1977), but do have a role in determining the length of the luteal phase, timing of coitus, and timing for various investigations and treatments, and as such are continued in many centres.

Coincident with the fall in percentage of patients with ovulatory dysfunction, there has been an increase in the percentage diagnosed as having tubal disease. This is due in some measure to the more regular use of laparoscopy to assess both tubal and pelvic factors. In 1966, laparoscopy was introduced into gynaecological practice in Australia and since then reports have appeared on its place in investigative gynaecology (Blunt, 1972; Correy, 1973). Even the senior author (J.F.C.), who in 1973 questioned the changing trend to laparoscopy instead of HSG in the investigation of infertility, considers that time has shown HSG is too unreliable in the determination of tubal disease and indeed this has been borne out by our own experience and the experience of others (Randolph, 1986; WHO Taskforce, 1986; Drake, 1980).

Attendance at the clinic

As can be seen from Table 1-3, the patients who ceased attendance of their own volition, as against those who moved from the state or were transferred from the general infertility clinic to the IVF clinic, remained steady at about 27 per cent to 30 per cent until 1981. However, from 1982–1987 the defaulters rate has fallen to 21 per cent and in 1986–87 10 per cent. Most of these have been patients seen at the Launceston clinic. We have considered that the basis of good infertility clinic care is the concept of day to day care, emotionally as well as with regard to the ongoing investigation and treatment. Since 1983 the Hobart clinic has had the services of a fulltime nurse coordinator who, with her staff, has come to know the patients very well and has provided a continuing seven days a week service, including counselling, to the couples. The authors consider that the fall in the rate of defaulters reflects the provision of this service. Since 1983 the services of the nurse coordinator have also extended to one of the author's (J.F.C.) private patients. Of 152 patients, only seven have defaulted, which is further evidence of the value of such a service.

Non-attendance is always a problem because it represents failed effort and a lack of communication and also a loss of investment by the health system, as well as a reduction in the potential for pregnancy. In 1986, Brodribb and his colleagues (Brodribb et al, 1986) were able to show that defaulters who had regular cycles had a pregnancy rate of 40 per cent, whereas the pregnancy rate for those continuing to attend the clinic was 55 per cent. Thus, non-attendance reduced the chance of pregnancy by a third. As has been shown in this series, about 30 per cent of patients attending the clinic achieve a spontaneous pregnancy (Table 1-5). The difference in pregnancy rate between clinic and defaulting patients almost certainly represents the pregnancies as a result of active treatment. Our figures for defaulting patients are higher than have been reported in other series (Thomas, 1980), but we believe this is changing.

The group which defaulted appears to have a similar spread of infertility factors as the clinic population as a whole. One might expect that this would be less in patients with ovulatory disorders, particularly associated with secondary amenorrhea, as the patients will have been advised of a better long term pregnancy prospect, and more with semen or tubal factors with their known lower pregnancy outcomes.

All that this implies is that there is far more involved in defaulting than simply the fertility disorder. Rather, it is a complex mixture of the effect of male and female psyche on personal and social expectations which, coupled with the technical aspects of fertility investigations, some of which involve considerable discomfort or embarrassment, not surprisingly affects couples to the extent that they choose not to continue (Menning, 1980). The authors consider that the fulltime support of a nurse coordinator is invaluable in helping patients and latterly there seems to be some support for this concept.

As infertility is said to afflict up to one in six couples during their reproductive life (Hull, 1985), the aim should be the maximum return on time and on money spent on expensive investigations and treatment.

Pregnancy outcome

As the actual dates of achieved pregnancy in many patients with spontaneous pregnancies was not known, cumulative pregnancy rates could not be ascertained. Therefore we can report only on the percentage of patients who became pregnant in each group and whether those pregnancies were spontaneous or as a result of treatment.

Table 1-5 sets out the percentage of pregnancies occurring: (a) overall, (b) spontaneously, and (c) during treatment cycles.

It can be seen that overall there is no increase in pregnancy rates in the last 22 years, with about 50 per cent of all patients achieving a pregnancy. It can be seen that quite a large proportion of pregnancies achieved are spontaneous and this includes those with oligomenorrhea and secondary amenorrhea, suggesting that the condition was transient in a proportion of patients. This has been discussed in the past by Schokman et al (1971) in relation to Clomiphene therapy, also Brodribb et al (1986) in relation to patients with regular menses.

During the period under review in the group with ovulatory disorders, there has been an increase in the pregnancy rate as a result of therapy, from 28 per cent to 46 per cent. This may partly be explained by the more recent use of bromocriptine, GnRH infusion and the development of ultrasound as an adjuvant to the treatment with pituitary gonadotrophins. The significantly lower pregnancy rate in patients with tubal disease is in line with other published reports, the spontaneous pregnancy rate being not much different than that obtained as a result of treatment. The pregnancy rate in patients with semen abnormalities shows no improvement.

Artificial insemination (AIH) using the "swim up" technique on the partner's semen has been used since October 1984 in a group assessed separately from the general infertility population. Artificial insemination was not used extensively prior to 1984 because of the cramps and shock associated with the use of unwashed semen. One hundred and forty-two patients have been treated, resulting in 36 pregnancies (25.4 per cent). Fourteen of these patients who did not become pregnant had, as well as semen abnormalities, tubal disease and endometriosis. If these are excluded, the pregnancy rate is 28 per cent. This is significantly higher than the overall spontaneous pregnancy rate of 16.3 per cent.

Patients with mucus factors had an overall pregnancy rate of 34 per cent for treated cycles. As the clinic did not provide, until 1983, a full week service, the assessment of mucus quality and the performance of AIH in the past is very likely to have been performed at a convenient time to the doctor rather than the right physiological time of the cycle. Indeed, in the 1986–87 period the pregnancy rate with treatment was 44.4 per cent.

The pregnancy rates in patients who had laparoscopy and HSG performed were similar in all groups (Table 1-7). This is not significant as these procedures were done as a first line investigation before referral to the clinics and without assessment of other infertility factors. As discussed elsewhere, these procedures are now being deferred until the ovulatory status has been determined and ovulatory dysfunction treated at least for several months.

Of the 227 patients who had both procedures performed, 19 (8.3 per cent) had normal laparoscopic findings and an abnormal HSG and 57 (25.1 per cent) had a normal HSG and abnormal laparoscopic findings. Thus, in 76 patients (33 per cent) the HSG was unreliable. Complacency in the presence of a normal HSG may lead to many months of unwarranted, time consuming and expensive investigations and treatment. Laparoscopy has the major advantage in that it allows visualisation of the pelvis for other factors (Randolph, 1986; Blunt, 1972; Drake, 1980; Kessler, 1986; Daly, 1986).

Hysterosalpingography will of course detect intrauterine abnormalities which may be pertinent to infertility such as submucous fibroids, intrauterine adhesions and congenital anomalies. Hysteroscopy in expert hands will not only detect these lesions but enable operative procedures via the hysteroscope to be performed.

The authors consider that HSG should only be performed in the following circumstances:

1. To determine tubal patency after tubal reconstructive surgery.
2. To determine tubal patency in known tubal disease.
3. Hysteroscopy is not available or lack of expertise in this procedure.
4. Failure to demonstrate tubal filling by laparoscopy in the presence of normal appearance of the tubes, probably as a result of leakage of dye around the cannula.

The procedure now followed as a routine is curettage, laparoscopy and hysteroscopy with instillation of methylene blue, having determined and corrected the ovulatory dysfunction.

The overall pregnancy rate in patients with ovulatory dysfunction only was 58 per cent (Table 1-5). The lower pregnancy rate (32 per cent) in ovulatory dysfunction associated with regular menses is explained by the higher proportion of tubal abnormalities (26 per cent as against 6 per cent to 15 per cent for the other groups) and also semen abnormalities (31.9 per cent as against 18.9 per cent, 26.7 per cent and 32.2 per cent) (Table 1-8). This is in keeping with the overall poorer pregnancy outcome in patients with tubal and semen factors. It has been our practice to assess the male and also ovulatory status early in investigations, leaving tubal assessment to later. However, because of the higher proportion of tubal disease in patients with regular menses, even if a patient has an ovulatory disorder, it may be justified to perform laparoscopy and hysteroscopy early in the investigative period. Patients with secondary amenorrhea and oligomenorrhea should have ovulation induced for two to four cycles before such investigations are undertaken (Correy, 1977).

Early pregnancy outcome

For all patients, 77 per cent were singleton, 4.4 per cent were twins, and 14.7 per cent were spontaneous abortion. The ectopic pregnancy rate of 2 per cent is a little higher than the Tasmanian rate overall of 1.6 per cent. Not surprisingly, tubal factors resulted in a high ectopic pregnancy rate (8 per cent). Ectopic pregnancy rate in the group which had semen abnormalities was 3.8 per cent. There does not appear to be a higher than expected incidence of tubal disease in this group and the authors are not aware of such an outcome being previously reported. However, because the numbers are small (two of 28 patients), this cannot be regarded as significant.

The spontaneous abortion rate of 14.7 per cent is higher than the 9.0 per cent incidence of clinical abortions in Tasmania (Correy, 1987). This may be explained by the higher incidence of pelvic disease in infertile patients and a higher incidence of biochemical pregnancies as pregnancy is confirmed earlier in patients undergoing treatment.

General protocol of management of patients

One

A semen analysis (SA), including autoantibodies, is performed unless this has been done within the preceding 12 months and was normal. Previously, it was considered that if the male had been responsible for a pregnancy or if a SA had previously been normal, there was no need to perform this assessment. It is now recognised that this is not so, as pregnancies do occur with very poor semen and this might explain a pregnancy in the past and the present infertility. Also the SA may very well alter in time (Poland, 1985).

Two

Assessment of ovulation (screening only) by use of BBT and serum progesterone seven days after presumed ovulation.

Three

If the semen count is >20 million/ml, motility > 50 per cent and normal forms > 60 per cent, with ovulation occurring, a curettage/hysteroscopy/laparoscopy with installation of methylene blue are performed in the luteal phase of the cycle. Couples are advised to use barrier contraception in that cycle. Thus, the cavity of the uterus is visualised, tubal problems or endometriosis are excluded, and the endometrial status in relation to the stage of the cycle is determined.

Four

Once pelvic disease has been excluded, more sophisticated tests to determine ovulatory defects and also a post coital test (PCT) are performed. This will involve "tracking" the follicle by ultrasound at around the time of ovulation and early into the luteal phase. The reasons for postponing these investigations until pelvic disease has been excluded are that if any abnormality is found, then valuable investigation time is lost correcting these abnormalities, whilst other factors might well be present and more significant. One cannot be concise in absolutely determining the sequence of the various investigations, but in general, in ovulating women, tubal assessment is done early, and in non-ovulating women, particularly in oligomenorrhea and secondary amenorrhea, this should be deferred until at least three ovulatory cycles have occurred. From our study, it appears that the investigation of women having regular cycles should include tubal assessment early, as there is a 25 per cent association with tubal abnormalities. The reason for deferring laparoscopy/hysteroscopy has been discussed earlier. A further reason why it is recommended that hysteroscopy/laparoscopy should be delayed for three ovulatory cycles is that most pregnancies will occur in the first three ovulatory cycles as a result of ovulation induction with CC (Correy, 1976).

Five

Prolactin, follicle stimulating and luteinising hormone levels are always determined if there is ovulatory dysfunction. If the prolactin is raised, thyroid stimulating hormone is assayed as a screening test to detect thyroid dysfunction and a CAT scan of the pituitary is performed. If a normal or borderline high prolactin level is found, a CAT scan is not performed unless there are clinical features to suggest a pituitary tumour. Drugs as an etiological cause for hyperprolactinaemia are excluded. Bromocriptine is given to non-ovulatory patients with high prolactin levels or to those patients with ovulatory defects if prolactin is raised.

Six

Anovulatory menstruation/luteal phase defects; normal prolactin; no evidence of metabolic problems; normal semen.

1. Clomiphene — if no pregnancy is achieved after three ovulatory cycles, a curettage/hysteroscopy/laparoscopy is performed. If this is normal, a PCT is performed to check that there is no adverse effect of CC on the mucus. If the mucus is poor, AIH is performed for several cycles.
2. If a luteal phase defect is present with CC or if the primary condition is a luteal phase defect, progesterone vaginal pessaries 50 mg at night are used from Day Four after ovulation for eight days.

3. If there is evidence of polycystic ovarian disease (PCO) by a raised LH/FSH ratio plus ultrasound evidence of polycystic ovaries and the above regimen is unsuccessful, the combined oral contraceptive pill is used for two months to effect pituitary suppression, or an LHRH analogue is used if available. Ovulation induction is then tried again. In the past, we have used FSH/HCG regimens but have had poor results in terms of pregnancy.
4. If there is still no success, all treatment is withheld to see if spontaneous ovulatory cycles occur. We have evidence in our clinic population that a proportion of patients with anovulatory cycles will ovulate spontaneously after cessation of CC and achieve a pregnancy.
5. The final step in management will be consideration of IVF or allied procedures.

Seven

Secondary amenorrhea/oligomenorrhea; prolactin normal; no evidence of a metabolic disorder; semen normal.

1. Clomiphene. This should establish ovulation in > 70 per cent of patients and once established, 70 per cent or more will become pregnant and of these the majority will achieve pregnancy in the first few ovulatory cycles.
2. If no pregnancy occurrs after three ovulatory cycles, a curettage/hysteroscopy/laparoscopy with pertubation is performed followed by CC and the performance of a PCT.
3. If there is poor mucus and PCT, continue with the CC plus AIH.
4. If still not ovulating and no pregnancy is achieved after six months, Human Menopausal Gonadotrophin with HCG (HMG/HCG) or GnRH infusion is used. If PCO is present, an LHRH analogue plus HMG/HCG is used.
5. IVF or allied procedures should be considered finally as larger amounts of HMG can be used without fear of problems related to ovarian hyperstimulation.

Eight

Poor mucus/semen defects; ovulation normal; pelvic disease excluded. AIH is used for six months, after which IVF will be attempted. If fertilisation occurs but no pregnancy, continue with IVF or allied procedures.

Nine

Female antisperm antibodies — use IVF.

Ten

Tubal problems/pelvic disease. Consideration is given to surgical procedures on the tubes to establish patency and to return the anatomy to normal. Distal tubal disease is an indication for early consideration of IVF as conception rates are low and ectopic pregnancy risks are high. Proximal tubal disease is better treated surgically initially as well as adhesive disease (Fredricsson, 1986; Semm, 1980). If the patient is not ovulating or if there are sperm/mucus problems with tubal patency present, it is probably reasonable to try measures that have been previously discussed, prior to IVF. Our results, however, suggest very low pregnancy rates, and IVF may give better results.

Eleven

Unexplained infertility. This is diagnosed by a process of exclusion and the criteria on which the diagnosis is made are as follows:

1. Regular ovulation confirmed by progesterone assays in two cycles with appropriate LH surges, normal ultrasound "tracking"of follicle developments and adequate luteal progesterone levels.
2. Normal parameters on semen analysis and the absence of IgG attachment to the sperm head.
3. Normal PCT and mucous production.
4. Absence of antisperm antibodies in the female.
5. A normal pelvis and appropriate endometrium in relation to the stage of the menstrual cycle.
6. Adequate timing of intercourse.
7. Continued attendance for at least six months.

There were very few patients in our series (17 out of 1535) who were diagnosed as having this problem. This is in contradistinction to other authors (Hull, 1985; Collins, 1983) who reported a considerably higher incidence of this group of patients. The authors are not convinced that bacteriological studies are helpful in this condition.

In vitro fertilisation is used in this group of patients after a prolonged period of infertility, not only in an attempt to achieve a pregnancy but also in an investigative manner, to assess whether fertilisation can be achieved (Trounson, 1980). In the future, salpingoscopy may prove valuable in the assessment of possible tubal factors in this condition (Brosens, 1982).

Conclusion

As a result of this study, there are a number of factors that may provide help in the management of patients with infertility. While the overall minimum pregnancy rate for the period of this survey was approximately 50 per cent, the pregnancy rates have been determined without excluding the defaulters. In reality, the pregnancy rates will be higher in each of the groups investigated. Information is not available regarding pregnancy rates in Tasmania prior to 1966, ie. the time of introduction of CC therapy, and therefore it is not possible to determine the effectiveness with certainty of this therapeutic modality. As only 16.4 per cent of patients with ovulatory dysfunction spontaneously became pregnant, it suggests that the use of ovulation induction with CC is in fact very effective. There has been no increase in the overall success rates throughout the period of this survey. This does not mean that treatment with modalities other than CC, such as Bromocriptine, GnRH infusion, have been ineffective as patients treated by these means form only a small fraction of the overall infertile population. Furthermore, the changing pattern of referral has meant that there is an increasingly higher proportion of patients with more difficult and often multiple problems in the clinic population.

We are able to counsel our patients that if they persist with attendance at the infertility clinic their pregnancy rate is likely to be 50 per cent higher than if they leave the clinic. This advice, coupled with the supportive attention of the nurse coordinator and her staff, will help to ensure that a larger proportion of patients continue with active treatment.

While there have been studies from other parts of Australia looking at the proportions of factors involved in infertility in local populations, this study has been of benefit to us in identifying the areas of need in our own community. In particular, we have identified particular subgroups such as those patients with regular menses in whom investigation protocols might be altered on the basis of associated infertility factors that have been demonstrated.

We have been able to confirm the experience of others with regard to the investigation of tubal factors, in that HSG's no longer play a significant role in the investigation of tubal disease in infertility.

Finally, the relatively steady rate of spontaneous pregnancy, even in documented tubal disease and semen abnormalities and the results of treatment with the various therapeutic modalities, have been helpful facts in the counselling of patients with regard to the possible outcome of treatment and the importance of postponing or expediting further management protocols.

Acknowledgements

The authors wish to acknowledge the continuing and efficient services of the nurse coordinator, Sister Gwen Gray and her staff, and to Sister Wendy Gray for obtaining the relevant information for patients in the Launceston clinic.

Table 1-1
Age distribution of infertility patients

	Primary infertility		Secondary infertility	
Age	No.	Per cent	No.	Per cent
Unknown	8	0.8	8	1.5
> 20	34	3.8	1	0.1
20–24	290	29.4	99	18.1
25–29	410	41.6	223	40.5
30–34	200	20.3	152	27.6
35–39	39	3.9	56	10.1
40+	4	0.4	11	2.0

Table 1-2
Infertility factors

	All (1535)		Primary (985)		Secondary (550)	
Causes	No.	Per cent	No.	Per cent	No.	Per cent
Ovulatory	1067	69.5	702	71.2	365	66.4
Tubal	280	18.2	168	23.9	112	20.4
Semen	437	28.5	311	31.5	126	22.9
Mucus	191	12.4	140	14.2	51	9.3
Endometriosis	80	5.2	61	6.2	19	3.4
Adhesions	52	3.3	38	3.8	14	2.5
Unexplained	17	1.1	9	0.9	8	1.4
Ovulatory/tubal	159	10.4	98	9.9	61	11.1
Ovulatory/semen	298	19.4	213	21.6	85	15.5
Tubal/semen	59	3.8	37	3.7	22	0.4

Table 1-3
Infertility factors grouped in years

Year Annual No.	1966–69 (62)	1970–73 (106)	1974–77 (289)	1978–81 (434)	1982–85 (498)	1986–87 (110)	All (1499)
	Per cent	Per cent	Per cent	Per cent	Per cent	Per cent	Per cent
Ovulatory	85.4	72.6	78.9	72.6	65.8	64.5	69.5
Tubal	6.5	7.5	12.8	18.2	24.7	23.6	18.2
Semen	22.5	31.1	29.4	24.6	32.1	27.3	28.1
Mucus	3.2	21.6	16.3	12.9	9.6	8.2	12.4
Endometriosis	0	4.7	2.1	7.1	5.8	4.5	5.2
Ovulatory/tubal	4.8	6.6	8.3	9.2	14.5	9.0	10.4
Ovulatory/semen	17.7	24.5	19.0	18.6	18.9	18.2	19.1
Ovulatory/tubal/semen	0	0.9	0.6	2.5	4.8	1.8	2.6
Tubal/semen	0	0.9	1.3	3.2	6.8	4.5	3.8

Table 1-4
Defaulters by years and infertility factors

Year Total	1966–69 (62)		1970–73 (106)		1974–77 (289)		1978–81 (434)		1982–85 (498)		1986–87 (110)		All (1499)	
Defaulters	23	[37]	38	[36]	79	[27]	139	[32]	116	[23]	11	[10]	406	[27]
Ovulatory	18	(78)	24	(63)	50	(63)	92	(66)	65	(56)	7	(63)	256	(63)
Tubal	0	(0)	2	(5)	12	(15)	24	(17)	31	(27)	0	(0)	69	(17)
Semen	7	(30)	12	(31)	22	(28)	41	(30)	44	(38)	3	(27)	129	(32)
Endometriosis	0	(0)	2	(5)	1	( )	11	(8)	5	(4)	0	(0)	19	(5)
Mucus	1	(4)	8	(20)	15	(19)	16	(11)	13	(11)	0	(0)	53	(15)

[ ] = per cent of year total ( ) = per cent of defaulters in year group for each infertility factor

Table 1-5
Percentage of completed pregnancies (a) overall, (b) spontaneous, and (c) treatment related

		1966–69	*1970–73*	*1974–77*	*1978–81*	*1982–85*	*1986–87*	*All*	*No.*
Overall	(a)	54.8	50.9	59.5	52.5	48.5	46.4*	51.9	
	(b)	30.6	26.4	20.1	21.8	19.6	14.5*	20.9	1499
	(c)	24.2	24.5	39.4	26.0	28.5	31.8*	31.0	
Ovulatory	(a)	58.4	55.8	64.9	57.2	54.5	59.1	58.4	
	(b)	30.1	23.4	15.8	16.4	13.7	12.6	16.4	1067
	(c)	28.3	32.5	49.1	40.8	40.8	46.4	41.9	
Secondary amenorrhea	(a)	65.2	67.7	58.3	43.1	56.0	59.3	56.2	
	(b)	21.7	29.0	15.5	20.6	12.0	3.7	16.5	274
	(c)	43.4	38.7	44.8	22.4	44.0	55.5	40.1	
Oligomenorrhea	(a)	60.0	54.5	71.6	74.5	59.7	47.4	64.8	
	(b)	46.6	31.8	16.6	15.3	16.4	10.5	19.0	247
	(c)	13.3	22.7	55.0	59.3	43.3	36.8	45.8	
Regular menses	(a)	44.4	37.8	51.6	38.7	38.9	33.3	40.6	
	(b)	44.0	18.9	22.0	22.1	22.4	14.5	21.8	707
	(c)	0	18.9	29.6	16.6	16.6	18.7	18.9	
Tubal disease	(a)	25.0	25.0	37.8	36.7	34.1	26.9	34.2	
	(b)	25.0	0	13.5	25.3	17.2	11.5	18.1	280
	(c)	0	25.0	24.3	11.4	17.2	15.4	16.3	

Table 1-5 (continued)

		1966–69	*1970–73*	*1974–77*	*1978–81*	*1982–85*	*1986–87*	*All*	*No.*
Abnormal semen	(a)	35.7	47.1	53.4	42.1	31.3	50.0	40.6	
	(b)	0	17.6	19.2	19.6	12.5	23.3	16.3	437
	(c)	35.7	29.4	34.2	22.4	18.7	26.6	24.4	
Ovulatory/tubal	(a)	33.3	42.8	45.8	40.0	36.1	50.0	39.7	
	(b)	33.3	0	12.5	27.5	11.1	10.0	15.4	159
	(c)	0	42.8	33.3	12.5	25.0	40.0	24.3	
Ovulatory/semen	(a)	45.5	50.0	61.8	44.4	37.2	55.0	46.7	
	(b)	27.2	15.4	16.3	17.3	7.5	15.0	13.9	298
	(c)	18.2	34.6	45.5	27.1	29.7	40.0	32.7	
Tubal/semen	(a)	0	0	50.0	50.0	29.0	40.0	36.2	
	(b)	0	0	25.0	28.5	11.7	20.0	17.2	59
	(c)	0	0	25.0	21.4	17.6	20.0	18.9	
Mucus	(a)	50.0	52.1	55.5	53.5	31.2	44.4	47.5	
	(b)	50.0	13.0	12.7	16.0	12.5	0	13.5	191
	(c)	0	34.7	42.5	37.5	18.7	44.4	34.1	
Endometriosis	(a)	0	40.0	33.3	48.3	44.8	0	42.1	
	(b)	0	0	16.6	35.4	34.5	0	28.9	80
	(c)	0	40.0	16.6	12.9	10.3	0	13.1	

* *There are a further 25 ongoing pregnancies in 1987 which have not been included in the detailed analysis. Overall pregnancy rate (1986–87) 56.3 per cent. Spontaneous pregnancy rate (1986–87) 20.7 per cent. Treatment related pregnancies 34.8 per cent. No correction has been made for any of the other factors presented in this table.*

Table 1-6
Outcome of completed pregnancies

	Clinic		Ovulatory		Tubal		Semen	
	No.	Per cent	No.	Per cent	No.	Per cent	No.	Per cent
	1535		*1067*		*280*		*437*	
Pregnancies	795	51.7	616	57.7	98	35.0	175	40.0
Single	554	76.9	437	78.0	66	75.8	119	76.2
Twin	35	4.4	25	4.2	0	0	10	6.4
Triplet	3	<1	2	<1	0	0	1	0.6
Ectopic	16	2.2	12	2.1	7	8	6	3.8
Miscellaneous	106	14.7	75	13.3	12	13.7	18	11.5

Table 1-7
Comparison of HSG and laparoscopy

	A		B		C		D	
	No.	Per cent	No.	Per cent	No.	Per cent	No.	Per cent
No.	106	(46.6)	19	(8.3)	57	(25.1)	45	(19.8)
Pregnant spontaneously	26	24.5	4	21.0	15	26.3	8	17.7
Treated	22	20.7	4	21.0	11	19.3	10	22.2
Single	39	81.2	8	10.0	20	74.1	11	61.1
Twin	2	4.1	0	0	0	0	0	0
Ectopic	0	0	0	0	0	0	1	5.5
Miscarriage	9	18.7	1	5.2	3	11.1	2	11.0
Unknown	7	0	0	0	6	0	6	0

( ) = per cent of the study group, 227
A: laparoscopy/HSG normal
B: laparoscopy normal/HSG abnormal
C: laparoscopy abnormal/HSG normal
D: laparoscopy/HSG abnormal

Table 1-8
Infertility factors and outcome according to nature of menstrual periods

	Secondary amenorrhea Category 2		*Oligomenorrhea Category 3*		*Regular cycles Category 4*		*Long cycles Category 5*	
	No.	*Per cent*	*No.*	*Per cent*	*No.*	*Per cent*	*No.*	*Per cent*
Total	274	[17.8]	247	[16.1]	707	[46.0]	180	[11.7]
Pregnant spontaneously	44	16.1	47	19.0	156	22.1	50	27.8
Treated	120	43.7	112	45.0	134	18.9	67	37.2
Ovulatory defects: No.	274	(100.0)	214	(86.6)	377	(53.3)	137	(76.1)
Pregnant spontaneously	44	16.1	34	15.8	60	15.9	26	18.9
Treated	120	43.7	103	48.1	123	32.6	65	47.4
Tubal defects: No.	17	(6.2)	29	(11.7)	184	(26.0)	28	(15.5)
Pregnant spontaneously	1	5.8	4	14.8	35	19.0	4	14.3
Treated	1	5.8	0	0	22	11.9	6	21.4
Semen defects: No.	52	(18.9)	66	(26.7)	226	(31.9)	58	(32.2)
Pregnant spontaneously	8	15.4	9	13.6	39	17.3	14	24.1
Treated	20	38.5	23	34.8	34	15.0	16	27.5

[ ] = per cent of study population
( ) = per cent of category

References

Blunt, A. The place of laparoscopy in 'normal' gynaecological practice. *Australian and New Zealand Journal of Obstetrics and Gynaecology*, 1972; 12: 194.

Brodribb, J.K.R., Correy, J.F., Schokman, F.C.M. Pregnancy outcome in patients with regular menses. *Asia-Oceania Journal of Obstetrics and Gynaecology*, 1986; 12 (1): 49.

Bronson, R., Coupers, G., Jort, T.H., Ing, R., Johns, W.R., Wang, S.X., Mather, F., Williamson, H.O., Rust, P.F., Fudenbert, H.H. Antisperm antibodies detected by agglutination immobilisation, microcytotoxicity and immunobead binding assays. *Journal of Reproductive Immunology*, 1985; 8 (4): 279.

Brosens, I., Boeckx, W., Delattin, Ph., Puttemans, P., Vasquez, G. Salpingoscopy: A new pre-operative disgnostic tool in tubal infertility. *British Journal of Obstetrics and Gynaecology*, 1987; 94: 768.

Collins, J.A., Wrixon, W., Jones, L.B., Wilson, E.H. Treatment-independent pregnancy among infertile couples. *New England Journal of Medicine*, 1983: 309: 1201.

Correy, J.F. Laparoscopy and loss of clinical acumen. *Australian and New Zealand Journal of Obstetrics and Gynaecology*, 1973; 13: 60.

Correy J.F., Schokman, F.C.M., An appraisal of clomiphene in the induction of ovulation. *Australian and New Zealand Journal of Obstetrics and Gynaecology*, 1976; 16: 40.

Correy, J.F., Schokman, F.C.M., Laparoscopy and hysterosalpingography in the diagnosis of infertility in patients with secondary amenorrhea and ovulatory disorder. *Australian and New Zealand Obstetrics and Gynaecology*, 1977; 17: 205.

Correy, J.F., Marsden, D.E., Allen, D.G. The implementation of a statewide gynaecology audit in Tasmania. *Australian and New Zealand Journal of Obstetrics and Gynaecology*, 1987; 27: 330.

Correy, J.F., Watkins, R.A., Bradfield, G.F., Garner, S., Watson, S., Gray, G. Spontaneous pregnancies and pregnancies as a result of treatment in an IVF programme terminating in ectopic pregnancies or spontaneous abortion. *Fertility and Sterility*, 1988; in press.

Cox, L.W., Infertility: A comprehensive programme. *British Journal of Obstetrics and Gynaecology*, 1975; 82 (1): 2.

Daly, D.C., Soto-Albors, C.E., Aversa, M.A. Hysteroscopic detection and treatment of adhesions at the tubal ostium/uterine junction in infertile patients. *Fertility and Sterility*, 1986; 46 (1): 138.

Drake, T.S., Grunert, G.M., Unsuspected pelvic factor in the infertility investigation. *Fertility and Sterility*, 1980; 34 (1): 27.

Fredricsson, B., Rosenborg, L., Surgical correction of female infertility. *Acta Obstetrica et Gynaecologica Scandinavia*, 1986; 65: 421.

Gemzell, C.A., Diczfalusy, E., Tillinger, G. Clinical effect of human pituitary follicle stimulating hormone (FSH). *Clinics in Endocrinology Metabolism*, 1958; 18: 1333.

Gomel, V., McComb, P. Unexpected pregnancies in women afflicted by occlusive tubal disease. *Fertility and Sterility*, 1981; 36 (4): 529.

Greenblatt, R.B. ' Chemical induction of ovulation. *Fertility and Sterility*, 1961; 12: 402.

Harding, A., Ing, R.M.Y., Jones, W.R. ' The immunobead test in the assessment of sperm autoimmunity in fertile males. *Proceedings of the Sixth Annual Scientific Meeting*, The Fertility Society of Australia, Sydney, Australia, 1987.

Hull, M.G.R., Glazener, C.M.A., Kelly, N.J., Conway, D.I., Foster, P.A., Hinton, R.A., Coulson, C., Lambert, P.A., Watt, E.M., Desai, K.M. Population studies of causes, treatment and outcome of infertility. *British Medical Journal*, 1985; 291: 1693.

Jeffcoate, T.N.A. *Principles of Gynaecology,* Second Edition, Butterworth, London, 1962, 572.

Kessler, I., Lancet, M. Hysterography and hysteroscopy: A comparison. *Fertility and Sterility,* 1986; 46 (4): 709.

Lenton, E.A., Weston, G.A., Cooke, I.D. Problems in using basal body temperature recordings in an infertility clinic. *British Medical Journal,* 1977; 1: 803.

Lillford, R.J., Dalton, M.E. Effectiveness of treatment for infertility. *British Medical Journal,* 1987; 295: 155.

Menning, B.E. The emotional needs of the infertile couple. *Fertility and Sterility,* 1980; 34 (4): 313.

Olive, D.L. Analysis of clinical fertility trials: A methodological review. *Fertility and Sterility,* 1986; 45 (2): 157.

Poland, M., Moghissi, K., Giblin, P., Ager, J., Olson, J. Variation of semen measures within normal men. *Fertility and Sterility,* 1985; 44 (5); 396.

Randolph, J.R., Ying, Y.K., Maier, D.B., Schmidt, C.L., Riddick, D.H. Comparison of real time ultrasonography, hysterosaloingography, and laparoscopy/hysteroscopy in the evaluation of uterine abnormalities and tubal patency. *Fertility and Sterility,* 1986; 46 (5): 828.

Schokman, F.C.M., Correy, J.F., Cusick, E.T. The investigation and treatment of patients with ovulation failure; with special reference to the problems arising from the use of clomiphene. *Australian and New Zealand Journal of Obstetrics and Gynaecology,* 1971; 11: 241.

Semm, K., Mettler, L. Technical progress in pelvic surgery via operative laparoscopy. *American Journal of Obstetrics and Gynecology,* 1980; 138 (2): 121.

Thomas, A.K., Forrest, M.S. Infertility: A review of 291 infertile couples over eight years. *Fertility and Sterility,* 1980; 34 (2): 106.

Trounson, A.O., Leeton, J.F., Wood, C., Webb, J., Kovacs, G. The investigation of idiopathic infertility by in vitro fertilization. *Fertility and Sterility,* 1980; 34 (5): 431.

W.H.O. Task Force, Geneva, Switzerland Comparative trial of tubal insufflation, hysterosalpingography, and laparoscopy with dye hydrotubation for assessment of tubal patency. *Fertility and Sterility,* 1986; 46 (6): 1101.

2
Unexplained infertility

J.P. Forsey and M.G.R. Hull

Introduction

Unexplained infertility, like any idiopathic diagnosis, is one of exclusion, and protracted investigations can add to the frustration often felt by the patient and clinician alike faced with this diagnosis. A thorough but efficient investigative approach is therefore essential. The fact that this diagnosis is reached so frequently is a reminder of our ignorance concerning much of the process of reproduction and the many factors which can affect it. Couples with unexplained infertility represent a heterogenous group with different subtle factors accounting for their subfertility, about which we know very little. The fact that it is unlikely that one common cause is responsible for the infertility seen in this group has led to many fascinating avenues of research, often however with divergent and apparently contradictory results. It would seem likely that until many of these areas are more thoroughly investigated, treatment will not change from the empirical approach that has largely prevailed today. Nevertheless, enough is now known on which to base clear advice about the investigations of critical importance, the chance of conception with or without therapy, and the effectiveness and selection of treatment.

Diagnostic criteria

The lack of uniformity in the diagnostic criteria for unexplained infertility has been a major complicating factor in the interpretation of results. Patient groups are frequently not comparable between different studies. For example, in a recent study by Haxton et al (1987) of 95 couples referred as having unexplained infertility, one third were subsequently found to have some abnormality.

Investigative facilities differ widely, limiting the information available for diagnosis. For instance, if laparoscopy is not freely available, important conditions such as endometriosis and peritubal adhesions can be missed (Drake et al, 1977). Some simple tests of importance, such as sperm-mucus interaction, may not be applied due to lack of daily facilities to ensure accurate timing. On the other hand, the application of sophisticated investigative procedures — for example detailed hormonal assessment of the ovarian cycle or hysteroscopy — may reveal apparent abnormalities that are in fact of no relevance to fertility. A final absurdity is that sometimes findings of great functional importance — for example antisperm antibodies in seminal plasma — are reported as occurring in "unexplained infertility" because of diagnostic prejudice confining assessment of male fertility to seminal microscopy.

Unexplained infertility is often defined as "infertility" occurring despite "ovulatory cycles", "patent fallopian tubes" and "normal sperm counts". Some authors have limited their practical requirements to a history of normal menstrual cycles, laparoscopy and standard seminal analysis (eg. Aitken et al, 1982). Yet all the terms in quotation marks need definition and qualification.

Infertility, subfertility, fertility

Infertility can only be defined by reference to normal fertility. Amongst normal couples of eventual proven fertility, the average chance of conception per ovarian cycle is 20 per cent (Spira, 1986); 10 per cent failed to conceive in their first year of trying and five per cent after two years (Tietze, 1956, 1968). Because of the chance nature of fertility, conception can never be guaranteed in advance; fertility is not an absolute condition.

On the other hand, infertility is seldom absolute, as when there is a premature menopause, bilateral tubal occlusion or azoospermia. It is mostly subfertility of varying degrees. Because 90 per cent of normal couples should conceive within one year, "infertility" is usually defined as failure to conceive after more than a year. Nevertheless, as time passes there is an increasing likelihood of a severe cause of infertility, which may or may not be discernible. Therefore unexplained infertility may be greatly affected by a definition based on varying duration, as will be seen later in this chapter.

When assessing the benefit of treatment for unexplained infertility, it is crucially important to take into account the chance of conceiving without treatment, therefore necessitating rigorously controlled prospective studies. The influence of duration of infertiity, and to a lesser extent, age, in addition to the diagnostic criteria applied in the first place, must all be considered.

Assessment of possible ovulatory disorder

Fertility obviously depends on normal ovulation, which implies not only follicular rupture but also the timing of rupture in relation to the LH surge and full functional maturation of the follicle. It has been suggested, based on inadequate hormonal and laparoscopic evidence, that failure of follicular rupture may be a common occurrence (Koninckx et al, 1978; Marik & Hulka, 1978). But ultrasound studies have shown this to be rarely the case when there is hormonal evidence of complete follicular maturation as suggested by normal midluteal progesterone levels (Coutts et al, 1982; Petos et al, 1987). Similarly, disruption in the timing of follicular rupture compared with the oestradiol and LH surges has also been found to occur rarely when midluteal progesterone levels are favourable (Polan et al, 1982).

The luteal phase (LP) seems to be a reliable reflection of preovulatory maturation of the follicle and rupture, the timing of test samples is easier and this is therefore where diagnostic attention is routinely focussed. The concept of LP deficiency leading to infertility is now almost 40 years old (Jones, 1949), but still remains a matter of controversy (Balasch & Vanrell, 1987).

There is no need in this short chapter to discuss the shortcomings of basal body temperature charting, which does not reflect progesterone levels quantitatively. Nor do we wish to debate the use of endometrial biopsy which, despite widespread use, has never been validated in terms of fertility by prospective study. In addition, endometrial biopsy does not lend itself to application repeatedly whereas it is essential to demonstrate that any abnormality found occurs persistently if it is to account for prolonged infertility, as discussed below.

Serum progesterone measurement can easily be done in several cycles, but there have been claims that it needs to be done daily to assess the early luteal pattern of rise, which would be difficult to repeat in several cycles. There are several possible different progesterone patterns of luteal phase defects (Figure 2-1). Whether the LP is short or of normal duration, low levels of progesterone (Figure 2-1, a and b) are easy to detect by single midluteal sampling. A normal rise to normal peak levels ending abruptly in a short LP (Figure 2-1c) seems a rare event of uncertain relevance and fairly easily recognisable. Of greatest practical concern is the possible occurrence of an abnormally slow early luteal progesterone rise eventually reaching normal peak values and normal duration (Figure 2-1d). It is assumed to be relevant because it tends to be the average pattern in infertility compared with conception cycles (Lenton et al, 1983), but it is not clear how persistent it is. Coutts (1985) noted this finding in some individual women with prolonged unexplained infertility, but of the five cases he illustrated, four could have been clearly distinguished by inadequate peak progesterone values in the midluteal phase.

If LP defects are to explain prolonged infertility they must be persistent. Smith et al (1984) found short LPs occur no more often in infertile than in normal women. Glazener et al (1988) found that neither mild nor severe LP deficiency, as indicated by midluteal progesterone levels, occurred any more often than in a normal control population, and during the course of six cycles persisted in only two per cent of cases (Table 2-1).

There is no convincing evidence that measuring serum oestradiol levels in the follicular or luteal phase contributes any information independent of luteal phase progesterone.

Assessment of tubal, pelvic and uterine factors

Only a brief review is possible or necessary in this short chapter. Gas insufflation of the fallopian tubes has long been discredited. Hysterosalpingography provides useful and occasionally unique information on the internal anatomy of the uterus and tubes and tubal patency. On the other hand, it may fail to provide crucial information about pelvic adhesions and endometriosis, and it can indicate false abnormalities of the uterine cavity.

Laparoscopy is essential to define pelvic adhesions and endometriosis, and in the latter case it may be necessary to aspirate the pool of fluid in the pouch of Douglas. It is also essential to examine the underside of the ovaries for endometriosis hidden there because it is now clear from prospective studies of fertility how great the influence of ovarian endometriosis is (Foster, Foulkes and Hull, unpublished observations). The significance of minimal endometriosis (as classified by the American Fertility Society) has often been ignored, but prospective comparison with couples with unexplained infertility and matched in all other respects seems to show marked reduction in conception rates (Figure 2-2).

Hysteroscopy remains of uncertain value for the routine investigation of infertility because the contribution of intrauterine polyps or adhesions is not known, as will be discussed later, and other abnormalities are rare.

Brosens et al (1987) have recently described salpingoscopy, the use of a fine endoscope to examine and biopsy the endotubal mucosa. Whether the technique will reveal otherwise unsuspected abnormalities to account for hitherto unexplained infertility remains to be seen. It seems likely, however, that if such abnormalities are a frequent cause there would have been relatively high rates of tubal ectopic pregnancy reported in women with unexplained infertility, but this does not seem to be the case.

Assessment of semen and sperm function

The interpretation of standard seminal analysis is contentious. The World

Health Organisation (WHO) suggests a minimum of 20 x 10^6/ml sperm, of which at least 40 per cent should be motile, 60 per cent alive and 50 per cent of normal form with no evidence of agglutination (WHO, 1980). Hewitt et al, (1985) have preferred to use a lower limit of 10 x 10^6/ml sperm, 20 per cent motility and 20 per cent normal forms, based on studies by Van Zyl et al (1975) and Bostofte et al (1984). Unfortunately, most of the studies have been retrospective, which allows definition of what seminal "counts" are possible to achieve pregnancy, not what is probable. Definition of a criteria for a normal chance of pregnancy requires prospective study. As described in the chapter by Wardle, Ford and Hull, the best criterion of normal derived from prospective studies of both natural conception and in vitro fertilisation is a motile normal sperm density (MNSD) greater than 4–6 x 10^6/ml. The MNSD is a product of the proportions of normally progressing and normally formed spermatozoa and overall density.

Nevertheless, those criteria provide, although significant, only weak power of prediction of pregnancy. Aitken et al (1982) found that of men with unexplained infertility, as indicated by standard seminal analysis alone, a third had lost the fertilising ability of their spermatozoa, as shown by the hamster egg penetration test. If it is accepted that many men with normal "sperm counts" are infertile (or severely subfertile), it must also be true than many men with low "counts" have normal fertility. It is now clear that standard seminal analysis is of little clinical value except when "counts" are extremely low, and assessment of sperm function is essential.

The first function required of spermatozoa is penetration of cervical mucus and survival for 24 hours or more in the female genital tract. These features can easily be tested by the delayed postcoital test (PCT), done about 12 hours after coitus in the immediate preovulatory phase when the cervical mucus is fully developed. The test is simple, but frequently mistimed, particularly in infertility services that do not function daily. The PCT has been shown in prospective studies to provide twice the predictive power of standard seminal analysis, particularly for severe subfertility (Glazener et al, 1987a). The PCT findings also correlate closely with in vitro fertilising ability both with the woman's oocytes (Hull et al, 1984; Wardle et al, 1985) and hamster oocytes (Schats et al, 1984).

In vitro testing of sperm-mucus penetration may give rise to misleadingly favourable results in a small proportion of cases due to testing only short term sperm survival, which is associated with poor fertilising ability (Hull et al, 1987). However, in general, the details of penetration at the sperm-mucus interface offer accurate indication of primary sperm dysfunction, antisperm antibodies or mucus "hostility" (Glazener & Hull, 1987). In addition, crossed testing can be undertaken using normal donor mucus and semen samples in order to distinguish the site of disorder, including occasional coital failure. More complex tests of sperm dysfunction are discussed in the chapter by Wardle, Ford and Hull.

Basic definition of unexplained infertility

From the discussion so far, the essential investigations and criteria required to make a basic diagnosis of unexplained infertility can be summarised as the following:

Normal menstrual cycles. Range 21–35 days. As luteal deficiency is so uncommon as a persistent occurrence in women with otherwise unexplained infertility, it is necessary to assess at least six cycles or it is not worth assessing any.

Normal post-coital sperm-mucus penetration and survival. At least one forward-progressing spermatozoon in every high power microscope field of mucus about 12 hours after coitus.

Normal laparoscopic pelvic findings. Exclude even minor adhesions and endometriosis.

Normal coital frequency. At least twice per week, or at least regular correct preovulatory timing by recognition of the mucus and/or LH surge.

Further refinements of uncertain or rare applicability will be considered later, but the definition above already goes beyond what is generally used and is sufficient for most practice and study. It is the definition used for the studies from our unit described in this chapter.

Epidemiology of unexplained infertility

Frequency

The reported frequency of unexplained infertility varies widely in world literature, with rates as high as 58 per cent (Smith and Horger, 1967). However, when applying more modern diagnostic criteria similar to those outlined above, most reported rates are 5-30 per cent of infertility. This large range probably reflects population differences, selective specialist referral and variations in diagnostic criteria.

The WHO multicentre clinic based investigation involving both developed and developing countries found the average frequency of unexplained infertility was 14 per cent, varying from 26 per cent in Asia to five per cent in Africa (Cates & Rowe, 1987). This last figure is surprising, as a high incidence could be expected in a country where diagnostic facilities are limited and laparoscopy not so frequently performed. However, Africa is unusual in its high proportion of secondary compared to primary infertility, due to the high frequency of puerperal and sexually transmitted infection leading to tubal disease. In a true population study confined to the local residents attending our clinics, we have found the proportion with unexplained infertility to be 28 per cent (Hull et al, 1985). This is similar to a rate of 24 per cent reported elsewhere in the United Kingdom (Templeton and Penney, 1982) but twice the rates reported from some clinics in the United States of America (Sher and Katz, 1976) and Australia (Pepperell and McBain, 1985).

Most studies agree that the majority of couples with unexplained infertility have primary infertility (73-88 per cent; Lenton et al, 1977; Templeton and Penney, 1982; Hull et al, 1985; Cooke et al, 1987).

Pregnancy rates

Pregnancy occurs not infrequently without treatment in couples with unexplained infertility and it has been difficult to demonstrate true benefit from any treatment. Older reports have suggested widely varying pregnancy rates (Southam, 1960; Warner, 1962; Lamb and Cruz, 1972), but diagnostic criteria were unreliable and these studies were poorly controlled, particularly with respect to durations of infertility and exposure during study. The chances of pregnancy are related to age, parity and the duration of infertility, and the subsequent cumulative chance of pregnancy is time dependent. Lenton (1977) found a cumulative conception rate of 36 per cent after seven years for the primary infertile group and 79 per cent for women with secondary infertility. A conception rate of 79 per cent was also found by Templeton and Penney (1982) in their patients with secondary infertility, but they found a more favourable outcome than did Lenton in those with primary infertility, 66 per cent conceiving by nine years. These results represent severe subfertility, given the prolonged time spans, although prognostically a little misleading because all the couples had by clinical definition failed to conceive during the first few years of exposure, which were included in the calculated durations reported.

Hull et al (1985) related subsequent pregnancy rates to the duration of infertility from the time of diagnosis and the woman's age at that time, as shown in Figures 2-3 and 2-4. The woman's age has little effect until after 35 years. This is in keeping with the observed trend seen in the fertile population (CECOS, 1982), in which the fall is irrespective of the reduction in coital frequency seen with age (MacLeod and Gold, 1953). It is unlikely that reduced coital frequency per se is a causal factor in unexplained infertility (Lenton et al, 1977).

Duration of infertility has a major effect. Couples with one to three years of infertility have an 84 per cent chance of conceiving in the next two years, which is not far short of normal, and suggests that the main explanation for the previous infertility had been adversity of chance — simple bad luck. There is little to be gained from treatment and none has been shown to be beneficial. It is natural, however, for women much older than 35 years to want active intervention because they feel they cannot afford to wait. On the other hand, whatever the woman's age, after five or more years of unexplained infertility, the chance of success is reduced to 30 per cent during the next two years, which seems as unrealistic hope, requiring treatment if possible. In such couples, there would seem to be a real unidentified cause of their infertility.

Reduced oocyte quality (Hertig, 1975) and more frequent anovulatory cycles (Brown et al, 1981) have been suggested, although without evidence. Whatever the cause related to age, it would appear to affect equally both fertile women and women with unexplained infertility.

Possible remaining etiological factors

Extra ovarian influences on follicular function

Disorder of the thyroid and adrenal endocrine systems, and possibly diabetes mellitus, can disrupt ovarian function in specific ways with recognisable disordered ovulation. When ovulation appears to be normal, however, there seems to be no reason to attribute infertility to endocrine disorder although it seems appropriate to undertake at least basic assessment, perhaps limited only to a symptom history.

Hyperandrogenism has long been associated tenuously with infertility (Steinberger et al, 1979), although without evidence of origin or effective treatment. Recent ultrasonographic evidence shows that polycystic ovaries can be found in about a quarter of apparently normal women, who can only be distinguished otherwise by slight menstrual irregularity (although within the normal range), a quarter of them having raised LH levels (Polson et al, 1988). There is no evidence yet that such women are subfertile, but the information links intriguingly with impaired fertilising ability of oocytes in women undergoing IVF treatment who have raised LH levels (Stanger & Yovich, 1985). An association with unexplained infertility has yet to be studied.

A premature LH surge has been postulated as the cause in some cases of unexplained infertility by Dodson et al (1975), who therefore used an LHRH analogue to suppress endogenous LH release. In five women so treated who then received ovulation induction with exogenous gonadotrophins, two conceptions did occur (Fleming et al, 1982). However, from this small study it is not possible to deduce to what extent, if any, these pregnancies can be attributed to therapy and the frequency with which premature LH surges occur has yet to be established in this group.

Hyperprolactinaemia has of course been associated with abnormal luteal function by many authors (see Balasch and Vanrell, 1987) and also with unexplained infertility in women with apparently normal luteal phase (Bahamondes et al, 1979).

However, well controlled studies have failed to demonstrate any beneficial effect of bromocriptine in unexplained infertility (Wright et al, 1979; McBain and Pepperell, 1982; Glazener et al, 1987b). The idea that follicular function might be impaired to a significant but undetectable degree affecting fertility, or that fertility might be affected directly, by relative hyperprolactinaemia within the normal range, or by borderline hyperprolactinaemia, has been explored in our unit. Glazener et al (1987c) studied prospectively conception rates and luteal progesterone levels related to bands of prolactin values throughout the normal range and above, in women with otherwise unexplained infertility, and found no difference (Table 2-2). It therefore seems clear that in women with normal menstrual cycles it is generally not worth measuring prolactin.

On the other hand, if hyperprolactinaemia is to be considered as a significant factor it would be necessary to test at least six cycles to demonstrate persistent luteal deficiency. Ben-David and Schenker (1983) described transient relative hyperprolactinaemia coincidental with the preovulatory oestradiol peak occurring in 94 per cent of cases with unexplained infertility, and an encouraging pregnancy rate following suppression of these prolactin rises with bromocriptine. However, the study of treatment was uncontrolled and a preovulatory prolactin rise has been described as normal phenomenon (Backstrom et al, 1982). There can be no justification yet for the daily measurement of prolactin required to make such a tentative unproven diagnosis.

Pelvic abnormalities

Anatomical abnormalities, such as septate or bicornuate uterus, although relevant to recurrent abortion, are no longer considered causes of failure to conceive and utriculoplasty has no place in the management of infertility in that respect. Likewise, surgical correction of uterine retroversion is only indicated because of dyspareunia, which may only indirectly affect fertility by reducing coital frequency. Cervical stenosis, such as that resulting from conisation, is seldom a barrier to the passage of spermatozoa, but destruction of endocervical glands can result in insufficient cervical mucus to facilitate sperm transport and storage. Postcoital testing is the key to investigating all those possibilities.

The finding of uterine fibroids, particularly subserous and intramural fibroids, remains of unclear relevance. Frequently dismissed as having no effect on conception, several small studies have however, indicated encouraging pregnancy rates following myomectomy in otherwise unexplained fertility (Garcia & Tureck, 1984; Rosenfeld, 1986). Those findings seemed to occur irrespective of symptoms such as menorrhagia directly referrable to the fibroids. On the other hand, these studies were uncontrolled and there are some features of the results which suggest the presence of the fibroids and myomectomy are both of no relevance. Rosenfeld's results showed that the chance of conceiving after myomectomy was closely related to the duration of infertility as occurs in unexplained infertility (Hull et al, 1985) and was unaffected by either the size or number of fibroids. The relevance of such fibroids therefore, seems very doubtful.

Tubocornual polyps detected on hysterosalpingography have been reported in association with infertility (David et al, 1981), but their significance has not been substantiated. Microsurgical removal has not improved the chance of pregnancy (Gordts et al, 1983) and recently Glazener et al (1987d) have shown by prospective study that conception rates are the same in otherwise unexplained infertility, whether polyps are present or not (Figure 2-5). Therefore, the finding of tubocornual polyps should not exclude diagnosis of unexplained infertility.

Laparoscopy often demonstrates abnormalities in women previously said to have unexplained infertility (El-Minawi et al, 1978; Cooke et al, 1987). However, as in the case of tubocornual polyps demonstrated by hysterosalpingography, the significance for fertility of any apparent abnormality needs to be considered. There is no information about the relevance of fimbrial cysts, nor of minor adhesions. If adhesions are found associated with a significantly raised antibody titre to Chlamydia trachomatis, however, it is likely there is also some endotubal damage (see below).

By contrast, prospective study appears to have clearly demonstrated the substantial importance of even minimal endometriosis (see Figure 2-2), which has also been shown to be associated with impaired fertilising ability of oocytes and presumably impaired follicular function (Wardle et al, 1985) as discussed earlier. Interestingly, Pepperell and McBain (1985) report finding endometriosis in 20 per cent of their patients with unexplained infertility in whom laparoscopy two years earlier had been normal. This suggests that the mechanism leading to reduced fertility in this group antedates the appearance of endometriosis and is not a result of it (at least when disease is minimal).

However, this does not wholly explain why the in vitro fertilisation (IVF) success rate in unexplained infertility patients without endometriosis is better than those with minimal disease if a similar initial underlying pathology is proposed. Changes in the intraperitoneal environment leading to an inflammatory process in the absence of visible abnormalities have been suggested as being causal in some cases of infertility (Olive et al, 1987).

The success of IVF in the treatment of patients with unexplained infertility has led to the hypothesis that endotubal damage, insufficient to cause occlusion but resulting in a failure of gamete transport, may be an underlying cause in cases of unexplained infertility. Some indirect evidence does exist to support this suggestion. Employing the sperm recovery test (SRT) as described by Asch (1976), several studies have reported a positive correlation between the finding of intraperitoneal spermatozoa following intrauterine insemination or coitus and subsequent pregnancy rates (Templeton and Mortimer, 1982; Murakami et al, 1985; Matsuura et al, 1987).

Templeton and Mortimer (1982) confined their study to patients with unexplained infertility and observed 12 pregnancies in 26 patients with a positive SRT and only two pregnancies in 21 patients with a negative SRT. Although the duration of infertility is not stated and two different insemination procedures were used, the differences would appear to be significant. This study did not indicate whether spermatozoa recovered were viable, but other studies have shown that motile sperm, and thus presumably potentially fertile sperm, can be recovered in this way. In Templeton and Mortimer's study, 21 of the 47 patients had a negative SRT (45 per cent), an incidence similar to that found by Stone (1983) who failed to find sperm in seven out of 15 similar patients (47 per cent), suggesting that occult tubal damage may be present in up to half of those women with unexplained infertility.

However, Matsuura et al (1987) found a negative SRT in only 5.7 per cent of their similar cases and, surprisingly, still found recovered sperm in over 90 per cent of women with abnormal pelvic anatomy. This finding would tend to suggest that abnormalities in sperm function rather than tubal disease are responsible for the incidence of negative SRT seen. If endotubal damage was an underlying factor, it might be expected that unexplained infertile patients would have more common serological evidence of past pelvic infection. In our clinic there is a strong association of high antibody titres to Chlamydia trachomatis and tubal damage (Conway et al, 1984). However, we do not see any increased frequency of antibodies to chlamydia in our patients with unexplained infertility compared with fertile controls (Forsey, Owen & Hull; unpublished data).

If endotubal malfunction was responsible for poor sperm transport, it would also be reasonable to predict that embryo transport might also be adversely affected with a resultant increase in the tubal ectopic pregnancy rate. Templeton and Penney (1982) did note one ectopic compared to 57 live births in their patients studied, but the data generally available are too few and the frequency of tubal pregnancy too low to be conclusive. However, the frequency of ectopic pregnancy is greater following IVF, and in our experience usually occurs in those patients with tubal disease but not with unexplained infertility.

The IVF results of Martinez and Trounson (1986) also suggest no increased frequency of ectopic pregnancy in unexplained infertility. In a large multicentre study of 1163 IVF pregnancies including 54 ectopics, Cohen et al (1986) failed to find any link between the indication for IVF and an ectopic outcome. Indeed, the fact that gamete intrafallopian transfer (GIFT) has proven as successful as IVF in the unexplained group (Leeton et al, 1987) would tend to suggest that tubal function is not usually damaged in women with unexplained infertility.

Intrauterine polyps and adhesions found by hysteroscopy remain of very doubtful relevance. Studies, for example by Taylor's group in Canada, showed that polyps occurred equally often (about 15 per cent) in women with primary and secondary infertility and infertile controls undergoing sterilisation, whereas adhesions occurred much more often in secondary infertiity (35 per cent) compared with primary infertility and fertile controls (11–19 per cent) (Cumming & Taylor, 1980), although not always.

Unfortunately, these studies were done using dextran 70 to distend the uterus and more recent studies by Taylor using CO_2 have given rise to findings of only one tenth the number of polyps and adhesions found before (Taylor et al, 1987; and see the accompanying chapter by Taylor, 1988). It would therefore seem that although adhesions may still be relevant, misleading artefacts are common and true adhesions could account very infrequently for unexplained infertility.

Subtle follicular disorders

We earlier showed in discussion that the luteal phase is in general an accurate guide to prior follicular maturation and rupture, even when assessed simply by midluteal progesterone measurement. Furthermore, evident abnormality in women with normal menstrual cycles is usually a random event that seldom persists. Detailed investigation of the ovarian cycle in women with prolonged unexplained infertility, by means of daily follicular ultrasonography and oestrogen, LH and progesterone measurements, has so far led to no new treatment or better selection of treatment with proven benefit.

Coutts et al (1985) have, however, claimed to identify by daily progesterone measurements a distinct treatable abnormality. They describe a reduced rate of progesterone rise in the early luteal phase that is distinguishable in individual women despite eventually reaching a normal peak value. On the basis of a single investigation cycle, Coutts achieved an encouraging number of pregnancies using combined LHRH analogue and gonadotrophin therapy in a small uncontrolled study. However, not only is a properly controlled trial of treatment needed, reliability of the original diagnosis needs to be properly established in the first place. Coutts claimed that only by daily progesterone measurement could the abnormality be recognised. Yet in four of the individual examples he cited, the peak progesterone value eventually reached was obviously reduced, and therefore the abnormality would appear to have been quite marked and could have been easily distinguished by a single midluteal progesterone measurement. Furthermore, Coutts did not show whether the abnormality he described was a persistent feature, necessary to account for prolonged infertility.

Another possibility is that subtle follicular disorder occurs as a common cause of prolonged unexplained infertility without usually being recognisable. In that case it may be appropriate to employ ovarian stimulation empirically in all cases. Glazener et al (1987e, as yet unpublished) studied the effect of clomiphene by means of a double blind placebo controlled crossover trial. Each treatment was given for three cycles with an untreated cycle interval at the crossover. The life table method was used to calculate conception rates in order to allow for those women who conceived during the study and therefore could not complete both courses of treatment. The women acted as their own controls in this study because of the crossover design, except again for those who conceived at an early stage. The results were compared in terms of luteal progesterone levels, as an index of ovarian function, and pregnancy rates; they are summarised in Table 2-3.

There was a substantial rise in progesterone after clomiphene, indicating the degree of ovarian stimulation, although not necessarily implying ovulatory improvement, as much of the increase would be accounted for by the contribution of the numerous subsidiary follicles stimulated. There was, however, a significant increase in the conception rate with clomiphene, unrelated to the degree of rise in progesterone. Most important, the increased conception rate was confined to the women with more than three years unexplained infertility. The increased conception rate in that group was still not as high as in the women with less than three years' infertility. Without clomiphene treatment, the chance of conception in the women with the longer duration of infertility was extremely low.

Those findings indirectly suggest that subtle follicular disorder is a common cause of prolonged unexplained infertility (not less than three years' duration) and can be partially overcome using clomiphene to stimulate follicular growth. The results at least encourage the use of more powerful stimulation by gonadotrophin therapy. Further encouragement for such treatment has been given by some favourable, but uncontrolled, reports of combined treatment with gonadotrophin and intrauterine insemination of sperm prepared in culture fluid (Serhal et al, 1988). But whether the benefit of treatment, if any, is due to the insemination or ovarian stimulation has yet to be determined.

These empirical therapeutic questions beg the essential question of what is the nature and cause of the underlying assumed follicular disorder, and whether the cause is follicular or extraovarian in origin. New understanding of paracrine control within the follicle (Hillier, 1987) focuses attention on intrafollicular factors. There may also be a gradual ageing process long before the menopause, as suggested by the distinct but unexplained reduction in fertility that affects women generally (CECOS, 1982), and it is also well known that in the years approaching the menopause there is already evidence of rising FSH levels, suggesting incipient ovarian failure (see Gindoff & Jewelewicz, 1986). These are questions remaining to be studied which may shed light on women with prolonged unexplained infertility. Meanwhile, although it may seem advisable to measure FSH routinely in the investigation of infertility it is rarely raised in those women with normal menstrual cycles (Conway et al, 1985).

Sperm dysfunction

Earlier, in discussing the basic criteria for fertility, we drew attention to the lack of diagnostic value of standard methods of seminal analysis and to the need to assess sperm function rather than numbers. We took sperm penetration of, and survival in, normal cervical mucus as the essential basic test of sperm function. In cases of prolonged unexplained infertility, other functions of sperm may possibly be disordered. After escaping from the seminal plasma into the cervical mucus, they must traverse the uterine cavity, penetrate the uterotubal opening, reach the tubal ampulla, survive possibly for 24–48 hours in the fallopian tube, undergo capacitation including adoption of "whiplash" flagellar action and the acrosome reaction, then penetrate between the cumulus cells of the egg, bind to the zona pellucida, penetrate the zona pellucida, and attach to the vitelline membrane of the egg cell. These are distinct steps on the way to fertilisation, any of which can go wrong. They are discussed in the chapter by Wardle, Ford & Hull.

All these functions have been explored to varying extents, and practical interest is focused on photographic assessment of movement characteristics of capacitated spermatozoa, biochemical assessment of sperm metabolism, and testing fertilising ability using human and hamster eggs. In all these instances, spermatozoa are tested after suspension in physiological culture medium, although usually only a simple artificial medium is required. Whether sperm function is tested in an artificial culture medium or in natural cervical mucus, it is important to appreciate that it is not tested in semen. We earlier referred to sperm "escaping" from seminal plasma and used the term intentionally. Paradoxical though it may seem, semen is not the place for sperm — or at least, not for long. Seminal plama is essentially a medium of transport for the spermatozoa. They are mixed with the several constituents of seminal plasma only at ejaculation, and successful spermatozoa must escape within a few minutes into cervical mucus. Fertilising ability is lost in proportion to the time spent in seminal plasma, and reduction is evident within 30 minutes (Rogers, 1985). It is therefore perhaps not surprising after all that counting sperm in semen is of such little value.

Aitken et al (1984) studied 68 couples with prolonged infertility in whom the women appeared normal and the man had normal sperm "counts" on standard seminal analysis. They compared conception rates with several semen parameters. Using multivariant discriminant analysis, they found that conventional semen analysis was not of significant value in discriminating the incidence of pregnancy but that the addition of post-capacitation movement characteristics in particular lateral head displacement did improve predictability. This could be further improved by including the results of zona free hamster egg penetration tests, which increased predictability to 76.5 per cent.

Check et al (1987), analysing the clinical role of the hamster egg test in determining male treatment in unexplained infertility, concluded that it was not on its own particularly useful for this purpose. Unfortunately, the hamster egg test shows a wide range of variation in both fertile and infertile men, leading to difficulties in interpreting results. Although Aitken's findings are encouraging because of their diagnostic value, the predictive power for fertilisation of human eggs in vitro and for natural pregnancy does not seem to be any greater than the much simpler tests of sperm-mucus penetration and survival (Glazener et al, 1987a). Direct comparison of these is needed.

Another fairly simple test is the recovery of sperm by their own motility into artificial culture medium and measurement of duration of survival in the medium. This test does away with the need for cervical mucus but requires greater technical provision. The results seem to correlate with fertilising ability, but proper comparison remains to be done.

Fertilisation and implantation

Hertig (1975) suggested that the ovulation of abnormal oocytes with reduced capacity for fertilisation may be a cause of infertility. It is known that fecundity in man is low compared to other animals (Short, 1979) and an increased frequency of abnormal gametes in man could be a cause. In vivo fertilisation rates in man appear to be high (> 80 per cent), but so is embryo wastage (Leridon, 1977). In vitro fertilisation and embryo transfer studies now enable the relative contributions of these factors to unexplained infertility to be assessed.

In a small early study, Trounson et al (1980a) suggested that fertilisation was impaired in unexplained infertility, compared with tubal infertility. A larger study by his group, however, later found only a slight reduction in the fertilisation rate (67 per cent), but the women were also relatively old (Mahadevan et al, 1983). Hull et al (1984) also seemed to find a slight reduction in fertilisation rate in unexplained compared with tubal infertility, but at that time minor endometriosis had not been excluded from the unexplained group because its significance was doubted. A larger study later by this group, however, showed significant loss of fertilising ability of oocytes associated with untreated endometriosis and no loss of fertilising ability in unexplained infertility (Wardle et al, 1985). Jones (1985) also found no reduction in fertilisation in unexplained infertility, nor any reduction in the implantation rate. Although not thoroughly studied yet, there does not seem to be any increased loss during early pregnancy after IVF and embryo transfer. Concerning in vivo conception, Pepperell and McBain (1985) found no increase in the appearance of beta-HCG in the luteal phase of women with unexplained infertility to suggest occult abortions.

It, therefore, appears that in general there is no impairment of fertilisation (given adequate assessment of basic sperm function) or implantation to account for unexplained infertility. It is too soon, however, to assess possible subtle effects of, for example, age, previous pregnancy and duration of infertility — at least not each independently. However, as discussed earlier and shown in Figure 2-3, it is clear that duration of infertility has a major effect on the chance of natural conception and we have, therefore, studied the effect on fertilisation in vitro, as follows.

It is important to appreciate that the following study (Forsey, Wardle and Hull, as yet unpublished), along with earlier studies from which this has been extended (Hull et al, 1984; Wardle et al, 1985), was done in carefully controlled conditions using standardised methods at all stages, including, particularly, treatment to stimulate the ovaries. Therefore, the results of IVF are properly comparable between all the groups and subgroups studied.

Figure 2-6 indicates no reduction in fertilising ability with increasing duration of unexplained infertility. This conclusion also implies that the fertilising ability of both oocytes and spermatozoa separately remain normal. It should also not be forgotten that in the cases studied, basic investigations had included a normal finding for sperm-mucus penetration and survival (a favourable PCT result). Although fertilisation rates remained constant, observation suggests a slight decline in the absolute number of embryos obtained, which may have been due to slight reduction in the numbers of eggs recovered with advancing duration of infertility. We suspect that is related primarily to age, although our results are as yet insufficient to be conclusive.

It should be appreciated that much of the data relating to fertilisation rates and implantation derived from IVF studies relates to the situation following exogenous ovarian stimulation. The situation as it appears in spontaneous cycles has yet to be determined.

Endometrial steroid receptor defects

A lack of endometrial steroid receptors, notably to progesterone, leading to endometrial dysfunction with suboptimal conditions for implantation, despite adequate corpus luteum function, has been suggested as a possible cause of some cases of unexplained infertility. In vitro studies by Maynard et al (1983) indicated a reduced nuclear uptake of progesteone by endometrial cells from 14 patients with unexplained infertility, although considerable overlap of values between fertile and infertile groups limit the discriminatory power of the assay. The recurrence of this abnormality in subsequent cycles was not tested. How commonly such intrinsic defects occur remains to be established. When cases due probably to inadequate follicular phase receptor stimulation are excluded, those occurring in a totally normal ovarian cycle would appear to be rare and at present remain untreatable.

Immunological factors

Immunological causes have been reported to account for 10 per cent of cases described as having unexplained infertility (Haas et al, 1980). Such cases have been attributed to antisperm antibodies present in either partner, cellular immunity to sperm, and antibodies to the zona pellucida of the oocyte. These factors appear to be able to interfere with sperm motility and transport, and sperm survival and fertilisation. Possible effects post-fertilisation on implantation are as yet however unsubstantiated.

Antisperm antibodies

Reduced conception rates have been found in association with antisperm antibodies in the male (Ayvraliotis et al, 1985) and female (Jones, 1980) in couples said to have "unexplained" infertility. However, in such cases antisperm antibodies invariably lead to an abnormal postcoital test, which thus provides a basic means of screening for locally secreted antibodies and should in any case disallow a diagnosis of unexplained infertility. Identification of the class of antibody responsible and its site of binding is possible by employing tests using antiglobulin conjugated to either polyacrylamide spheres (immunobeads; Bronson et al, 1981) or latex particles (Comhaire et al, 1987). This is important as it appears that only antibodies directed against the head of the spermatozoa inhibit fertilisation in vitro (Mandelbaum et al, 1987).

The significance of complement dependent antisperm antibodies in cervical mucus has been questioned (Jager et al, 1984), although it is well established that antibodies of the IgA class lead to the shaking phenomenon seen in cervical mucus tested in vitro (Jager et al, 1977) and a negative postcoital test (Clarke et al, 1984). As both IgG and IgA class antibodies in serum have been shown to reduce fertilisation rates in vitro (Ackerman et al, 1984; Yovich et al, 1984; Clark et al, 1986; Daitoh et al, 1986) it would thus be necessary to perform assays for antisperm antibodies on both serum and cervical mucus in the woman as well as semen if the postcoital test is not routinely employed in order to rule out immunological causes. Whereas a positive postcoital test makes it very unlikely that circulating levels of antisperm antibodies exist, as most studies have shown higher levels of local antibody production (Moghissi et al, 1980; Menge et al, 1982; Clarke et al, 1984). Thus although a potential cause for infertility, antisperm antibodies should be identified by basic investigation prior to a diagnosis of unexplained infertility being made.

There is, however, a possible exception to that rule. When antisperm antibodies are present in the woman, it is possible that in some cases immobilisation of the spermatozoa may be prevented at the cervix by complement inhibitors present in seminal plasma, allowing a positive postcoital test, whilst higher up the female tract inhibition lysis could occur (Bronson et al, 1984). Tubal secretion of antibodies has been demonstrated and IgA in particular may be secreted in higher concentrations than appear in the serum (Ping, 1979). Another situation where serum antisperm antibodies may not be detected may arise under conditions of relative antigen excess where all antibody present form circulating immune complexes which are not detectable by routine methods (Witkin et al, 1984).

Anti-zona pellucida antibodies

Specific antibodies to the zona pellucida of the oocyte have been shown in animals to inhibit sperm-zona binding and penetration (Shivers et al, 1972; Tsunoda and Chang, 1978) and may prevent implantation if fertilisation does occur (Aitken et al, 1981). Antibodies to porcine zona pellucida have been shown to inhibit human fertilisation in vitro (Trounson et al, 1980b). Immunisation in some species has been reported to reduce natural fertility (Aitken and Richardson, 1980). Several workers looking for similar antibodies in women with unexplained infertility reported their presence in approximately 30 per cent of cases (Shivers and Dunbar, 1977; Mori et al, 1978). However, other workers have also reported finding antibodies in 30 per cent of fertile women and men (Sacco and Moghissi, 1979; Kurachi et al, 1984) whilst Nayudu et al (1981), using a different assay method, failed to find similar antibodies in sera or follicular fluid of infertile women. Thus it remains very doubtful that antibodies to porcine zona pellucida antigens are an important factor in women with unexplained infertility. Whether or not antibodies specific to different human zona pellucida antigens exist, and their importance, remains to be found.

Cell mediated immunity

The role of cell mediated immunity to spermatozoa in the genesis of infertility is much less clear than the situation relating to humoral immunity. The female reproductive tract is immunologically competent in dealing with foreign antigens, and cellular immune mechanisms are probably important in the normal removal of dead or dying sperm. However, whether those mechanisms involve recognition of antigens only, expressed by damaged spermatozoa due to membrane changes or intracellular release after breakdown, remains unclear. Early reports of high levels of anti-HLA antibodies in patients with unexplained infertility (Stolp et al, 1973) have not been confirmed by others (Fellous and Dausset, 1973; Lindblom et al, 1972). There appears to be no evidence for increased HLA sharing or histo-incompatibility, as measured by the mixed lymphocyte reaction (Norlander, 1983). In vitro studies evaluating the cell mediated response to sperm of lymphocytes derived from women with unexplained infertility have demonstrated both increased responses (Lewis et al, 1978; McShane et al, 1985) associated with reduced conception rates (Soffer et al, 1976) and unchanged responses (Tait et al, 1976; Mettler and Schirwani, 1975). Clearly more work is needed to determine if cell mediated immune mechanisms have a role in the etiology of otherwise unexplained infertility.

Cervical mucus

Given a positive postcoital test, ie. the presence of forward progressing spermatozoa in most high power microscope fields of cervical mucus about 12 hours after intercourse, little more is usually done to assess cervical mucus further. It is not known whether subtle differences exist in mucus quality in women with unexplained infertility. Although the quality is enough to allow sperm penetration and survival to some degree, it is not known whether that is reduced compared with fertile women. Assessment of cervical mucus has largely been on morphological grounds and its study is difficult due to the need for accurate timing in relation to ovulation in order to ensure optimal mucus collection.

Despite the poor correlation of mucus quality and peak preovulatory oestrogen levels (McBain, 1980) exogenous oestrogens have been widely used empirically with little justification. Pharmacological doses usually lead to disruption of ovulation or anovulation. It is yet to be established whether the success claimed by the use of gonadotrophin therapy in patients with unexplained infertility is in part due to changes in cervical mucus resulting from the higher follicular phase levels of endogenous oestrogen achieved. At present, any possible etiological role of cervical mucus in unexplained infertility (which by our definition requires a positive postcoital test) requires further investigation.

Occult infection

Occult infection with mycoplasma organisms, in particular Ureaplasma urealyticum, has been found in association with infertility. Gnarpe and Friberg (1972, 1973) demonstrated the organism in 85 per cent of men and 91 per cent of women with apparently unexplained infertility, compared to just over 20 per cent in normal men and their pregnant wives. Stray-Pedersen et al (1978) also reported a higher frequency of Ureaplasma within cervical and endometrial specimens in their unexplained patients. However, other authors have pointed out the high frequency with which mycoplasma species can be recovered from semen and cervical mucus of fertile couples and so question the significance of these organisms when found (DeLouvois et al, 1974).

A more recent careful study by Cassell et al (1983) at the time of laparoscopy in infertile women and fertile women undergoing sterilisation revealed no difference after culturing the endocervix, uterine washings and endometrial tissue; about 40 per cent were found to have Ureaplasma. The only significant finding was that, within the infertile group Ureaplasma was isolated much more frequently in the women whose husbands had seminal abnormality (74 per cent) than any other subgroup (42 per cent overall), suggesting that the only real association is with male infertility. Therapeutic studies using doxycycline to eradicate the organism have been poorly controlled and results are contradictory (Gnarpe and Frieberg, 1973; Harrison et al, 1975). The only controlled prospective study suggested that clearance of mycoplasma from men benefitted more the outcome of pregnancy rather than achieving pregnancy. In many cases the problem had been recurrent miscarriages rather than infertility (Toth et al, 1983).

The association of Chlamydia trachomatis infection and tubal damage is well established, but the significance of past infection in unexplained infertility, particularly on aspects such as fertilisation and implantation, is unclear. Rowland et al (1985) in England found that the success of IVF and embryo transfer in women with serological evidence of past chlamydial infection was half that of those who were seronegative. However, Torode et al (1987) failed to find such an association in their IVF and GIFT patients despite a high incidence of seropositive patients (42 per cent). One explanation might be that the serological tests used reflect only prior exposure to chlamydia and not concurrent infection or carriage of the organism within the genital tract, which might be of greater importance. The patients studied in England might thus have had a higher incidence of the organism still within the genital tract compared with those in the Australian study. The greater awareness of this organism in recent times and continental differences in prescribing may have led to more of the women in the more recent Australian series having had antibiotic therapy and so eradication of the organism.

Chlamydia has always been difficult to culture from the endocervix despite active tubal disease and it would be hoped that newer monoclonal antibody techniques will allow better detection of the organism from endocervical and endometrial samples. At present, there is no information on the recovery rate of the organism from the female genital tract in women with unexplained infertility. From serological evidence we find no evidence of an increased incidence of antichlamydial antibodies in our patients with unexplained infertility and none is apparent in the 69 patients with idiopathic infertility included in the study by Torode et al (1987).

Psychological factors

Hypothalamic amenorrhea resulting from psychological or emotional causes is a well recognised entity, but the effects of such factors on normally menstruating women have been difficult to assess. Much has been written on possible psychological causes for infertility (Noyes and Chapnick, 1964; Mozley, 1976), but presented with an infertile couple, it is difficult to differentiate cause and effect. More recent reviews assessing psychological, emotional and behavioural factors in patients presenting with infertility have failed to show any significant difference in those women with normal ovulatory patterns (Seibel and Taymor, 1982).

Harrison et al (1981), using psychological and biochemical (prolactin) assessments of stress, did report, however, the identification of a subgroup of unexplained infertile patients who were unusually stressed, and attempted to reduce stress levels within this subgroup by relaxation therapy (O'Moore et al, 1983) and by inhibiting prolactin rises with bromocriptine (Harrison et al, 1979). Despite evidence that both techniques were effective at reducing stress and prolactin rises, pregnancy rates were no better than with placebo. The role of psychotherapy and emotional support, although essential in any form of patient management, do not appear to be significant in the development of unexplained infertility.

Advanced investigation and definition of unexplained infertility

From the above discussion of possible etiological factors in unexplained infertility, are there any investigations that might be appropriate in addition to the basic tests previously described, particularly when infertility has lasted a long time (more than three years)? The question would be better put: what investigations might usefully be applied? Investigations would be useful if they at least explained the cause of infertility with reasonable confidence; and better still if they led to specific effective treatment.

Put that way, consideration could only be given — yet only tentatively —

to two possibilities: first, finding of extensive intrauterine adhesions by hysteroscopy, and secondly, serological finding of antisperm antibodies in the woman despite normal sperm-mucus penetration and survival. Yet what evidence is there that division of intrauterine adhesions leads to a better chance of conception? As for circulating antisperm antibodies in the woman, there is no convincing evidence yet that immunosuppressive therapy improves fertility despite lowering antibody levels, in men or women. More extensive studies are needed than have been possible to date of in vitro fertilisation and embryo transfer. It may be found that fertilisation is successful if the woman's serum can be avoided; the outcome of implantation seems difficult to predict.

Thus, if there is virtually no investigation that leads either to convincing explanation of the cause of infertility — despite the finding of an apparent abnormality — or to any specific treatment, we are left with an approach to treatment that is both general and empirical, and unfortunately still often of unproven benefit.

Treatment

Many empirical therapeutic approaches to unexplained infertility have been tried and much anecdotal evidence to support empirical treatment has been amassed. However, few well controlled prospective studies have been undertaken. This rather disappointing reality is in fact hardly surprising as the problems in mounting such studies are daunting. Patients selected need to be comparable, particularly for duration of infertility and the diagnostic criteria used. Because pregnancy rates per cycle are low, large numbers and prolonged exposure are needed, giving rise to practical and statistical difficulties. Patients with prolonged unexplained infertility are seldom prepared to accept unproven treatment or act as controls for any suitable length of study without resorting to active treatment including IVF or GIFT.

Unexplained infertility of short duration

Figure 2-3 shows that couples with less than three years unexplained infertility have an 84 per cent chance of conceiving without treatment during the next two years. Their monthly chance of conceiving is five to 10 per cent. That means that compared with the highest claims for any treatment (up to 25 per cent but usually much less), natural intercourse gives them as good a chance of conceiving within about three months as a single cycle of what is often intensive, invasive, stressful and costly treatment. Therefore, such couples should be dissuaded against any form of treatment.

That is not to say they cannot or should not be offered any help. Explanation and encourgagement are the key. They must be made to understand the chance nature of fertility and the statistics of their own condition. Showing them the relevant graphs is very helpful. They can also be given advice about self-recognition of the preovulatory cervical mucus surge in order to ensure accurate timing of intercourse in every cycle, thereby optimising their chance of conceiving. Some couples, particularly when the woman finds it difficult to recognise her mucus surge (despite its occurrence as demonstrated in the diagnostic process), feel more confident and encouraged by testing for the LH surge.

When the woman is aged in her late 30s or older, couples cannot take a long term view of putting their fertility to the test as suggested above. They may therefore press reasonably for active treatment, just as a couple with longer infertility might do. In their case, however, the only rational choice should be treatment with a proven record of success. At present IVF and probably preferably GIFT are the only treatment that meet those requirements.

Prolonged unexplained infertility (more than three years)

As Figure 2-3 shows, without treatment the chance of conception is now only one to two per cent each cycle. Although the cumulative chance of conceiving amounts to about 30 per cent during the course of the next two years, after five years' infertility or more, that seems an unrealistic hope. The balance of choice is now undoubtedly in favour of active treatment. The choice of treatment, however, is not clear cut. It ranges from the simple but only moderately effective (clomiphene), to more complex treatments that are still optimistic and unproven (intrauterine or intraperitoneal insemination, or superovulation therapy using gonadotrophins, or a combination), to proven but highly complex treatment by IVF or GIFT.

Using clomiphene in standard dosage (100 mg daily, days two to six of the menstrual cycle) the results from the controlled study by Glazener et al (1987e, unpublished data) shown in Table 2-3 demonstrate an increase in the monthly chance of conception from about one per cent to five per cent. The cumulative pregnancy rate after three months treatment was 14 per cent. That is about the same as can be achieved by one cycle of IVF, although much more easily. In any case, the overall management of an IVF cycle spans more than a month. Whether further treatment with clomiphene beyond the three cycles studied would continue to be as effective remains unproven, but it is a reasonable assumption to make. There would seem to be no good reason not to continue clomiphene therapy at the same dosage indefinitely. The only precautions advisable in practice are to ensure, by appropriate testing occasionally, that favourable luteal progesterone levels are maintained and that there is no interference by the clomiphene with postcoital sperm-mucus penetration and survival.

Ovarian stimulation using gonadotrophins have been suggested to be beneficial without any other treatment (Wang and Gemsell, 1979), with artificial insemination (Melis et al, 1987) and in combination with intrauterine insemination (IUI; Dodson et al, 1987; Serhal et al, 1988) or intraperitoneal insemination (IPI) (Forrler et al, 1986). IPI has not been properly studied and has not been taken up with much enthusiasm. Gonadotrophin treatment with IUI has led to pregnancy rates of about 20 per cent per cycle in the favourable studies reported, but the efficacy of this treatment has yet to be established by controlled trials. It is not without risk and considerable expense and cannot as yet be recommended without further evidence, although it seems reasonable to try as a compromise between clomiphene therapy on the one hand and IVF or GIFT on the other. Selection of such treatment as a compromise may seem more attractive after an attempt at IVF has at least confirmed fertilising ability.

Nor have IVF and GIFT been subjected yet to properly controlled trials in the treatment of unexplained infertility but, unlike IUI, there is a large mass of data accumulated from several centres demonstrating a consistent pregnancy rate far in excess of the expected rate without treatment. There can be no doubt that pregnancy occurs as a direct result of the treatment each time. Early reports showed IVF and GIFT techniques to be equally effective in the unexplained group (Leeton et al, 1987) but recent large series reported suggest consistently higher pregnancy rates using GIFT (Craft et al, 1988) than generally reported with IVF although the two treatments have not been properly compared.

The final choice and plan of treatment is likely to depend very much on emotional reasons for the patients, such as duration of infertility and age, and on medical philosophical opinion. In our view, we are strongly inclined towards IVF as a primary step after more than three to five years of properly defined unexplained infertility, partly for the diagnostic information provided by the fertilisation rate. Given a good or at least acceptable fertilisation rate, although pregnancy may fail to occur, there is powerful encouragement for the couple, not necessarily to persist with IVF (indeed GIFT would then be the better choice), also to consider any of the other more speculative treatments already discussed.

Table 2-1
Frequency of luteal phase deficiency* (and severe deficiency†) in unexplained infertility compared with normal (Glazener et al, 1988)

Occurrence of luteal deficiency	*Infertile patients*	*Normal control*
1. In individual cycles	17% (4%+)	15% (3%+)
2. In at least 2 of 3 cycles	13%	12%
3. In at least 4 of 6 cycles	2%	5%

** Deficiency = midluteal progesterone <28 nmol/l*
† Severe deficiency = midluteal progesterone <14 nmol/l

Table 2-2
Midluteal progestrone levels and cumulative conception rate related to prolactin levels in unexplained infertility without treatment (Glazener et al, 1987c)

Prolactin (mU/1)	*No. of Patients*	*Mean Progesterone (nmol/1)*	*Conception rate after 12 months (± SE)*
<200	47	40	41% ± 10%
201–400	100	42	49% ± 6%
401–600	18	44	58% ± 17%
601–800	16	36	26% ± 18%
>800*	7*	42	62% ± 22%

** including four patients with PRL>1000, one >3000mU/1*

Table 2-3
Clomiphene treatment of unexplained infertility compared with placebo in a double blind crossover study (Glazener et al, 1987e) (unpublished data)

Outcome	*Number of patients*	*Treatment*		*Proportional increase*
		Placebo	*Clomiphene*	
Mean progesterone (nmol/1)		43	71	+0.66 $p<0.001$
Conception rate after 3m.				
Total group	118	15%	22%	+0.53 $p<0.05$
Duration infertility				
< 3 yrs	82	20%	26%	Not significant
> 3 yrs	36	3%	14%	+4.97 $p<0.05$

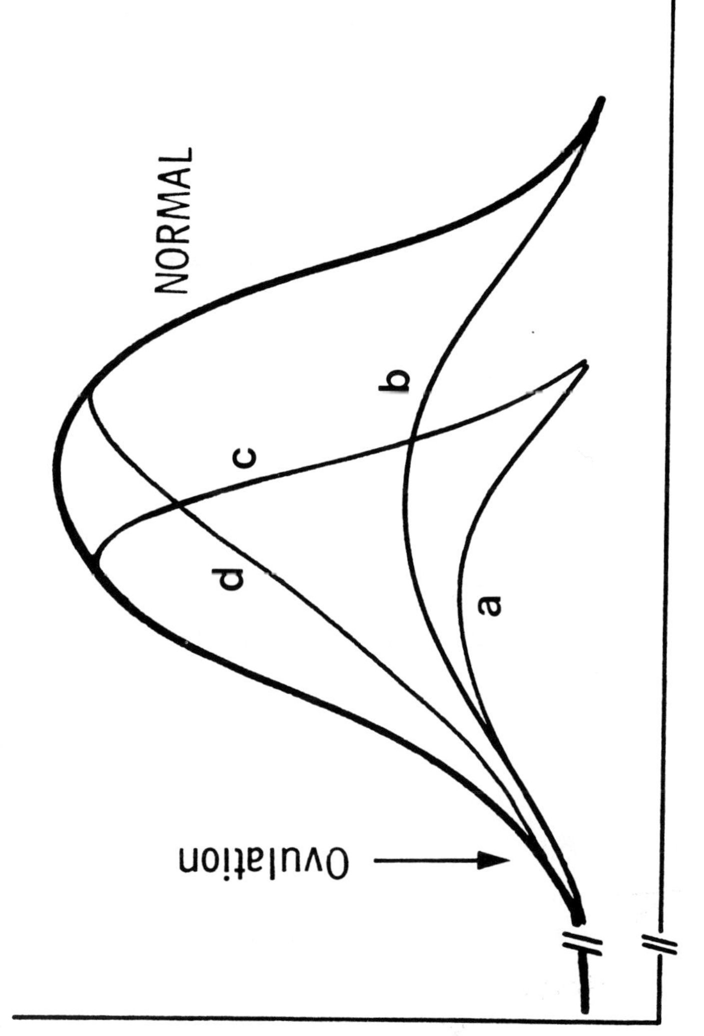

Figure 2-1
Possible different patterns of serum progesterone through the luteal phase in defective cycles (a, b, c, d) compared with normal.

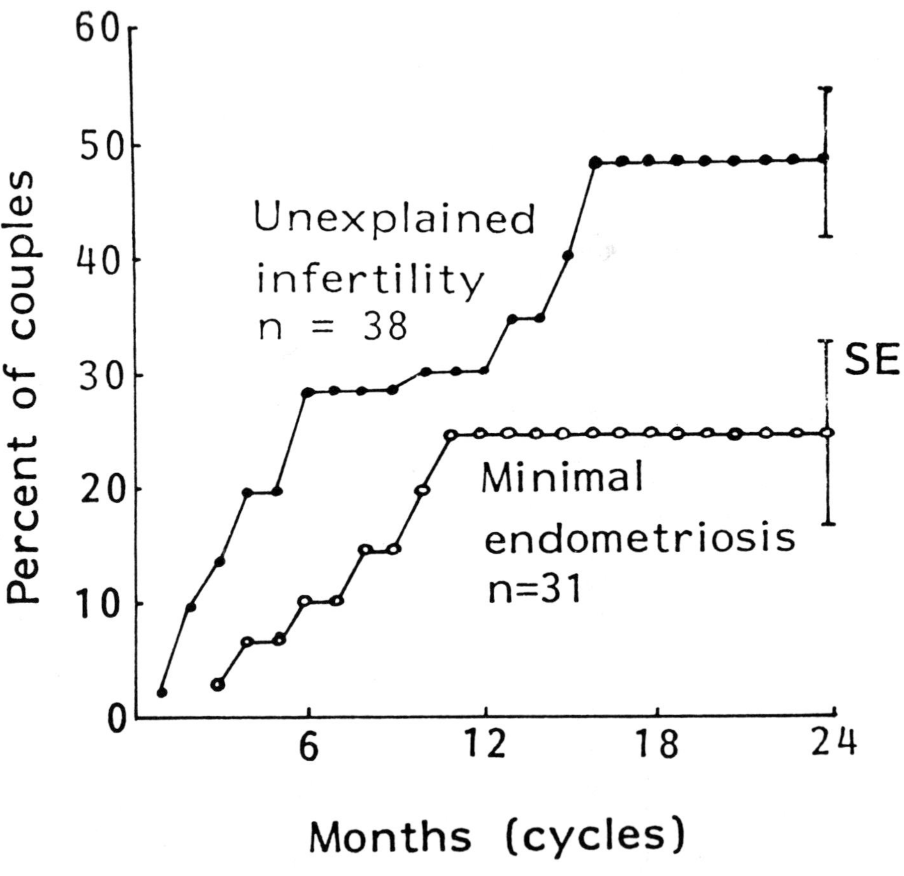

Figure 2-2
Cumulative conception rates from the time of diagnostic laparoscopy in couples with minimal endometriosis compared with others with unexplained infertility similar in all other respects.

Source: Foster, Foulkes & Hull, unpublished data.

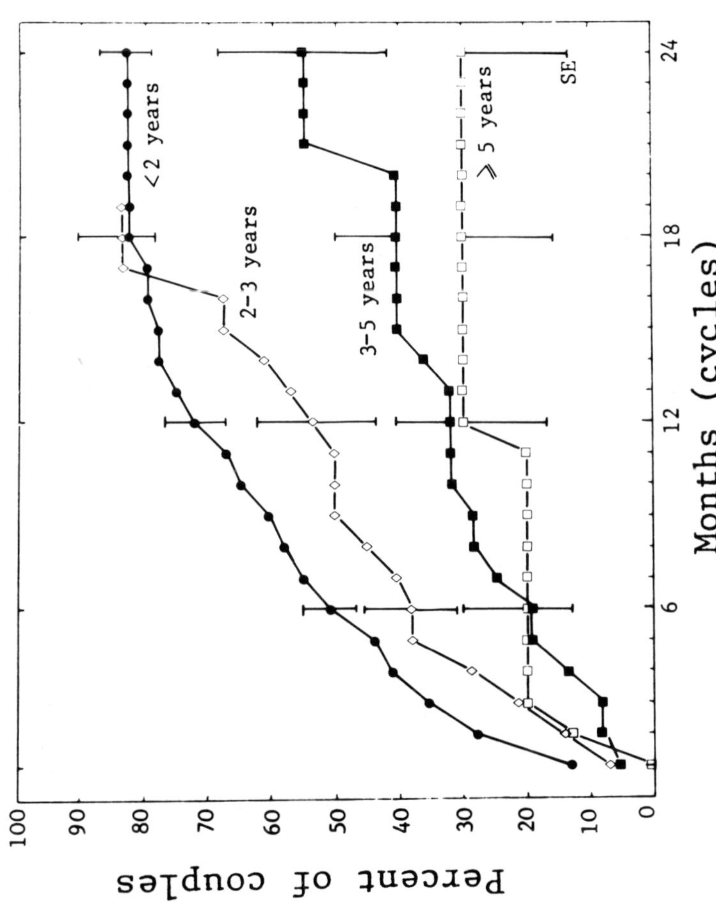

Figure 2-3

Cumulative conception rates without treatment in couples with unexplained infertility from the time of diagnosis related to the previous duration of infertility.

Source: From Hull et al, 1985.

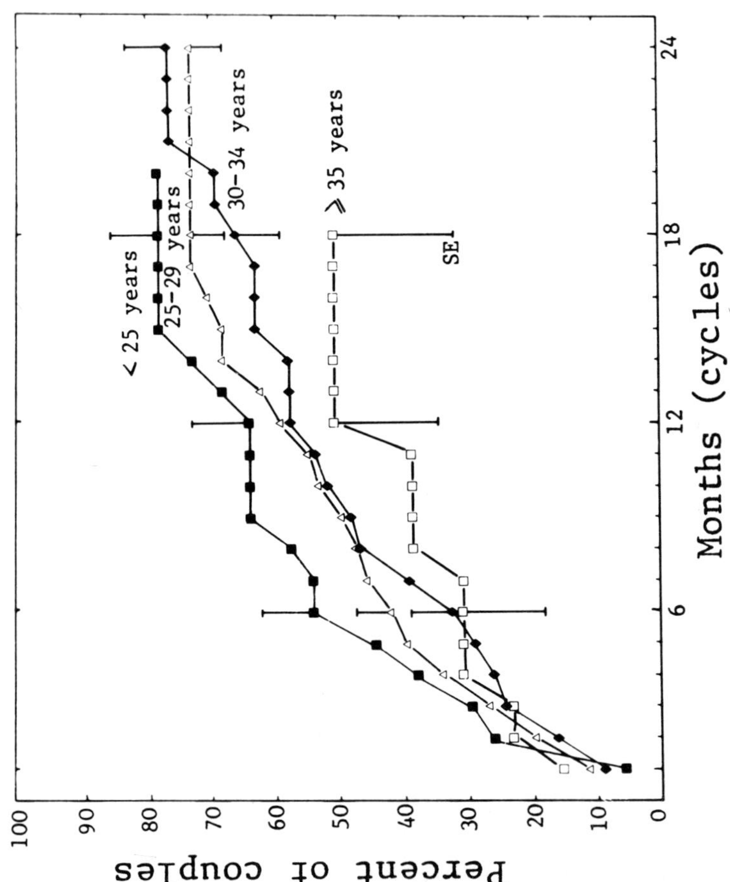

Figure 2-4

Cumulative conception rates in couples as in Figure 2.3 related to the woman's age at diagnosis of unexplained infertility.

Source: From Hull et al, 1985.

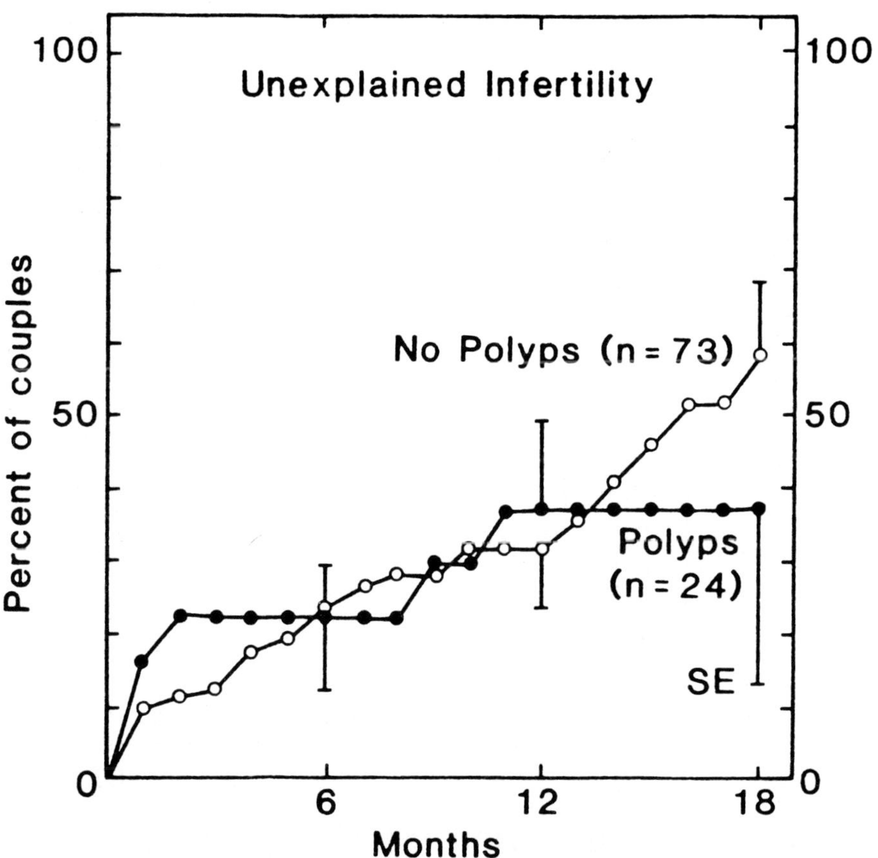

Figure 2-5
Cumulative conception rates related to the presence or absence of tubocornual polyps in couples with otherwise unexplained infertility.
Source: Reproduced with permission from Glazener et al, 1987.

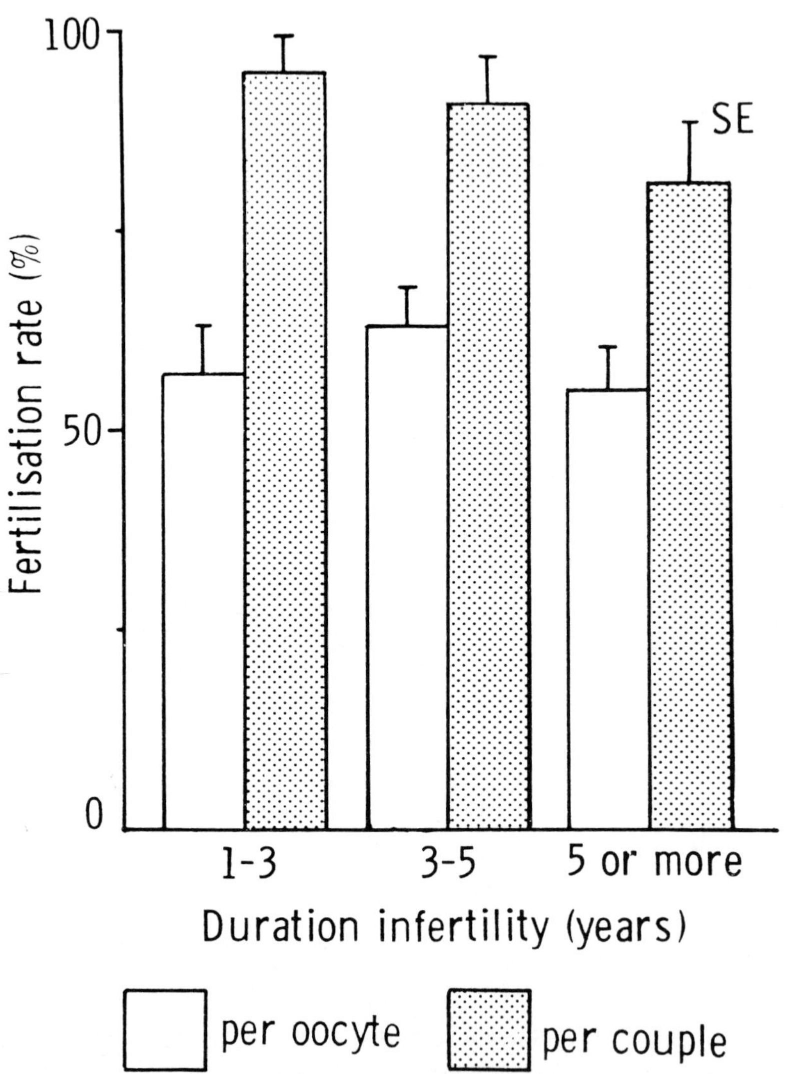

Figure 2-6
In vitro fertilisation rates related to duration of unexplained infertility.
Source: Forsey, Wardle & Hull, unpublished data.

References

Ackerman, S.B., Graff, D.Van, Clem, J.F., Swanson, R.J., Veekc, L.L., Acosta, A.A., Garcia, J.E. Immunologic infertility and in-vitro fertilisation. *Fertility and Sterility,* 1984; 42: 474.

Aitken, R.J., Best, F.S.M., Richardson, D.W., Djahanbakhah, O., Mortimer, D., Templeton, A. & Lees, M.M. An analysis of sperm function in cases of unexplained infertility: Conventional criteria, movement characteristics and fertilising capacity. *Fertility and Sterility,* 1982; 38: 212.

Aitken, R.J., Best, F.S.M., Warner, P. & Templeton, A. A prospective study of the relationship between semen quality and fertility in cases of unexplained infertility. *Journal of Andrology,* 1984; 5: 297.

Aitken, R.J., Richardson, D.W. Immunization against zona pellucida antigens. In Hearn, J.P. (Ed), *Immunological Aspects of Reproduction and Fertility Control,* University Park Press, Baltimore, 1980; 173.

Aitken, R.J., Rudak, E.A., Richardson, D.W., Dor, J., Djahanbahkah, O., Templeton, A.A. The influence of anti-zona and anti-sperm anti-bodies on sperm-egg interactions. *Reproduction and Fertility,* 1981; 62: 597.

Asch, R.H. Laparoscopic recovery of sperm from peritoneal fluid in patients with negative or poor Sims-Huhner tests. *Fertility and Sterility,* 1976; 27: 1111.

Ayvraliotis, B., Bronson, R., Rosenfeld, D., Cooper, G. Conception rates in couples where autoimmunity to sperm is detected. *Fertility and Sterility,* 1985; 43: 739.

Backstrom, C.T., McNeilly, A.S., Leask, A.S., Baird, D.T. Pulsatile secretion of LH, FSH, prolactin, oestradiol and progesterone during the human menstrual cycle. *Clinical Endrocrinology,* 1982; 17: 29.

Bahamondes, L., Saboaa, W., Tambascia, M., Trevisdan, M. Galactorrhoea, infertility and short luteal phases in hyperprolactinaemic women: Early stage of amenorrhoea-galactorrhoea. *Fertility and Sterility,* 1979; 32: 476.

Balasch, J., Vanrell, J. Corpus luteum insufficiency and fertility: A matter of controversy. *Human Reproduction,* 1987; 2: 557.

Ben-David, M., Schenkar, J.G. Transient hyperprolactinaemia: A correctable cause of idiopathic female infertility. *Journal of Clinical Endocrinology and Metabolism,* 1983; 57: 442.

Bostofte, E., Serup, J., Rebbe, H. Relation between number of immobile spermatozoa and pregnancies obtained during a twenty-year follow-up period. *Andrologia,* 1984; 16: 136.

Bronson, R., Cooper, G.W., Rosenfeld, D.L. Membrane-bound sperm-specific antibodies: Their role in infertility. In Vogel, H. and G. Jagiello (Eds), *Bioregulators in Reproduction,* New York, Academic Press, 1981: 521.

Bronson, R., Cooper, G., Rosenfeld, D. Sperm antibodies — their role in infertility. *Fertility and Sterility,* 1984; 42: 171.

Brosens, I., Boeckx, W., Delattin, Ph., Puttemans, P.G., Vasquez, G. Salpingoscopy: A new pre-operative diagnostic tool in tubal infertility. *British Journal of Obstetrics and Gynaecology,* 1987; 94: 768.

Brown, J.B., Harrison, P., Smith, M.A., Burger, H.G. Correlations between mucus symptoms and the hormonal markers of fertility throughout reproductive life. in *Monograph,* Advocate Press, Melbourne, 1981; 1.

Cassell, G.M., Yonger, J.B., Brown, M.B., Blackwell, R.E., Davis, J.K., Marriott, P., Stagno, S. Microbiologic study of infertile women at the time of diagnostic laparoscopy. Association of ureaplasma urealyticum with a defined populations. *New England Journal of Medicine,* 1983; 308: 502.

Cates, Jr W., Rowe, P.J., The prevalence of infertility: Measures and causes. *Proceedings of the 12th World Congress on Fertilty and Sterility, Singapore 1986.* In Ratnam, S.S. and Teoh E.S. (Eds), *Advances in Fertility and Sterility Series,* Parthenon Press, Carnforth, Lancs, UK, 1987; 93.

CECOS Federation, Schwartz, D., Mayaux, M.J. Female fecundity as a function of age. *New England Journal of Medicine,* 1982; 306: 404.

Check, J.H., Wu, C.H., Adelson & Liss, J. The clinical usefulness of the hamster ovum penetration test in unexplained infertility. In Ratnam, S.S. and Teoh E.S. (Eds), *Advances in Fertility and Sterility,* Parthenon Press, Carnforth, Lancs., UK, 1987; 4: 211.

Clark, G.N., Lopata, A., Johnston, W.I.H., Effect of sperm antibodies in females on human in-vitro fertilisation. *Fertility and Sterility,* 1986; 46: 435.

Clarke, G.N., Stojanoff, A., Cauchi, M.N., McBain, J.C., Speirs, A.L., Johnston, W.I.H. Detection of antispermatozoal antibodies of IA class in cervical mucus. *American Journal of Reproductive Immunology,* 1984; 5: 61.

Cohen, J., Mayaux, M.J., Guihard-Moscato, M.L., Schwartz, D. In-vitro fertilisation and embryo transfer: A collaborative study of 1163 pregnancies on the incidence and risk factors of ectopic pregnancy. *Human Reproduction,* 1986; 1: 255.

Comhaire, F.H., Hinting, A., Vermeulenl, Schoonjans, F., Goethals, I. Evaluation of the direct and indirect mixed antiglobulin reaction with latex particles for the diagnosis of immunological infertility. *International Journal of Andrology,* 1987; 11: 37.

Conway, D., Glazener, C.M., Caul, O.E., Hodgson, J., Hull, M.G.R., Clarke, S.K.R., Stirrat, G.M. Chlamydial serology in fertile and infertile women. *Lancet,* 28 January 1984; 191.

Conway, D.I., Glazener, C.M., Kelly, N., Hull, M.G.R. Routine measurement of thyroid hormones in infertility not worthwhile. *Lancet,* 1985; 977.

Cooke, I.D., Dunphy, B., Lenton, E.A. Unexplained infertility — Frontiers in fertility, presented to the Royal College of Obstetricians and Gynaecologists, London, September 1987.

Coutts, J.R.T., Adam, A.H., Fleming, R. The deficient luteal phase may represent an anovulatory cycle. *Clinical Endocrinology,* 1982; 17: 389.

Coutts, J.R.T. The abnormal luteal phase. In Jeffcoate, S.L. (Ed), *The Luteal Phase,* Wiley, Chichester, 1985; 101.

Craft, I., Ah-Moye, M., Al-Shawaf, T., Fiamanya, W., Lewis, P., Robertson, D., Serhal, P., Shrivastav, P., Simons, E., Brinsden, P. Analysis of 1,071 GIFT procedures — the case for a flexible approach to treatment. *Lancet* 1988; i: 1094.

Cumming, D.C., Taylor, P.J. Combined laparoscopy and hysteroscopy in the investigation of the ovulatory infertile female. *Fertility and Sterility,* 1980; 33: 475.

David, M.P., Ben-Zwi, D., Langer, L. Tubal intramural polyps and their relationship to infertility. *Fertility and Sterility,* 1981; 35: 526.

Daitoh, T., Kamanda, M., Mori, T. Studies on biological actions of sperm immobilising antibody on human fertilisation in vitro. *Acta Obstetrica et Gynaecologica,* Japan, 1986; 38: 1057.

DeLouvois, J., Harrison, R.F., Blades, M., Hurley, R., Stanley, V.C. Frequency of mycoplasma in fertile and infertile couples. *Lancet* 1974; i: 1073.

Dodson, K.S., MacNaughton, M.C., Coutts, J.R.T. Infertility in women with apparently ovulatory cycles. *British Journal of Obstetrics and Gynaecology,* 1975; 82: 602.

Dodson, W.C., Easley, H.A., Whitesides, D.B., Haney, A.F., Hughes, C.L. Superovulation with intrauterine insemination in the treatment of infertility: A possible alternate to gamete intrafallopian transfer or in-vitro fertilisation. *Fertility and Sterility,* 1987; 48: 441.

Drake, T.S., Tredway, T.S., Buchanan, G.C., Takaki, N., Daane, T. Unexplained infertility — a reappraisal. *Journal of Obstetrics and Gynaecology,* 1977; 50: 644.

El-Minawi, M.F., Abdel-Hadi, M., Ibrahim, A.A., Wahby, O. Comparative evaluation of laparoscopy and hysterosalpingography in infertile patients. *Obstetrics and Gynaecology*, 1978; 51: 29.

Fellous, M., Dausset, J. Histocompatibility antigens on human spermatozoa. In Bratanov, K., Edwards, R.G., Vulchanov, V.R., Dikov, V., Somlev, B. (Eds), *Immunology of Reproduction*, Sofia Bulgarian Academy of Science Press, 1973; 332.

Fleming, R., Adam, A.H., Barlow, D.H., Black, W.P., MacNaughton, M.C., Coutts, J.R.T. A new systematic treatment for infertile women with abnormal hormone profiles. *British Journal of Obstetrics and Gynaecology*, 1982; 89: 80.

Forrler, A., Dallenbach , P., Nisand, I., Moreau, L., Crauz, C.L., Clavert, A., Rumpler, Y. Direct intraperitoneal insemination in unexplained and cervical infertility. *Lancet* 1986; ii: 916.

Garcia, C.R., Tureck, R.W. Submucosal leiomyomas and infertility. *Fertility and Sterility*, 1984; 42: 16.

Gindoff, P.R., Jewelewicz, R. Reproductive potential in the older woman. *Fertility and Sterility*, 1986; 46: 989.

Glazener, C.M.A., Hull, M.G.R. The sperm-mucus interface: Patterns of disorder in the diagnosis of specific causes of penetration failure causing infertility. *Human Reproduction*, 1987; 2: 673.

Glazener, C.M.A., Kelly, N.J., Davis, J.S.C., Cornes, J.S., Hull, M.G.R. The diagnosis of male infertility — prospective time specific study of conception rates related to seminal analysis and postcoital sperm-mucus penetration and survival in otherwise unexplained infertility. *Human Reproduction*, 1987a; 2: 665.

Glazener, C.M.A., Kelly, N.J., Hull, M.G.R. Borderline hyperprolactinemia in infertile women: Evaluation of the prolactin response to thyrotropen releasing hormone and double-blind placebo-controlled treatment with bromocriptine. *Gynaecological Endocrinology*, 1987b; 1: 373.

Glazener, C.M.A., Kelly, N.J., Hull, M.G.R. Evaluation of prolactin measurement in the investigation of infertility in women with a normal menstrual cycle. *British Journal of Obstetrics and Gynaecology*, 1987c; 94: 535.

Glazener, C.M.A., Loveday, L.M., Richardson, S.J., Jeans, W.D., Hull, M.G.R. Tubo-cornual polyps: Their relevance in subfertility. *Human Reproduction*, 1987d; 2: 59.

Glazener, C.M.A., Coulson, C., Lambert, P.A., Watt, E.M., Hinton, R.A., Kelly, N.J., Hull, M.G.R. Clomiphene treatment for women with unexplained infertility: Placebo controlled study of hormonal responses and conception rates, submitted for publication, 1987e.

Glazener, C.M.A., Hull, M.G.R., Kelly, N.J. Luteal deficiency not a persistent cause of infertility. *Human Reproduction*, 1988; 3: 2.

Gnarpe, H., Friberg, J. Mycoplasma and human reproductive failure. I: The occurrence of 7 different mycoplasmas in couples with reproductive failure. *American Journal of Obstetrics and Gynecology*, 1972; 114: 727.

Gnarpe, H., Friberg, J. T-mycoplasmas as a possible cause for reproductive failure. *Nature*, 1973; 242: 120.

Gordts, S., Boeckx, W., Vasquez, G., Brosens, I. Microsurgical resection of intramural tubal polyps. *Fertility and Sterility*, 1983; 40: 258.

Haas, G.G. Jr., Cines, D.B., Schreiber, A.D. Immunological infertility: Identification of patients with antisperm antibody. *New England Journal of Medicine*, 1980; 303: 722.

Harrison, R.F., Blades, M. DeLouvois, J., Hurley, R. Doxycycline treatment and human infertility. *Lancet* 1975; i: 605.

Harrison, R.F., O'Moore, R.R., McSweeney, J. Idiopathic infertility. A trial of bromocriptine versus placebo. *Irish Medical Journal*, 1979; 72: 479.

Harrison, R.F., O'Moore, A.M., O'Moore, R.R., McSweeney, J. Stress profiles in normal infertile couples. Pharmacological and psychological approaches to therapy. In Insler V., Bettendorf G. and Geissler K.H. (Eds), *Advances in Diagnosis and Treatment of Infertility*, New York: Elsevier, North Holland, 1981; 143.

Haxton, M.J., Fleming, R., Hamilton, M.P.R., Yates, R.W., Black, W.P., Coutts, J.R. Unexplained infertility — results of secondary investigations in 95 couples. *British Journal of Obstetrics and Gynaecology*, 1987; 94: 539.

Hertig, A.J. Implantation of the human ovum. In Behrman S.J. & Kistner, R.W. (Eds), *Progress in Infertility*, Little, Braun & Co, Boston, 1975; 435.

Hewitt, J., Cohen, J., Krishnaswamy, V., Fehilly, C.B., Steptoe, P.C., Eurof Walters, D. The treatment of idiopathic infertility, cervical mucus hostility, and male infertility: Artificial insemination with husband's semen or in-vitro fertilisation. *Fertility and Sterility*, 1985; 44: 350.

Hillier, S.G. Paracrine control in the ovaries. *Research in Reproduction*, 1987; 19: 1.

Hull, M.G.R., Glazener, C.M.A., Kelly, N.J., Conway, D.I., Foster, P.A., Hinton, R.A., Coulson, C., Lambert, P.A., Watt, E.M., Desai, K.M. Population study of causes, treatment and outcome of infertility. *British Medical Journal*, 1985, 291: 1693.

Hull, M.G.R., Joyce, D.N., McLeod, F.N., Ray, B.D., McDermott, A. Human in-vitro fertilisation, in-vitro sperm penetration of cervical mucus and unexplained infertility. *Lancet* 1984; ii: 245.

Hull, M.G.R., Glazener, C.M.A., Wardle, P.G., McLaughlin, E.A., Sykes, J.A. Male infertility: Sperm penetration of mucus related to natural and in-vitro fertility. *Proceedings of the 12th World Congress on Fertility and Sterility, Singapore, 1986*. In Ratnam, S.S., and Teoh E.S. (Eds), *Advances in Fertility and Sterility Series*, Parthenon Press, Carnforth, Lancs, UK, 1987; 31.

Jager, S., Kremer, J., DeWilde-Janssen, I.W. Are sperm immobilising antibodies in cervical mucus an explanation for a poor postcoital test? *American Journal of Reproductive Immunology*, 1984; 5: 56.

Jager, S., Kremer, J., Kuiken, J., Van Slochteren-Draaisma, T. Immunologlobulin class of sperm antibodies in cervival mucus. In Boettcher, B. (Ed), *Immunological Influence of Human Fertility*, Academic Press, Sydney, 1977; 289.

Jewelewicz, R. Management of infertility resulting from anovulation. *American Journal of Obstetrics and Gynecology*, 1975; 122: 909.

Jones, G.S. Some newer aspects of the management of infertility. *Journal of American Medical Association*, 1949; 141: 1123.

Jones, H.W. The selection of patients for in-vitro fertilisation. *Proceedings of the Twelfth Study Group of the Royal College of Obstetricians and Gynaecologists, November 1984*, In *In-vitro Fertilisation and Embryo Transfer*. London Royal College of Obstetricians and Gynaecologists, 1985; 189.

Jones, W.R. Immunologic infertility — fact or fiction? *Fertility and Sterility*, 1980; 33: 577.

Koninckx, P.R., Sole, P., Den Bourke, W., Brosens, I.A., New aspects of the pathophysiology of endometriosis and associated infertility. *Journal of Reproductive Medicine*, 1978; 24: 257.

Kurachi, I., Wakimoto, H., Sakumeto, T., Aono, T., Kurachi, K. Specific antibodies to porcine zona pellucida detected by quantitative radioimmunoassay in both fertile and infertile women. *Fertility and Sterility*, 1984; 41: 265.

Lamb, E.J., Cruz, A.L. Data collection and analysis in an infertility practice. *Fertility and Sterility*, 1972; 23: 310.

Leeton, J., Healy, D., Rogers, P., Yates, C., Caro, C. A controlled study between the use of gamete intrafallopian transfer (GIFT) and in vitro fertilisation and embryo transfer in the management of idiopathic and male infertility. *Fertility and Sterility*, 1987; 48: 605.

Lenton, E.A., Laurence, G.R., Coleman, R.A., Cooke, I.D. Individual variation in gonadotrophin and steroid concentrations and in the lengths of the follicular and luteal phases in women with regular menstrual cycles. *Clinical Reproduction and Fertility*, 1983; 2: 143.

Lenton, E.A., Weston. G.A., Cooke, I.D. Long-term follow-up of the apparently normal couple with a complaint of infertility. *Fertility and Sterility*, 1977; 28: 919.

Leridon, H. *Human Fertility: The Basic Components.*, University of Chicago, Chicago, USA, 1977.

Lewis, W.R., Lincoln, P.M., Dattner, A.M. Sperm-induced lymphocyte activation. *Lancet* 1978; i: 937.

Lindblom, B., Friberg, J., Hogman, C. HLA haplotypes and unexplained infertility. *Tissue Antigens*, 1972; 2: 351.

Macleod, J. Gold, R. Z. The male factor in infertility. VI: Semen quality and certain other factors in relation to ease of conception. *Fertility and Sterility*, 1953; 4: 10.

Mahadevan, M.A., Trounson, A.O., Leeton, J.F. The relationship of tubal blockage, infertility of unknown cause, suspected male infertility, and endometriosis to success of in-vitro fertilisation and embryo transfer. *Fertility and Sterility*, 1983; 40: 755.

Mandelbaum, S.L., Diamond, M.P., De Cherney, A.H. Relationship of antisperm antibodies to oocyte fertilisation and cleavage in in-vitro fertilisation. *Fertility and Sterility*, 1987; 47: 644.

Marik, J., Hulka, J. Luteinized unruptured follicle syndrome: A subtle cause of infertility. *Fertility and Sterility*, 1978; 29: 270.

Martinez, F., Trounson, A. An analysis of factors associated with ectopic pregnancy in a human in-vitro fertilisation program. *Fertility and Sterility*, 1986, 45. 79.

Matsuura, S., Inoue, M., Kobayashi, Y., Hondai, Fujii, A. In Ratnam, S.S. and Teoh E.S. (Eds), *Advances in Fertility and Sterility*, Parthenon Publishing Group, Carnforth, Lancs, UK, 1987; 2: 137.

Maynard, P.V., Baker, P.N., Symonds, E.M., Sant-Cassia, L.J., Johnson, J., Selby, C. Nuclear progesterone uptake by endometrial tissue in cases of subfertility. *Lancet* 1983; ii: 310.

McBain, J.C. The timing of ovulation for AID. In Wood, C., Leeton, C., Kovacs, G. (Eds), *Artificial Insemination*, Brown Prior Anderson, Melbourne, 1980; 50.

McBain, J.C., Pepperell, R.J. Use of bromocryptine in unexplained infertility. *Clinical Reproduction and Fertility*, 1982; 1: 145.

McShane, P.M., Schiff, I., Trentham, D.E. Cellular immunity to sperm in infertile women. *Journal of American Medical Association*, 1985; 253: 3555.

Melis, G.B., Baoletti, A.M., Stringi, F., Fabris, F.M., Canale, D., Fioretti, P. Pharmacologic induction of multiple follicular development improves the success rate of artificial insemination with husband's semen in couple with male related on unexplained infertility. *Fertility and Sterility*, 1987; 47: 441.

Menge, A.C., Medley, N.E., Mangione, C.M., Dietrich, J.W. The incidence and influence of antisperm antibodies in infertile human couples on sperm-cervical mucus interactions and subsequent fertility. *Fertility and Sterility*, 1982; 38: 439.

Mettler, L., Schirwani, D. Macrophage migration inhibitory factor in female sterility. *American Journal of Obstetrics and Gynecology*, 1975; 121: 117.

Moghissi, K.S., Sacco, A.G., Barin, K. I: Cervical mucus antibodies and postcoital test. *American Journal of Obstetrics and Gynecology*, 1980; 136: 941.

Mori, T., Nishimoto, T., Kitagawa, M., Noda, Y., Nishimura, T.A., Oikawa, T. Possible presence of autoantibodies to zona pellucida in infertile women. *Experimentia*, 1978; 34: 797.

Mozley, P.D. Psychophysiologic infertility: An overview. *Clinics in Obstetrics and Gynaecology*, 1976; 19: 407.

Murakami, M., Inoue, M., Kobayashi, Y., Honda, I., Fuji, A. Clinical significance of sperm recovery from peritoneal fluid at diagnostic laparoscopy. *Archives of Gynaecology*, 1985; 237 (suppl) 50.

Nayudu, P.L., Freeman, L.E., Trounson, A.O. Zona pellucida antibodies in human sera. *Journal of Reproduction and Fertility*, 1981; 65: 77.

Nordlander, C., Fuchs, T., Hammarstrom, L., Eovard Smith, C.I. Human leukocyte antigens group A in couples with unexplained infertility. *Fertility and Sterility*, 1983; 40: 60.

Noyes, R.W., Chapnick, E.M. Literature on psychology and infertility. *Fertility and Sterility*, 1964; 15: 543.

Olive, D.L., Haney, A.F., Brice Weinberg, J. The nature of the intraperitoneal exudate associated with infertility: Peritoneal fluid and serum lysozyme activity. *Fertility and Sterility*, 1987; 48: 802.

O'Moore, A.M., O'Moore, R.R., Harrison, R.F., Murphy, G., Carruthers, M. Psychosomatic aspects in idiopathic infertility. Effective treatment with autogenic training. *Journal of Psychosomatic Research*, 1983; 27: 145.

Pepperell, R.J., McBain, J.C. Unexplained infertility: A review. *British Journal of Obstetrics and Gynaecology*, 1985; 92: 569.

Petos, P., Mamtora, M., Ratcliffe, A., Anderson, D.C. Inadequate luteal phase usually indicates ovulatory dysfunction: Observations from serial hormone and ultrasound monitoring of 115 cycles. *Gynaecological Endocrinology*, 1987; 1: 37.

Ping, W.W. Sperm antibody activity in human fallopian tube fluid. *Fertility and Sterility*, 1979; 32: 681.

Polan, M.L., Totora, M., Caldwell, B.V., De Cherney, A.H., Haseltine, F.P., Kase, N. Abnormal ovarian cycles as diagnosed by ultrasound and serum estradiol levels. *Fertility and Sterility*, 1982; 37: 342.

Polson, D.W., Wadsworth, J., Adams, J., Franks, S. Polycystic ovaries — a common finding in normal women. *Lancet* 1988; i: 870.

Rogers, B.J. The sperm penetration assay: Its usefulness re-evaluated. *Fertility and Sterility*, 1985; 43: 821.

Rosenfeld, D.L. Abdominal myomectomy for otherwise unexplained infertility. *Fertility and Sterility*, 1986; 46: 328.

Rowland, G.F., Forsey, T., Moss, J.R., Steptoe, P.C., Hewitt, J., Darougar, S. Failure of in-vitro fertilisation and embryo replacement following infection with chlamydia trachomatis. *Journal of In-Vitro Fertilisation Embryo Transfer*, 1985; 2: 151.

Sacco, A.G., Moghissi, K.S. Anti-zona pellucida activity in human sera. *Fertility and Sterility*, 1979; 31: 503.

Schats, R., Aitken, R.J., Templeton, A.A., Djahanbakham, O. The role of cervical mucus-semen interaction in infertility of unknown aetiology. *British Journal of Obstetrics and Gynaecology*, 1984; 91: 371.

Seibell, M.M., Taymor, M.L. Emotional aspects of infertility. *Fertility and Sterility*, 1982; 37: 137.

Serhal, P.F., Katz, M., Little, V., Woronowake, H. Unexplained infertility — the value of Pergonal superovulation combined with intrauterine insemination. *Fertility and Sterility*, 1988; 49: 602.

Sher, G., Katz, M. Inadequate cervical mucus — a cause of 'idiopathic' infertility. *Fertility and Sterility*, 1976; 27: 886.

Shivers, C.A., Dudkiewicz, A.B., Franklin, L.E., Fussell, E.N. Inhibition of sperm egg interaction by specific antibody. *Science*, 1972; 178: 1211.

Shivers, C.A., Dunbar, B.S. Autoantibodies to zona pellucida: A possible cause for infertility in women. *Science*, 1977; 197: 1082.

Short, R.V. When a conception fails to become a pregnancy. *Ciba Foundation Symposium No. 64: Maternal Recognition of Pregnancy*. Excerpta Medica, Amsterdam, 1979; 337.

Smith, H.E., Horger, R.C. Critical analysis of outpatient sterility studies. *American Journal of Obstetrics and Gynecology*, 1967; 99: 985.

Smith, S.K., Lenton, E.A., Landgren, B., Cooke, I.D. The short luteal phase and infertility. *British Journal of Obstetrics and Gynaecology*, 1984; 91: 1120.

Soffer, Y., Marcus, Z.H., Bukovsky, I., Caspi, E. Immunological factors and postcoital tests in unexplained infertility. *International Journal of Fertility*, 1984; 121: 89.

Southam, A.L. What to do with the 'normal' infertile couple. *Fertility and Sterility*, 1960; 11: 543.

Spira, A. Epidemiology of human reproduction. *Human Reproduction*, 1986; 1: 111.

Stanger, J.D., Yovich, J.L. Reduced in-vitro fertilisation of human oocytes from patients with raised basal luteinising hormone levels during the follicular phase. *British Journal of Obstetrics and Gynaecology*, 1985; 92: 385.

Steinberger, E., Smith, K.D., Tcholakian, R.K., Rodriguez-Rogau, L.J. Testosterone levels in female partners of infertile couples. Relationship between androgen levels in the woman, the male factor and the incidence of pregnancy. *American Journal of Obstetrics and Gynecology*, 1979, 133: 133.

Stolp, W., Bachner, U., Muller, N., Schneider, J. Hat das Histokompatibilitatssystem eine Bedeutung fur die weibliche sterilitat? *Fortschr. Med.*, 1973; 91: 1055.

Stone, S.C. Peritoneal recovery of sperm in patients with infertility associated with inadequate cervical mucus. *Fertility and Sterility*, 1983; 40: 802.

Stray-Pedersen, B., Eng, J., Reikvan, T.M. Uterine T-mycoplasma colonisation in reproductive failure. *American Journal of Obstetrics and Gynecology*, 1978; 130: 307.

Tait, B.D., Barrie, J.U., Johnston, I., Morris, P.J. Cellular immunity to lymphocyte antigens in human infertility. *Fertility and Sterility*, 1976; 27: 389.

Taylor, P.J., Lewinthal, D., Leader, A., Pattinson, H.A. A comparison of Dextran 70 with carbon dioxide as the distention medium for hysteroscopy in patients with infertility or requesting reversal of a prior tubal sterilisation. *Fertility and Sterility*, 1987; 47: 861.

Templeton, A.A., Mortimer, D. The development of a clinical test of sperm migration to the site of fertilisation. *Fertility and Sterility*, 1982; 37: 410.

Templeton, A.A., Penney, G.C. The incidence characteristics and prognosis of patients whose infertility is unexplained. *Fertility and Sterility*, 1982; 37: 175.

Tietze, C. Statistical contributions to the study of human fertility. *Fertility and Sterility*, 1956; 7: 88.

Tietze, C. Fertility after discontinuation of intrauterine and oral contraception. *International Journal of Fertility*, 1968; 13: 385.

Torode, H.W., McPetrie, R.A., Wheeler, P.A., Medcalf, S.C., Saunders, D.M., Ackerman, V.P. The role of chlamydial antibodies in an in-vitro fertilisation program. *Fertility and Sterility*, 1987; 48: 987.

Toth, A., Lesser, M.L., Brooks, C., Labriola, D. Subsequent pregnancies among 161 couples treated for T-mycoplasma genital tract infection. *New England Journal of Medicine*, 1983; 308: 505.

Trounson, A.O., Leeton, J.F., Wood, C., Webb, J., Kovacs, G. The investigation of idiopathic infertility by in-vitro fertilisation. *Fertility and Sterility*, 1980a; 34: 431.

Trounson, A.O., Shivers, C.A., McMaster, R., Lopata, A. Inhibition of sperm binding and fertilisation of human ova by antibody to porcine zona pellucida and human sera. *Archives of Andrology*, 1980b; 4: 29.

Tsundoda, Y., Chang, M.C. Effects of antisera on fertilisation of mouse, rat and hamster eggs. *Biological Reproduction*, 1978; 18: 468.

Van Zyl, J.A., Menkveld, R., Van Kotze, J.J., Reteif, A.E., Van Niekerk, W.A. Oligozoospermia: A seven year survey of the incidence, chromosomal abberrations, treatment and pregnancy rate. *International Journal of Fertility*, 1975; 20: 129.

Wang, C.F., Gemzell Pregnancy following treatment with human Sgonadotrophins in primary unexplained infertility. *Acta Obstetrica et Gynaecologica Scandinavia*, 1979; 58: 141.

Wardle, P.G., Mitchell, J.D., McLaughlin, E.O., Ray, B.D., McDermott, A., Hull, M.G.R. Endometriosis and ovulatory disorder: Reduced fertilisation in vitro compared with tubal and unexplained infertility. *Lancet* 1985; i: 236.

Warner, M.P. Results of twenty-five year study of 1553 infertile couples. *NY State Journal of Medicine*, 1962; 62: 2663.

Witkin, S.S., Bongiovanni, A.M., Berkley, A., Ledger, W.J., Toth, A. Detection and characterisation of immune complexes in the circulation of infertile women. *Fertility and Sterility*, 1984; 42: 384.

World Health Organisation (1980) Laboratory Manual for the examination of human semen and semen-cervical mucus interaction. In Belsey, M.A., Moghissi, K.S. et al. (Eds), *World Health Organisation Special Programme of Research and Development and Research Training in Human Reproduction*, Singapore Press Concern, 1980.

Wright, C.S., Steele, S.J., Jacobs, H.S. Value of bromocryptine in unexplained primary infertility: A double-blind controlled trial. *British Medical Journal* 1979; i: 1037.

Yovich, J.L., Stanger, J.D., Kay, D., Boeticher, B. In-vitro fertilisation of oocytes from women with serum antisperm antibodies. *Lancet* 1984; i: 369.

3
Polycystic ovarian disease

R. Fox and M.G.R. Hull

Introduction

In the context of infertility, the results of treatment of polycystic ovarian disease (PCOD) to induce ovulation are relatively poor (Hull, 1987). PCOD, the commonest cause of ovulatory disorder, remains elusive both to treat reliably and to understand. Existing treatments are almost entirely empirical. Recent therapeutic developments have often been based on unsound principles and their effectiveness has yet to be properly established.

In this chapter, we shall, in addition to practical discussion of diagnosis and treatment, focus attention on the nature of PCOD. We highlight aspects of the pathophysiology and range of clinical presentation. While recognising the heterogeneity of PCOD, we aim to simplify and clarify more general concepts of ovulatory disorders.

Chereau first recorded the finding of sclerocystic change of the ovary in 1844 (see Futterweit, 1984a), but it was the report by Stein and Leventhal (1935) of the association between absent or infrequent menstrual cycles, hirsutism, obesity and enlarged cystic ovaries that firmly established the association with ovarian dysfunction. This classic description defined a small group of women with the syndrome of anovulation and hyperandrogenism (polycystic ovary syndrome; PCOS).

Data from autopsy reports suggested that the prevalence of polycystic ovaries was greater than expected on clinical grounds alone (Sommers and Wadman, 1956). Later, a broad spectrum of clinical presentation came to be recognised (Goldzieher and Green, 1962), and it is now clear that many women have PCOD in the absence of one or two of the triad of hirsutism, obesity and anovulation (Goldzieher, 1981). It seems the syndrome Stein and Leventhal identified characterises only a small fraction of a much larger population of patients with polycystic ovaries (Goldzieher and di Zerega, 1985) and so the name was changed from polycystic ovary syndrome to polycystic ovarian disease. Recent studies have shown that PCOD is by far the commonest cause of ovulatory disorder presenting with oligomenorrhea (Adams et al, 1986; Hull, 1987). Also polycystic ovaries (as opposed to PCOD) are frequently present in healthy women with only slight irregularity of otherwise normal menstrual cycles (Polson et al, 1988), usually without hirsutism or raised LH.

Pathophysiology

Comprehension of the fundamental cause of disease is the key to effective therapy. Unfortunately, despite extensive research into PCOD, the basic defect remains ill-defined (Jacobs, 1987). Nevertheless, much insight has been gained into the pathophysiological mechanisms involved in the derangement of function of the hypothalamic-pituitary-ovarian (H-P-O) axis and, in turn, of the place of PCOD in the context of ovulatory failure. It now seems clear, as will emerge from the following discussion, that from an ovarian standpoint, there are only three types of ovarian condition to account for oligo- and amenorrhea:

1. Primary ovarian failure, from whatever cause, characterised by oestrogen deficiency and raised FSH levels due to ovarian inactivity.
2. Secondary ovarian failure due to hypothalamic or pituitary disorder or failure, characterised by oestrogen deficiency due to ovarian inactivity but normal FSH levels.
3. Polycystic ovaries, characterised by oestrogenisation and normal FSH levels, and often without the "typical" features of hirsutism or raised LH.

Characteristic features

The ovaries are usually, but not always, enlarged to a few times their normal size due to the great number of small active antral follicles up to five or 6mm in diameter lying in the cortex. As a result, the ovaries have a smooth surface unbroken by the usual wrinkles or protruding dominant follicles, and there is a blue mottled appearance due to the numerous follicles just below the surface. The cut surface of the ovary shows the follicles arranged around the periphery like an arcade, which on ultrasonography produces the characteristic "necklace" pattern.

Histology reveals hyperplasia of the theca interna and the ovarian stroma. There appears to be a distinct capsule to the ovary, which gave rise to the old fashioned description of "sclerocystic ovaries" and the idea that a thickened capsule interfered with ovulation. This is clearly not the case.

"Polycystic" ovaries is an unfortunate misnomer. They are really polymicrofollicular. They need to be distinguished from "multifollicular" ovaries

(Franks et al, 1985) which are typified by fewer follicles evenly distributed throughout the ovary and may abutt closely, being thin walled, without intervening stromal tissue. Multifollicular ovaries are relatively inactive, being found in childhood, early puberty and in hypothalamic amenorrhea. In PCOD, no inherent defect in the individual elements of the ovary, pituitary or hypothalamus has been defined. There is no structural or ultrastructural (Green & Goldzieher, 1965) or enzyme defect (Wilson et al, 1979) of any of the ovarian components, and the functional potential of the granulosa cells remains intact (Erickson et al, 1979). In vitro studies on granulosa cells, Erickson et al (1979) have demonstrated a lack of potential to produce oestrogen, but no less than follicles of the same small size from normal ovaries, and provision of FSH for sufficient time to induce aromatase activity leads to normal oestrogen production. Despite typically raised LH levels and relatively reduced FSH, steroid feedback mechanisms, both negative and positive, affecting pituitary gonadotrophin secretion remain intact (Rebar et al, 1976; Baird et al, 1977).

The ovarian abnormalities in PCOD may simply represent the expected response to an inappropriate gonadotrophin environment resulting from a vicious cycle of endocrine disorder as explained below. But it is perhaps not so simple; there may be abnormality of the architectural configuration of the ovarian elements including the stroma, which may be inherent or secondary to disorder of the adrenals or insulin metabolism (discussed later).

Hyperandrogenism is the primary functional feature of PCOD, excess androgen production originating from the ovaries (see Figure 3-1: Chang et al, 1983a) and often also from the adrenal cortex (see Figure 3-2: Chang et al, 1983a; Lachelin, 1984). Testosterone levels, particularly of unbound testosterone, are typically elevated (de Vane et al, 1975) but there is wide variation and overlap with values in normal women (Vejlsted & Albrechsten, 1976; Givens et al, 1976). But despite almost invariable hyperandrogenaemia, the women are not always hirsute. In this respect there is marked racial variation, hirsutism being very uncommon, for example, in Japanese women despite PCOD (Aono et al, 1977).

The active expression of hyperandrogenaemia depends on peripheral conversion of testosterone to dihydrotestosterone (DHT) within androgen dependent cells in, for instance, hair follicles. Thus, levels in serum of 3 alpha-androstanediol glucuronide, the major metabolite of DHT, clearly distinguish between hirsute and nonhirsute women with PCOD (Lobo et al, 1983).

Oestradiol production by the ovary is reduced (Serio et al, 1976) and circulating levels are usually in the mid-follicular phase range (Franks et al, 1985). However, availability of oestradiol is increased by reduction in sex hormone binding globulin (Lobo et al, 1981) and there is often increased peripheral production of oestrone (Yen, 1980) due to both the increased androgen pool and obesity, which is a common feature. Thus, patients, including those with amenorrhea and hirsutism, are usually demonstrably oestrogenised (Hull et al, 1979a).

Although its clinical presentation may be varied, recognition that PCOD is expressed in a wide spectrum of severity now helps to greatly simplify the classification of ovarian abnormalities accounting for ovulatory disorder and infertility, as is discussed later.

Hypothalamic-pituitary-ovarian interaction

Most authors have attempted to explain the dual disturbance in pituitary and ovarian physiology by proposing that a self-perpetuating cycle of events exists between pituitary and ovary (Yen, 1980; Goldzieher, 1981; Lachelin, 1984; Franks et al 1985). There is no general agreement about the exact mechanism involved and, indeed, the mode of onset and maintenance may differ from patient to patient. In essence, there appears to be an imbalance in ovarian steroidogenesis with increased production of androgen (predominantly androstenedione and testosterone) by theca cells under the influence of LH (Haney et al, 1986). Their conversion to oestrogen within the follicle by granulosa cells is greatly reduced, because of a relative deficiency of FSH, and the excess enters the circulation.

Aromatisation of this androgenic surplus to oestrogen, which occurs continuously in adipose tissue (Sitteri and MacDonald, 1973) independently of FSH (James et al, 1982), leads to a relatively constant oestrogen production with a larger proportion than usual of oestrone (Baird et al, 1977). It is advocated that acyclic formation of oestrogen, particularly when unopposed by progesterone (Futterweit, 1984c), results in abnormal feedback on the pituitary suppressing the release of FSH and promoting increased secretion of LH. The resulting disparate gonadotrophin profile in turn distorts ovarian steroidogenesis further by accentuating theca cell hyperfunction and suppressing granulosa cell aromatase activity (Rajaniemi et al, 1980). A vicious cycle is thus created (Figure 3-3). This model is perhaps simplistic. The true mechanism may involve other factors such as alterations in inhibin production and the generation of peptides responsible for the local (paracrine) control of ovarian function (Franks et al, 1986).

The crux of this hypothesis concerns the effect of sustained moderate elevation of oestrogen production on the pituitary. Mennin and Gorski (1975) demonstrated that injection of oestradiol valerate in rats induces a condition similar to PCOD. Evidence for a similar effect of oestrogens on the human pituitary is lacking. Chang et al (1982) were able to show that oestrone administration enhances the disparity of gonadotrophin secretion in women with PCOD but does not induce such a state in normal controls, though it is perhaps not surprising that exogenous oestrogens cannot mimic the dynamic interplay between ovary and pituitary in PCOD.

Etiology

How the vicious cycle is generated is difficult to explain. Evidence that H-P-O interrelationships although disrupted, are qualitatively normal led to speculation that PCOD merely represents a spontaneous aberration of pituitary homeostatic control sequence at puberty (Hosseinian et al, 1976). If this is the case one might expect that escape from pituitary/ovarian quiescence induced by combined oestrogen/progestogen preparations or LHRH agonists would be followed by the commencement of cyclical ovarian activity in a proportion of cases. Almost invariably, however, hormone concentrations quickly return to their former level and acyclic ovarian activity promptly resumes (Kirschner et al, 1970; Calogero et al, 1987). These data suggest that PCOD is not a random malfunction of ovarian control but rather that a defect is present which prevents the establishment of normal ovarian cycles.

Futterweit (1984d) proposed that PCOD develops in two stages: a generating phase in which a factor or factors within or without the H-P-O axis promote the initial disruption, and an effector stage in which the disturbance is propagated throughout the system and thereby amplified. Unfortunately the disease is propagated in such a way that neither the nature nor the site of action of the generating factor(s) is easily determined.

PCOD is manifestly a heterogenous condition (Lobo, 1985). Although this variation can be partly explained by a spectrum of severity ranging from idiopathic hirsutism (Adams et al, 1986) to ovarian hyperthecosis (Futterweit, 1984e), there are data from studies examining adrenal function (Carmina et al, 1986) and prolactin levels (Falaschi et al, 1980) in PCOD that point to the existence of a number of subgroups. Franks et al (1985) have concluded that PCOD is not one distinct nosological entity but rather that the polycystic ovary simply represents a non-specific response of the H-P-O axis common to a number of stimuli.

Hypothalamus and pituitary

The findings described above are most easily explained by a lesion affecting the hypothalamus or the pituitary, the ovarian dysfunction being secondary to the abnormal gonadotrophin secretion with the LH-dependent theca cell compartment being hyperstimulated at the expense of the FSH-dependent granulosa cells. Wortsman et al (1981) proposed a hypothalamic origin of the PCOD, but there is no conclusive evidence to support this. LH-RH pulse frequency is normal (Kazer et al, 1987), and the increase in LH-pulse amplitude (Rebar et al, 1976) probably represents hypersensitivity of the pituitary gonadotroph to LH-RH (Mortimer et al, 1978) rather than increased release of LH-RH. In contrast, pituitary physiology is overtly disturbed as evidenced by disordered gonadotrophin release (Rebar et al, 1976) and sometimes, hyperprolactinaemia (Luciano et al, 1984). Some authorities believe that a disturbance of pituitary function is the primary event (Pehrson et al, 1986).

On the other hand, evidence that the ultrasound features of PCOD may be found in the presence of a non-functioning pituitary (Stanhope et al, 1987), and that ovarian morphology is not significantly altered by prolonged pituitary suppression with LH-RH agonists (MacLeod, 1986) suggest ovarian dysfunction is not entirely dependent upon a central lesion. Jacobs (1987) proposed there is an abnormality intrinsic to the ovary. This is supported by the recent observation that aberrant response of the polycystic ovary to gonadotrophin therapy persists despite suppression of endogenous gonadotrophin release following pituitary desensitisation with superactive LH-RH analogues (Charbonnel et al, 1987; Coutts et al, 1988).

Although these findings are consistent with an inherent abnormality of the ovary, they could be equally explained by factors without the H-P-O axis acting upon the ovary; the resulting dysfunction affecting an otherwise normal pituitary. A further possibility is that a single extraneous factor could affect the function of both the ovary and the pituitary independently of each other. Evidence that ovarian wedge resection induces cyclical ovarian activity without any discernible change in pituitary function (Judd et al, 1976) supports the idea that a single factor may be acting through two very similar but nevertheless independent pathophysiological mechanisms. Hyperinsulinaemia, an endocrinopathy associated with PCOD (Figure 3-4: Chang et al, 1983b) and a possible etiological factor (Chang and Geffner, 1985), influences the function of both ovarian theca (Barbieri et al, 1984) and pituitary gonadotroph (Adashi et al, 1981) cells in culture, amplifying the action of their respective trophic hormones.

Hyperprolactinaemia and PCOD

Isolated hyperprolactinaemia is a common cause of anovulation, accounting for perhaps one quarter of patients with amenorrhea. Prolactin levels have also been said to be elevated in approximately 25 per cent of patients with PCOD (Pehrson et al, 1986). However, this may be a spurious observation brought about by failure to recognise that the normal distribution of prolactin has a skew with a long upper tail to at least 800 mU/l (Jeffcoate, 1978). In Hull's (1987) study of 112 cases, although the average prolactin level was higher than in women with hypothalamic disorders, it was never raised above 800 mU/l in any individual.

Occasionally, by chance, polycystic ovaries are found in women with prolactin-secreting pituitary adenomas (Futterweit and Krieger, 1979). Although Futterweit and Krieger suggested the abnormal steroid milieu of PCOD promotes the formation of pituitary adenomas, this relatively rare combination probably represents nothing more than the chance association of two common conditions. The presence of the ovarian abnormality in such cases is in fact masked by the effect of the hyperprolactinaemia on gonadotrophin secretion, being exposed only when the prolactin level has been suppressed by bromocriptine or surgery.

The more common association of apparently mildly elevated prolactin and PCOD may be a real entity. In contrast to patients with true hyperprolactinaemia who have depressed LH levels and oestrogen deficiency, those with PCOD and raised prolactin are demonstrably oestrogenised and their LH levels are usually elevated. Moreover, there is an exaggerated release of prolactin in response to TRH in women with PCOD (Falaschi et al, 1980) whereas in women with primary hyperprolactinaemia, the rise is attenuated.

The nature of the relationship between hyperprolactinaemia and PCOD is not clear. It has been suggested that hyperprolactinaemia may disrupt the H-P-O axis, thus promoting the generation of PCOD, by stimulating adrenal androgen production. Dehydroepiandrosterone-sulphate (DHEA-S), which is produced almost exclusively by the adrenal gland (Hatch et al, 1981), is present in increased amounts in hyperprolactinaemic women (Giusti et al, 1977) and there are some data to show that DHEA-S levels fall following suppression of prolactin. Furthermore, Thorner and colleagues (1975) in an uncontrolled study appeared to demonstrate improved ovarian function following suppression of prolactin with bromocriptine. However, not all patients with PCOD and elevated prolactin levels have evidence of adrenal dysfunction (Carmina et al, 1986).

Other workers have suggested that hyperprolactinaemia associated with PCOD may occur as a secondary phenomenon. Falaschi et al (1980) have proposed that it is the result of the effect of the sustained oestrogen excess. Interestingly Kandeel et al (1977) has shown that exogenous oestrone but not oestradiol produces a rise in prolactin concentrations. How hyperoestrogenaemia affects the function of the lactotrophs is not fully understood. It may be a direct effect, inducing lactotroph hyperplasia (Corenblum & Taylor, 1982; Futterweit & Krieger, 1979) or an indirect mechanism influencing the concentration of the prolactin inhibitory factor dopamine within the hypothalamus (Quigley et al, 1981). Although more information is required to help elucidate the nature of hyperprolactinaemia associated with PCOD, indeed whether it is a true condition, it seems clear at least that pharmacological manipulation of prolactin release has no part in the treatment of PCOD.

The adrenal gland and PCOD

The association between adrenal dysfunction and PCOD was first noted in 1937 when Broster found evidence of adrenal hyperplasia in a woman with polycystic ovaries (see Goldzieher & di Zerega, 1985). Kirschner and Jacobs (1971) subsequently studied ovarian and adrenal function in hirsutism using selective adrenal and ovarian vein sampling. Other groups later examined adrenal steroid and ACTH levels both basally (Abraham et al, 1975; Lachelin et al, 1979; Chang et al, 1982; Hoffman et al, 1984) and after adrenal suppression and provocation with dexamethasone and ACTH respectively (Givens et al, 1975a; Lachelin, 1982). The interpretation of these studies is made difficult by the use of different criteria to categorise hirsutism and PCOD and they have not been verified by studies using ultrasonography. Nevertheless they strongly suggest that adrenal dysfunction and PCOD are commonly associated. More recent work using stricter criteria has confirmed this association (Carmina et al, 1986).

In rare cases, a discrete abnormality such as 21-hydroxylase deficiency (Lobo and Goebelsmann, 1980) or Cushing's syndrome (Korth-Schutz et al, 1974) may be identified. In the majority of cases, all that is found is a selective hyper-responsiveness of the androgen secreting cells of the adrenal cortex to ACTH (Devesa et al, 1987) with an exaggerated androgen rise but normal glucocorticoid response. Basal measurements reveal elevated levels of the androgenic steroid DHEA-sulphate (DHEA-S), which is synthesised almost exclusively by the adrenal, but normal, ACTH and cortisol levels (Lachelin et al, 1979). Furthermore these findings are unaffected by complete suppression of ovarian activity using LH-RH analogue therapy to desensitise the pituitary (Figure 3-2: Chang et al, 1983a).

It has therefore been postulated that a Cortical Androgen Stimulating Hormone (CASH) exists (Parker et al, 1983). It is further postulated that CASH selectively modulates the effect of ACTH on adrenal androgen production.

Interestingly β-endorphin, which is thought by some to be CASH (Ruutiainen et al, 1985), is present in increased concentrations in PCOD (Aleem et al, 1984), apparently produced by developing follicles (Aleem et al, 1987). As Figure 3-2 shows, however, suppression of follicular activity does not lead to a fall in DHEA-S levels (Chang et al, 1983a).

Other workers have suggested that prolactin, which is said to be elevated in over one third of PCOD patients (Luciano et al, 1984), affects adrenal function, proposing that prolactin has a specific action on the synthesis of androgens by the adrenal cortex (Giusti et al, 1977). Successful suppression of prolactin release by bromocriptine may be associated with a reduction in DHEA-S levels, but not all PCOD patients with raised prolactin levels have evidence of adrenal dysfunction and many of those with high DHEA-S levels have normal prolactin concentrations (Carmina et al, 1986).

Lobo (1984) has demonstrated reduced 3β-hydroxysteroid-dehydrogenase activity in PCOD patients with high DHEA-S levels but Anderson and Yen (1976) have shown that this is an acquired deficiency secondary to elevated oestrogen production and not a primary defect of adrenal metabolism.

It seems clear that adrenal dysfunction is present in only a proportion of cases of PCOD and that the mechanism of the disturbance is varied. The relationship between PCOD and the adrenal gland is less well known. Even though the physiology of the two glands are delicately intertwined, manipulation of one affects the function of the other. Despite evidence that sustained elevation in oestrogen can influence adrenal function (Anderson and Yen, 1976), the fact that suppression of the H-P-O axis with LH-RH agonists fail to lower DHEA-S levels (Chang et al, 1983a) suggests that any derangement in adrenal activity seen in PCOD is unlikely to be secondary to disruption of ovarian function.

In contrast there is strong evidence to support the hypothesis that alterations in adrenal androgen production influence the ovary. Hoffman and Lobo (1985) have shown that the ovarian response to clomiphene is poorer in patients with higher DHEA-S levels. Daly et al (1984) demonstrated in a similar group of patients that suppression of adrenal androgen production with dexamethasone appears to improve the response to clomiphene. Glucocorticoids have been shown to have a direct effect on the function of granulosa cells in culture (Danisova et al, 1987) but it seems improbable that this phenomenon could operate in vivo at the doses used in Daly's study. The most plausible explanation for improved ovarian responsiveness to clomiphene is an indirect effect through suppression of adrenal androgen synthesis, although a direct effect on LH secretion cannot be discounted (Melis et al, 1987).

How adrenal androgens disrupt the hypothalamic-pituitary-ovarian axis is open to question. In vitro study of Marmoset granulosa cells incubated with and without testosterone at physiological concentrations suggests that androgenic steroids have an inhibitory effect on aromatase activity. It seems odd, however, that the substrate of a cell's major enzyme system is able to suppress the activity of that enzyme. It is even more difficult to understand how moderate elevation in the circulating androgen pool are able to affect granulosa cell function in vivo when the concentration at the theca/granulosa interface of androgens produced by the theca cells is likely to be several orders of magnitude higher. Granulosa cell hypofunction is a recognised feature of PCOD (Goldzieher and Axelrod, 1963) but this is perhaps more likely to be related to the generation of inhibitory peptides such as epidermal growth factor (Mason et al, 1986), known to be present at increased concentrations in the follicular fluid of patients with PCOD (Franks et al, 1986).

A second hypothesis stems from the observation that androgen secreting tumours promote a rise in LH levels and suppression of FSH (Dunaif et al, 1984) and it has been proposed that androgens directly regulate gonadotrophin release. The administration of DHEA to neonatal rats induces a condition similar to PCOD (Mahesh, 1980) but the LH levels are low. In addition, both acute and chronic administration of testosterone to primates (Billiar et al, 1985) and to women (Dewis et al, 1985) failed to induce changes in gonadotrophin levels that would explain the genesis of PCOD.

A more attractive hypothesis is the idea that peripheral conversion of the androgens, released by the adrenal gland, to oestrogen leads to sustained positive and negative feedback on the pituitary. This in turn promotes the secretion of LH and inhibits the release of FSH. The resulting imbalance in plasma gonadotrophin levels disrupts the balance between the theca and granulosa cell compartments raising the androgen level further, and a vicious circle is created (Figure 3-3). As indicated above, there is no direct evidence to show that oestrogen can have such an effect on pituitary function but it is interesting to note that in Mahesh's study the conversion of DHEA to oestrogen was a prerequisite for the various effects observed.

Hyperinsulinaemia and PCOD

Hyperinsulinaemia is another endocrinopathy commonly associated with PCOD (Figure 3-4: Chang et al, 1983b; Barbieri and Ryan, 1983). A relationship between glucose, insulin and testosterone has been recognised for many years (Lewis et al, 1950) but Givens et al (1974a) was the first to identify the syndrome of marked insulin resistance, elevated insulin levels, hyperandrogenism and acanthosis nigricans. Kahn (1976) shortly afterwards noted that a proportion of these patients had bilaterally enlarged multicystic ovaries. Studies showing insulin concentrations to be proportional to androgen levels (Burghen et al, 1980) led to the proposal that a causal relationship existed between the two. It was initially proposed that androgens induced the insulin resistance.This was supported by reports of young boys with aplastic anaemia being treated with the synthetic androgen oxymetholone developing insulin resistance (Woodard et al, 1981), and a case report describing a return to normal insulin sensitivity following ovarian suppression with an oestrogen/progestogen preparation in a patient with ovarian hyperandrogenaemia (Cole and Kitabchi, 1978). Realisation that the mechanism of insulin resistance differed from case to case, despite a single proposed cause (Bar et al, 1978), cast doubt upon the hypothesis. The idea that endogenous androgens affect glucose metabolism was discounted when Geffner et al (1986) demonstrated that insulin resistance persists following pituitary desensitisation with LH-RH agonists even though testosterone levels fall to castrate levels.

The patients described in these initial reports were severely obese and it was suggested that marked adiposity altered insulin-insulin receptor interaction and, through an independent mechanism, also caused ovarian dysfunction (Pasquali et al, 1982). Drastic weight loss in obese patients with PCOD and severe insulin resistance fails to restore insulin concentrations to normal (Pasquali et al, 1986). Moreover Chang et al (1983b) and Jialal et al (1987) showed that non-obese PCOD patients often had hyperinsulinaemia as well, thus refuting the hypothesis.

A third hypothesis to explain the link between insulin and testosterone levels in plasma proposes that insulin directly influences ovarian steroidogenesis (Chang and Geffner, 1985), although how it might achieve this was not immediately obvious. In vitro experimentation with porcine theca cell cultures has provided a model (Barbieri et al, 1983). These studies, using control media, media with added LH alone, and media with insulin with and without added LH, revealed that insulin promotes testosterone production but to a lesser degree than LH. When present with LH, however, insulin appears to greatly amplify testosterone formation. Comparable results were later obtained by Barbieri et al (1984) investigating the effect of insulin on incubated human ovarian theca fragments from a patient with hyperandrogenism and insulin resistance. Similar studies using mouse Leydig cells seem to indicate that insulin augmentation of LH-stimulated testosterone production is a dose-dependent effect (Jacobs, 1987).

It should be remembered that these are in vitro phenomena and may not represent a true physiological entity. More recently, however, various groups have produced data from in vivo studies to support the hypothesis that insulin affects ovarian function. Using a high dose insulin infusion to artificially induce hyperinsulinaemia and an infusion of glucose to maintain euglycaemia, a rise in androgen levels was induced in both normal and hyperandrogenic women. Smith et al (1987) gave five hirsute women with severe insulin resistance and seven normal female controls a 75gm oral glucose load to induce an endogenous insulin rise. At three hours, both androstenedione and testosterone concentrations had risen significantly in the hirsute group whereas the levels in the control group fell. DHEA-S levels fell in both the study group and the controls indicating an ovarian source for the androgen rather than adrenal.

These collected data point to insulin playing an important part in the disruption of ovarian function seen in PCOD. Poretsky and Kalin (1987) have even suggested that insulin is not only an important factor in ovarian dysfunction but also in normal ovarian physiology, together with various paracrine growth factors such as insulin-like growth factor I (Adashi et al, 1985). He cites the observation that insulin-dependent diabetes mellitus, a state of insulin deficiency, is associated with ovarian hypofunction. Although his arguments are attractive his proposal is no more than conjecture. Nevertheless, it seems likely that the relationship between hyperinsulinaemia and PCOD is one of cause and effect.

The primary lesion appears to be an abnormality of the insulin receptor which renders it resistant to the insulin molecule. This may be an inherited condition (Kahn et al, 1976). To compensate for the insensitivity to insulin, in order to maintain euglycaemia, the pancreas releases more insulin and circulating insulin levels rise. The mechanism of action of hyperinsulinaemia on the ovary probably starts with amplification of LH-induced androgen synthesis by theca cells. As previously described, the excess androgen is converted peripherally to oestrogen which in turn is thought to augment the pituitary responsiveness to LH-RH. Insulin itself may also directly augment the release of LH (Adashi et al, 1981). By whatever means it is elevated, LH further disrupts ovarian steroidogenesis (Baird et al, 1977). Although insulin receptors have been detected in ovarian tissue (Ladenheim et al, 1984) insulin probably exerts its effect on ovarian steroidogenesis by binding to the IGF I receptor (Poretsky and Kalin, 1987). The proportion of patients with PCOD who have hyperinsulinaemia is not known.

It remains to be established whether the previously described ill-defined adrenal hypersensitivity to ACTH and theca cell hypersensitivity to LH outlined above are separate endocrinopathies with distinct etiologies or two facets of a single pathological entity. Both phenomena appear to be an augmented response of a target organ to its trophic hormone and they may reflect a common mechanism. As with the ovary, adrenocortical function is thought to be controlled by locally produced peptides (Baird and Walicke, 1987). Theoretically, hyperinsulinaemia could influence the action of ACTH on the adrenal cortex in a manner similar to its effect on LH-dependent theca cell steroidogenesis. Smith et al (1987) have shown however, that plasma DHEA-S and peak insulin levels following a glucose load are inversely proportional when one would expect a positive correlation. This work suggests that there are two subgroups of patients with PCOD; one with adrenal hyperandrogenism but normal insulin levels, the other with hyperinsulinaemia but normal adrenal function.

Obesity and PCOD

Opinions about the role diet plays in the development of PCOD vary. Obesity was originally thought to be one of the cardinal features of the clinical syndrome and crucial to the pathogenesis of the condition, but it is now recognised that many patients with PCOD have a normal body habitus (Goldzieher and di Zerega, 1985).

Obesity is known to depress sex hormone binding globulin levels (Plymate et al, 1981), increasing the proportion of testosterone available for peripheral conversion to oestradiol. In addition, there is evidence to suggest that a disproportionately high body fat content causes a rise in extra-ovarian aromatase activity (Edman and MacDonald, 1978), thus increasing the rate of conversion of androgen to oestrogen. It is also well established that the obese develop hyperinsulinaemia as a consequence of their body size (see above) and it has been reported that obesity adversely effects adrenal function (Feher and Halmy, 1975). In both instances, these reactions to dietary excess are mild and it is important to realise that although overweight women more commonly have menstrual disturbance (Rogers and Mitchell, 1952), the vast majority have normal ovarian function (Hartz et al, 1979).

Overall, it appears that the effects of obesity on the reproductive endocrine system are small, but nevertheless there is little doubt that diet may have a critical effect on ovarian function. There is undoubtedly also a relationship between PCOD and bodyweight, but this is not truly one of cause and effect. Rather, diet determines the expression of the condition. Weight reduction should be advised where necessary. Even if it fails to promote the return to cyclical ovarian activity it may improve the response to therapy.

Diagnosis

The importance of defining PCOD in infertility practice lies in the selection of effective treatment to induce ovulation. The unreliability of clinical findings alone requires more sensitive diagnostic techniques. Ovarian visualisation and biopsy by laparotomy or laparoscopy are unnecessarily and unacceptably invasive. Accuracy of ovarian imaging by ultrasonography depends on mechanical capability, technical skill and inherent difficulties such as obesity. The increasing availability and reliability of hormone assays has led to a continuing search for indirect diagnostic criteria based on hormonal findings.

Ultrasonography

The development of high-resolution ultrasonography, by enabling non-invasive visualisation of pelvic anatomy, offers an attractive method of investigating ovarian dysfunction. Many researchers have shown that the ovarian morphology typical of PCOD (multiple small follicular cysts in combination with an expanded stromal compartment) can be displayed ultrasonographically (Parisi et al, 1982; Orsini et al, 1985; Adams et al, 1985), although these findings have yet to be validated by histological studies. The ultrasound criteria of PCOD described by Adams et al (1985, 1986) are 10 or more cysts two to eight mm in diameter associated with an increase in ovarian stroma, and in most cases the ovarian volume is at least nine ml, which is greater than the upper normal limit.

In a study of 76 patients with anovulation and/or hirsutism, Adams et al (1985) also demonstrated that it is possible to distinguish not only normal and polycystic ovaries but a third type, also with a multicystic appearance. In contrast to the polycystic variety, there were usually fewer follicles, not distributed peripherally, and no increased stromal content could be identified. They termed these multifollicular ovaries. The three groups of patient categorised according to ovarian appearance (normal, polycystic and multifollicular) differed significantly in terms of body habitus, hormone profile and, when associated with anovulatory cycles, response to ovulation induction therapy. Patients with multifollicular ovaries all had a history of weight loss, a normal serum LH level and a good response to therapy while those with polycystic ovaries tended to be overweight, had a high LH level and an unsatisfactory response to ovulation induction.

In the study by Adams, it seems that the ovaries were displayed in every patient, suggesting that ultrasonography is a highly reliable diagnostic method. This is not everyone's experience, however. Orsini et al (1985) failed to display either ovary in 12 per cent of patients with PCOD diagnosed on clinical and biochemical criteria, and in the remainder they identified four different ultrasonic ovarian patterns, two of which were indistinguishable from patterns seen in women with normal menstrual cycles. Hann and co-workers (1984) found that only 71 per cent of cases with suspected PCOD had evidence of the condition on scan. The reasons for these discrepancies are not clear. They may reflect nothing more than differences in patient groups but are perhaps more likely to represent differences in ultrasound equipment and operator skill. These difficulties may be overcome with the introduction of transvaginal endosonography, which facilitates detailed examination of pelvic anatomy (Barlow et al, 1988) and in our experience we have found it greatly superior to transabdominal scanning for defining the ovarian details.

Apart from any limitation of ultrasonography in the definition of the morphology of the ovaries it must also be recognised that the method is limited to the morphology of the ovaries. In the diagnosis of ovulatory disorders and/or hirsutism extra-ovarian causes must be sought. Most commonly, this involves the exclusion of hypothalamic disorders, hyperprolactinaemia and thyroid dysfunction, but a number of rarer biochemical and neoplastic conditions can be present in an identical fashion to PCOD (Futterweit, 1984b), mimicking not only the clinical features of PCOD but the ovarian appearances as well. Polycystic ovarian change has been seen in cases of congenital adrenal hyperplasia (Stevens and Goldzieher, 1968; Hague et al, 1986) and in conjunction with adrenal and ovarian tumours (Givens et al, 1975b). Ultrasonography is therefore unlikely to be a reliable method of differentiating between the various causes of hyperandrogenaemia. In contrast, endocrine testing is able to determine the level and likely source of androgen production, thereby indicating when a search for inherited enzyme disorder (Benjamin et al, 1986) or occult tumour is warranted (Hatch et al, 1981; Meldrum and Abraham, 1979).

Even though ultrasonography has proved to be a useful research tool, it seems obvious that the imaging quality and degree of skill necessary to distinguish between the different types of multicystic ovary (Franks et al, 1985) do not lend this method to widespread use. Moreover, ultrasonography can play only a small part in a complex diagnostic process. The drawbacks of ultrasonography mean that in general hormonal assessment, as discussed below, is of greater clinical value.

Endocrine evaluation

As described above (in "Characteristic features"), hyperandrogenism is the primary endocrine feature but it is not reliably distinguished biochemically. In serum, unbound testosterone is usually raised, but not as readily measured as total testosterone, which varies widely in its levels with marked overlap of the normal range. Hirsutism, when clearly defined, is a reliable index of hyperandrogenism, but in many women hyperandrogenaemia is not expressed by evident hirsutism due to lack of peripheral conversion of testosterone to DHT in the androgen-dependent end-organs (Lobo et al, 1983).

Other endocrine features have therefore been employed for diagnosis. Kletsky et al (1975) made a presumptive diagnosis of PCOD in amenorrhoeic women who were demonstrably oestrogenised and had a raised LH level in the absence of hirsutism. That assumption is strongly supported by a recent study by Hull (1987) of women with "functional" oligo- or amenorrhea. As shown in Figure 3-5, he found that the hirsute women, who were mostly demonstrably oestrogenised (by their menstrual response to progestogen), were closely resembled by non-hirsute oestrogenised women in terms of raised LH and to a lesser extent body mass and (not shown in the figure) responsiveness to clomiphene. This was in contrast to women with presumed hypothalamic disorder or hyperprolactinaemia (which causes ovarian failure through hypothalamic disorder: Polson et al, 1986), who were oestrogen deficient, had normal LH levels, smaller body mass, and seldom responded adequately to clomiphene.

The presumptive diagnosis of PCOD based on oestrogenised state and raised LH has now been confirmed by comparison with ultrasonographic findings as shown in Table 3-1 (Fox, Corrigan and Hull, unpublished data from a continuing study). These show close association between PCOD and oestrogenisation, with overall accuracy of 90 per cent. The occasional finding of polycystic ovaries (PCO) in amenorrhoeic oestrogen deficient women with hyperprolactinaemia or hypothalamic disorder should not be surprising, as polycystic ovaries can be found at ultrasound scan in 23 per cent of apparently normal women (Polson et al, 1988) and the effect of the PCO would be masked by the overriding disorder leading to suppression of ovarian activity.

On the other hand, the occasional oestrogenised amenorrhoeic woman will be recovering from hypothalamic disorder instead of having PCOD (as in the exceptional case in Table 3-1). Another occasional exception is the occurrence of oestrogen deficiency with PCOD but in our study this only occurred in hirsute women and may be due to greater severity of hyperandrogenism in those cases. The greater severity of disorder in the women with hirsutism is suggested by reduced responsiveness to clomiphene. Hull (1987) found that 45 per cent of hirsute women had a regular ovulatory response, compared with 84 per cent of women with PCOD but without hirsutism.

Thus it appears that in oligo- or amenorrhoeic women, combined assessment of oestrogen state and hirsutism gives 96 per cent accuracy in the individual diagnosis of PCOD, the errors being due to overriding unrelated disorders. This is in contrast to the diagnostic accuracy of LH measurement due to the extensive overlap between PCOD and normal ranges. Studies of the LH ranges in both oligo-amenorrhoeic (Figure 3-5: Hull, 1987) and normal women (Adams et al, 1986) show that serum LH is only distinctly raised at a level of 12 iu/l or greater, with a diagnostic accuracy of 74 per cent. The LH:FSH ratio is only distinctly raised at 2.5 or greater, (Figure 3-5: Hull, 1987) with a diagnostic accuracy of 58 per cent; but is anyway an unattractive parameter, being an artificial index compounding the errors in measuring the two hormones and hiding heterogeneous relations between these hormones at different orders of concentration, particularly when relatively low.

Allowing for the expected temporary masking of PCO by overriding presenting conditions, the endocrine features most reliable in the positive diagnosis of PCOD as the primary cause of oligo- or amenorrhea in individual women are summarised in Table 3-2.

Although 23 per cent of women with apparently normal menstrual cycles and no hirsutism have polycystic ovaries on scan, in infertility, accurate diagnosis of PCOD is only necessary when there is evident ovulatory disorder. After excluding the need to treat other conditions, for example, weight loss, thyroid disorder and hyperprolactinaemia specifically, or hypothalamic disorders empirically using pulsed LH-RH, a diagnosis of PCOD indicates the need to try clomiphene persistently before turning to gonadotrophin therapy or occasionally glucocorticoids (see later).

Epidemiology of PCOD

Recent studies using the ultrasonographic and endocrine criteria described above have enabled accurate determination of the prevalence of PCOD in representative populations of women. In amenorrhoeic women Adams et al (1986) using ultrasonography and Hull (1987) using endocrinology found 26 per cent and 37 per cent respectively had PCOD or presumed PCOD. In oligomenorrhoeic women the rates were 87 per cent and 90 per cent respectively.

When menstrual cycles were in the normal range of 21-35 days, the Polson group (Polson et al, 1988) found that in those women with only slight irregularity (individual cycle length range varying by more than four days), the prevalence of polycystic ovaries (PCO) on scan was 96 per cent. In contrast, amongst women with very regular cycles (individual variation no more than four days), the prevalence of PCO was only 7 per cent. The overall prevalence of PCO in women with apparently normal cycles was 23 per cent. The only endocrine abnormality found in this apparently normal group with PCO was raised LH in 25 per cent; LH was raised in only two per cent of those with normal ovaries. It also seems that some of the women with PCO had evident hirsutism but none had felt it sufficient to complain about. Thus it appears that PCO is a common abnormality, although usually minor in degree, and any possible adverse effect, for example on fertility, has yet to be studied.

As far as infertility associated with PCOD presenting with oligo- or amenorrhea is concerned, study of a defined resident population by Hull Hull et al, 1985; Hull, 1987) shows that it accounts for 15 per cent of all infertility, and the annual incidence to be expected is 180 cases per million of the general population (including men and children). Of those, 22 per cent (40 cases annually per million population) failed to respond adequately to clomiphene and required gonadotrophin therapy. More than half the women with hirsutism (55 per cent) needed gonadotrophin therapy, compared with only 16 per cent of the non-hirsute women, emphasising the range of severity of PCOD not only in its clinical presentation but in its therapeutic requirement. The prevalence of severe PCOD represents a major burden due to the difficulty in controlling treatment and cost involved, and a major challenge to therapeutic research.

Infertility

Sterility was a common feature of the patients described by Stein and Leventhal and PCOD is one of the leading diagnoses in women attending subfertility clinics as described above. Analysis of conception rates for patients with PCOD receiving ovulation induction therapy indicates that the most important contribution to the infertility was their failure to ovulate (Jacobs, 1987). However, failure to induce ovulation and conceive may not be the only reason for childlessness in women with PCOD. In those who do conceive there is said to be a high risk of early pregnancy loss (Jacobs, 1987). Possible reasons for the high spontaneous abortion rate include formation of abnormal oocytes and endometrium hostile to the implanting embryo.

Oocyte maturation is thought to be affected by high LH levels and analysis of fertilisation rates from in vitro fertilisation programmes support this (Stanger et al, 1985). Jacobs has recently presented data from pregnancies in PCOD patients showing a higher abortion rate in women with LH levels above 10 than those with levels below (Jacobs, 1988). He also seemed to demonstrate that suppression of LH using an LH-RH agonist during exogenous gonadotrophin therapy was associated with improvement in pregnancy outcome. This has not been the experience of Coutts' group in Glasgow however (personal communication). Previously, Sarris et al (1978) had seemed to reduce the abortion rate associated with biochemically demonstrable hyperandrogenism by glucocorticoid therapy. Unfortunately there is as yet no conclusive evidence of treatment leading to reduced risk of abortion.

The endometrium is frequently hyperplastic in PCOD (Chamlian and Taylor, 1970). Endometrial hyperplasia is the response to prolonged exposure to endogenous oestrogen unopposed by progesterone (Paterson et al, 1980). It has been assumed that induction of a withdrawal bleed by a short course of progestogen will provoke the abnormal endometrium to be shed and allow the regeneration of a more favourable endometrium (Franks et al, 1985). Recently published data (Randolph et al, 1987) suggests that insulin alters endometrial physiology and this effect may not be counteracted by progestogen therapy, thus preventing the formation of a favourable environment for implantation despite endometrial shedding. On the other hand, Homburg et al (1988) described a seemingly favourable response to progestogen therapy both in terms of subsequent improved ovulatory response and conception rates with clomiphene, but they attributed the benefit to modulation of pituitary sensitivity to LH-RH leading to reduction in LH levels and pulse frequency.

The endometrium may also be adversely affected by agents used to induce ovulation. Clomiphene, for instance, by virtue of its anti-oestrogenic properties, is thought to affect the endometrial response to oestrogen, ultimately rendering it atrophic but only during treatment (Kokko et al, 1981). This effect probably plays no more than a small part in spontaneous abortion, however, as clomiphene is associated with a higher fetal wastage rate in PCOD patients than those receiving it for other indications (Garcia et al, 1977). One other potential cause for the higher abortion rate is the increased proportion of multiple pregnancies seen after ovulation induction (Huppert, 1979) but again, this is unlikely to be the major factor.

Induction of ovulation

The ideal agent for ovulation induction would be inexpensive, convenient to use (for both patient and physician), and associated with a low incidence of side effects and no inherent anti-fertility effects. In addition, in inducing normal ovulation it should lead to a high conception rate but low incidence of multiple pregnancy. No agent currently used for PCOD fulfills all of these criteria. In particular, there is no drug that is both simple to use and reliably effective. Some authors have advocated tests such as oestrogen provocation test (Shaw et al, 1975) to help predict which patients will respond to clomiphene, but they are not reliable. Hull (1981) has advocated a therapeutic trial of clomiphene in all cases. A sequential programme starting with the simplest protocol and trying each agent in turn until a satisfactory response is achieved seems to be practically the most logical approach, albeit empirical. A key factor in treatment is the use of adequate criteria for the ovulatory response, which is particularly important with PCOD due to the hormonal contribution to circulating levels from the numerous subsidiary follicles.

Clomiphene

Clomiphene, one of a group of oestrogen receptor blockers, is first line therapy for induction of ovulation in women with PCOD. Its mode of action is poorly understood but it almost certainly involves a reduction in oestrogen mediated negative feedback on the pituitary (Adashi, 1984) and consequently an increase in LH and FSH. The rise in FSH levels stimulates follicular growth. The majority of patients with PCOD respond to clomiphene; MacGregor (1968) reported that 76 per cent of a series of 827 patients with PCOS including hirsutism responded but with a much reduced pregnancy rate. Hull (1987), using stricter criteria for defining a satisfactory response, found 78 per cent of his group of PCOS responded adequately, but only 45 per cent of those with hirsutism, with corresponding pregnancy rates.

When ovulation fails to occur in response to clomiphene, treatment should simply be tried again, for at least three cycles. There is no convincing evidence of any benefit from increasing the dose above 100 mg/day except in extremely obese women (Lobo et al, 1982). Responsiveness is unpredictable, often being only intermittently satisfactory, but because alternative treatments with gonadotrophins are so much more difficult and costly, an adequate response to clomiphene in only some cycles may be acceptable enough.

For the 22 per cent who fail to respond adequately to clomiphene alone, some centres advocate the addition of hCG at a set time but this is of unproven value (Yen, 1978). Failure to ovulate with clomiphene is usually due to failure of folliculogenesis which hCG is unlikely to benefit. Even if follicular development occurs, hCG given blindly is likely to be administered at an inappropriate time. Serial oestradiol measurements and ultrasound scans may help to time the injection of hCG (O'Herlihy et al, 1982), but their greater value is in detecting impaired follicular development. Initially, there is no need for detailed cycle monitoring; clomiphene is safe to use, with little risk of multiple pregnancy greater than twins (Futterweit, 1984f).

Pulsatile LH-RH therapy

The value of the hypothalamic releasing factor for patients with a hypothalamic cause for their amenorrhea is well established (Tan and Jacobs, 1985). Its application to patients with PCOD is in many ways illogical, as there is no conclusive evidence of hypothalamic dysfunction and test doses of LH-RH lead to an exaggerated rise in LH (Rebar et al, 1976) of which there is already an excess. The results of therapy do not entirely bear out the illogicality but are nevertheless disappointing with an ovulatory response in only 40 per cent of cycles and an even smaller proportion eventually conceiving (Adams et al, 1985). The same group noted that a much better result was achieved in those with a body mass index of no more than 20 (Jacobs, 1987).

The attraction of pulsatile LH-RH therapy, and its great advantage over exogenous gonadotrophin therapy, is that in a successful cycle a single follicle usually dominates (Franks et al, 1985). Even so, a triplet pregnancy has been associated with its use in a woman with PCOD (Fillicori et al, 1986). A further benefit of the single follicular response is the reduced need for serial monitoring in comparison with exogenous gonadotrophin therapy. The disappointing results achieved limit the application of this treatment in PCOD but its use should be considered in slimmer patients who have difficulty attending for the more intensive monitoring required for exogenous gonadotrophin therapy.

Exogenous gonadotrophin therapy

In women with infertility and amenorrhea generally, gonadotrophin therapy results in a normal conception rate (Hull et al, 1979b). However, the original studies were largely confined to patients with hypogonadotrophic amenorrhea in whom the use of human menopausal gonadotrophins (hMG) represents a simple form of hormone replacement therapy (Lunenfeld and Insler, 1978). In cases of PCOD resistant to clomiphene, hMG is given to patients with active pituitaries in effect to redress the imbalance between FSH and LH. Moreover, it is being used in patients who probably have an inherent ovarian disorder. Not surprisingly, the responses of the two groups is quite different. Wang and Gemzell (1980) reported only 28 per cent pregnancy rate despite 76-95 per cent apparent ovulation rate, with a greater propensity for multiple follicular development and consequently greater risk of ovarian hyperstimulation syndrome and high-order multiple pregnancy.

Those results were achieved, however, using only oestrogen measurements to assess the follicular response. It is now clear that such monitoring is very inaccurate in PCOD compared with hypothalamic disorders because of the much greater number of follicles stimulated and the large contribution of the numerous subsidiary follicles to the circulating pool of oestrogens and, in the luteal phase, progesterone. In PCOD much higher levels of oestrogens are frequently required before a dominant follicle reaches maturity, as indicated using ultrasonography, which is therefore the primary method of monitoring required in this condition. Unfortunately, there may be too many mature follicles and treatment with hCG to induce follicular rupture must be avoided for safety. This led to a search for a more selective form of treatment, either in the type of drug used or greater refinement in the control of dosage.

hMG is a mixture of FSH and LH but it has been shown that follicular growth can be induced by FSH without added LH (Shaw et al, 1987). Presumably this particularly applies to PCOD, which is characterised by high endogenous LH concentrations. Berger and colleagues (1972) suggested that additional LH is associated with hyperstimulation. It has also been suggested that the LH activity within hMG may add to the risk of premature luteinisation (Franks et al, 1985). To overcome these problems, purified FSH preparations have been formulated. The initial results from a small group of patients were encouraging (Raj et al, 1977) and analysis of human follicular fluid suggests the FSH results in reduced androgen concentrations when compared with hMG (Polan et al, 1986). More recent work doubts the practical benefits of FSH (Garcea et al, 1985; Jacobs, 1987). It may be that giving LH along with FSH as in hMG or not makes no significant difference due to the already large amounts of endogenous LH present. There have been preliminary reports of purified FSH treatment leading to suppression of endogenous LH but proper evaluation is awaited (Jones et al, 1985).

LH-RH agonists and superimposed exogenous gonadotrophin therapy

When employing hMG or FSH therapy in patients with PCOD it is not uncommon for an endogenous, often attenuated, LH surge to occur before follicular maturation (Gemzell et al, 1978). Combined with the effect of raised basal LH levels, the resulting premature luteinisation probably results in a failure to ovulate or the release of an abnormal oocyte (Stanger et al, 1985). To overcome these problems, Fleming and co-workers (1985) suppressed endogenous LH production by pituitary desensitisation with superactive LH-RH agonists and then induced ovulation by superimposing hMG therapy. The resulting ovarian response is little different (Coutts et al, 1988) but premature luteinisation is prevented and the pregnancy rate appears tentatively to be improved. This regimen is expensive, however, both because of the cost of the LH-RH agonist and because the dose of exogenous gonadotrophin required to induce follicular growth is greater, and the advantages if any have yet to be determined.

Glucocorticoid therapy

Of all the treatments used to induce ovulation in PCOD, glucocorticoid therapy has perhaps been the most misunderstood and consequently the least favoured. It is generally agreed that they are the treatment choice for the small group of anovulatory women with congenital adrenal hyperplasia (Chrousos et al, 1982) with the apparent added benefit in that group of reducing the risk of abortion (Sarris et al, 1978). However, their value alone or in combination with clomiphene, for the majority of patients with PCOD has been variably accepted. The dichotomy of opinion that prevails possibly reflects their indiscriminate use, often combined with ovulation induction agents.

Recent studies indicate that combined clomiphene/dexamethasone therapy is only of benefit to those patients with evidence of adrenal hyperfunction (Daly et al, 1984). Only one group have shown apparent improvement in ovulation and conception rates using hMG after the addition of small doses of dexamethasone, but in an uncontrolled study (Evron et al, 1983). The most likely beneficial effect of glucocorticoids, if any, is a reduction in adrenal androgen production leading to changes in ovarian and pituitary function. Glucocorticoids may have direct effects on the ovary (Danisova et al, 1987) and pituitary (Melis et al, 1987) but probably not at the doses used in these studies. Nevertheless, these data indicate that glucocorticoids offer a cheap, simple and apparently effective adjunct to clomiphene and gonadotrophin therapy and their selective use warrants proper consideration.

Ovarian wedge resection

Stein's group (1949) noticed that diagnostic ovarian biopsy was often followed by the commencement of ovulatory menstrual cycles in a substantial proportion of patients and wedge resection was quickly adopted as a treatment of anovulatory infertility associated with PCOD. A review of 1079 cases by Goldzieher and Green (1962) showed that 80 per cent developed regular menstrual cycles and 63 per cent conceived. The pregnancies were nearly all singleton and Cohen (1979) found a miscarriage rate of only 6 per cent. Wedge resection also provides the opportunity to confirm the diagnosis histologically and exclude occult intra-ovarian neoplasia.

Despite all these seeming advantages, wedge resection fell out of favour. Its effects are only temporary, meaning the chances of a second pregnancy are slim (Buttram and Vaquero, 1975). Secondly, and perhaps more importantly, there is a high risk of pelvic adhesion formation and consequent tubal infertility (Buttram and Vaquero, 1975). Two recent developments have renewed interest in surgical treatment of PCOD. First of all, microsurgical techniques have been shown to limit adhesion formation after wedge reection (Eddy et al, 1980) and more recently still Gjonnaess (1984) described the successful use of laparoscopic ovarian electrocautery as a method of ovulation induction. Pregnancy occurred in 69 per cent of PCOD patients troubled by infertility and it has been suggested that the incidence of postoperative adhesions will be lower than following wedge resection but this awaits verification.

The mechanism by which wedge resection and electrocautery induces regular ovulatory cycles is not known. The main effect seems to be a reduction in plasma androgen levels without any significant change in basal gonadotrophin levels (Judd et al, 1976); Aakvaag & Gjonnaess, 1985). Gjonnaess has postulated that ovulation is triggered by changes in the intravarian environment. One theory is that the removal of a wedge of stroma including thecal tissue lowers the androgenic capacity of the ovary allowing the reorganisation of intra-ovarian control mechanisms.

A surgical approach to ovulation induction for PCOD holds many attractive advantages for patients over gonadotrophin therapy because of cost in money, time and effort. Its use as second line therapy in those resistant to clomiphene deserves careful reassessment.

"Medical wedge resection"

"Medical" wedge resection is the concept of reducing the volume of androgenic stromal and thecal tissue using pharmacological agents rather than surgery. Such a technique would potentially have all the advantages of surgical wedge resection without the risk of adhesion formation. Unfortunately the agents used to date have failed to achieve this aim (Givens et al, 1974b; Calogero et al, 1987), possibly because the primary aim has been suppression of LH production. Fleming et al (1987) suggest that LH is not the cause of the increased rate of follicular recruitment seen in PCOD, and the observation that stromal hypertrophy is a feature of ovarian hyperthecosis in the absence of high LH levels (Nagamani et al, 1981) also points against LH being the agent directly responsible for the expansion of stromal tissues.

Hyperinsulinaemia is a common feature of classical PCOD and ovarian hyperthecosis (Nagamani et al, 1986) suggesting that insulin may be involved in the genesis of the stromal hypertrophy. Insulin is certainly a potent mitogen in vitro for many cell types, possibly acting through the IGF I receptor (Hill & Milner, 1985) and these authors have speculated that insulin is a physiological growth factor. Hyperinsulinaemia, a feature of PCOD, is known to be associated with disordered somatic growth such as acral hypertrophy (Flier et al, 1980). Poretsky and Kalin (1987) have proposed that insulin behaves as any trophic hormone within the ovary. We therefore hypothesise that insulin plays a significant part in hypertrophy of ovarian stromal tissues. We infer from this that a reduction of circulating insulin levels will allow the hypertrophic tissues to regress and thus a return to normal ovarian structure and function.

Somatostatin is a peptide hormone known to inhibit the release of insulin from the pancreas (Alberti et al, 1973). An orally active somatostatin analogue has now been formulated that inhibits insulin release without any adverse effect on glucose tolerance. It has been shown to retard the growth of growth factor dependent tumours and we propose that the application of a somatostatin analogue together with a superactive LH-RH agonist might allow ovarian recovery and, after withdrawal, the commencement of normal menstrual cycles.

Table 3-1
Comparison of ultrasonographic ovarian findings and hormonal features in women with functional disorders of the hypothalamic-pituitary-ovarian axis presenting with oligo- or amenorrhea

Hormonal category (and diagnosis)	*Number of patients*	*Oestrogenised*	*Ultrasonographic ovarian finding*		
			Normal	*Multi-follicular*	*Polycystic*
Hirsute (PCOD)	19	17 (89%)	0	0	19 (100%)
"Functional"/oestrogenised (? PCOD)	7	7 (100%)*	1	0	6 (86%)
Hyperprolactinaemia	5	0	4	0	1 (20%)
"Functional"/oestrogen-deficient (hypothalamic disorder)	8	0*	4	3	1 (13%)

* *result by definition*
Source: Fox, Corrigan & Hull, unpublished data.

Table 3-2
Accuracy of hormonal criteria in the diagnosis of ultrasonically confirmed PCOD as the primary cause* of oligo- or amenorrhea in individual women

Hormonal criterion	*Single test*	*Combined tests*
1. Oestrogenised state (normal menstrual response to progestogen challenge	92%	} 100% (1 and 2)
2. Hirsutism	73%	
3. Serum LH ≥ 12iu/l	60%	No added benefit
4. LH:FSH ratio		
(a) ≥2.5	60%	No added benefit
(b) ≥3.0	44%	No added benefit

* *There are a few additional cases of suppressed or latent PCOD, overridden by the primary cause of oligo- or amenorrhea, such as hyperprolactinaemia or hypothalamic disorder.*
Source: Fox, Corrigan and Hull: unpublished continuing study.

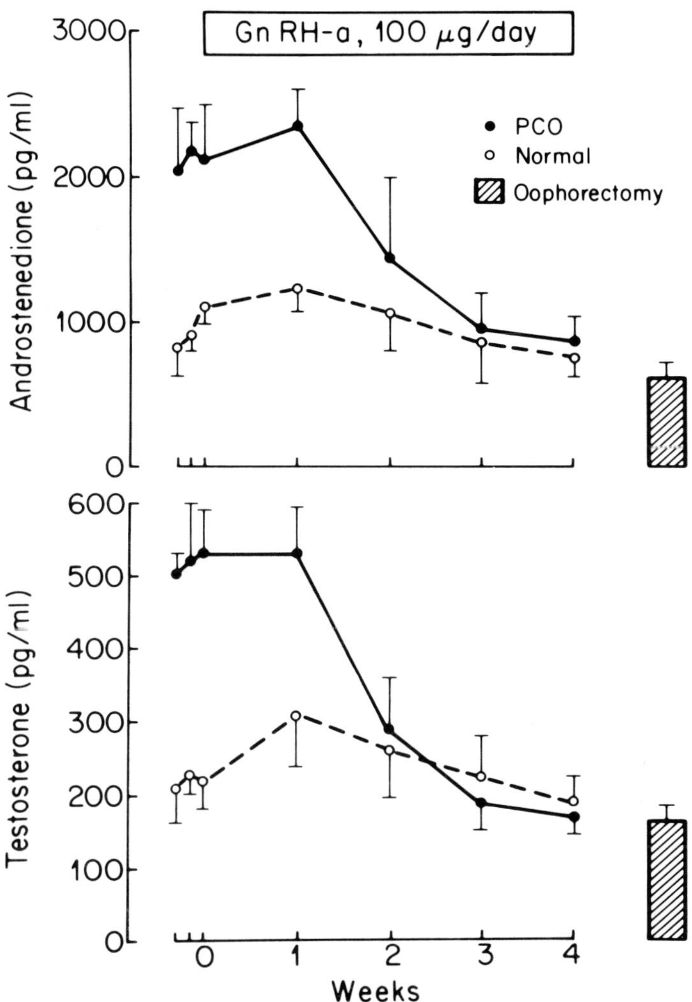

Figure 3-1
Effect on androgen levels of suppressing pituitary gonadotrophin secretion in women with PCOD compared with controls, demonstrating the primary ovarian origin of excess androstenedione and testosterone in PCOD.

Source: Reproduced with permission from Chang et al, 1983a.

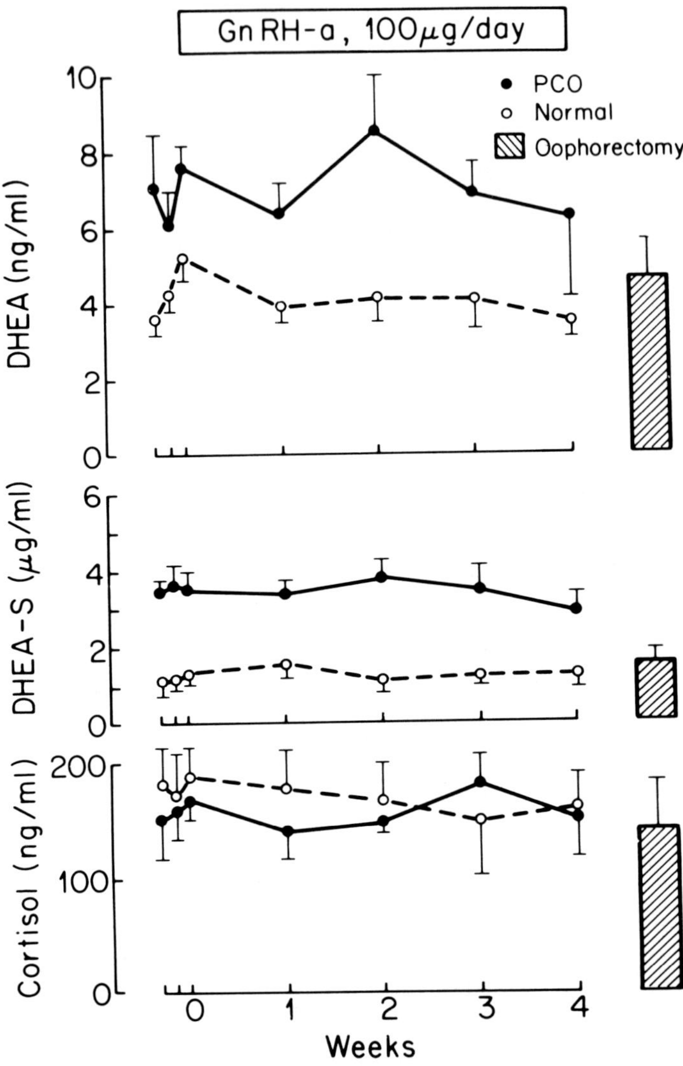

Figure 3-2

Results of treatment as in Figure 3-1, demonstrating the primary adrenal origin of excess dehydroepiandrosterone (DHEA) and DHEA sulphate (DHEA-S), despite normal production of cortisol, in PCOD.

Source: Reproduced with permission from Chang et al, 1983a.

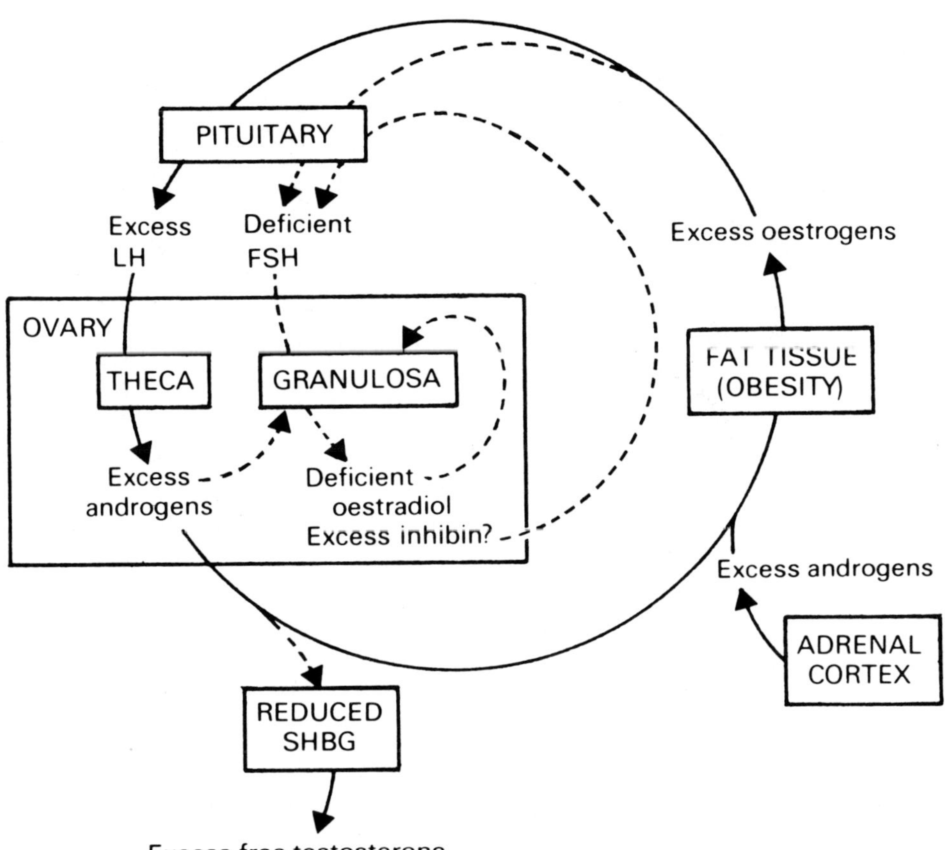

Figure 3-3
Illustration of vicious circle(s) involved in pathogenesis of PCOD. Continuous lines indicate stimulatory and broken lines inhibitory effects. In addition the extraneous influence of hyperinsulinaemia and possible intrafollicular paracrine influence of growth factors may be important factors, as discussed in the text.

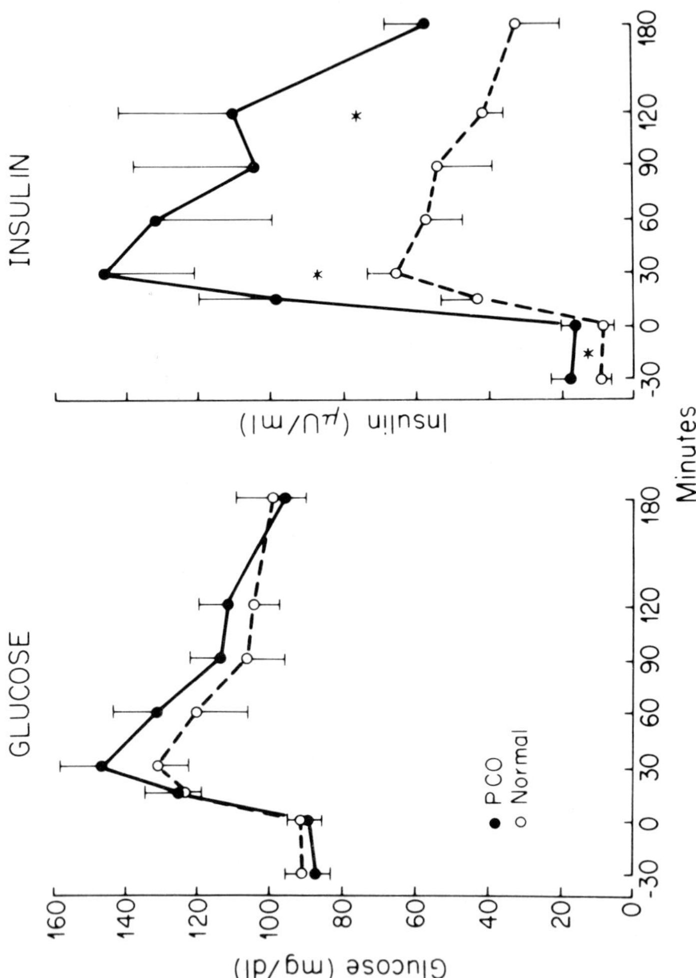

Figure 3-4

Response to oral glucose load in women with PCOD compared with controls, demonstrating glucose tolerance and compensatory hyperinsulinaemia due to insulin resistance in PCOD.

Source: Reproduced with permission from Chang et al, 1983b.

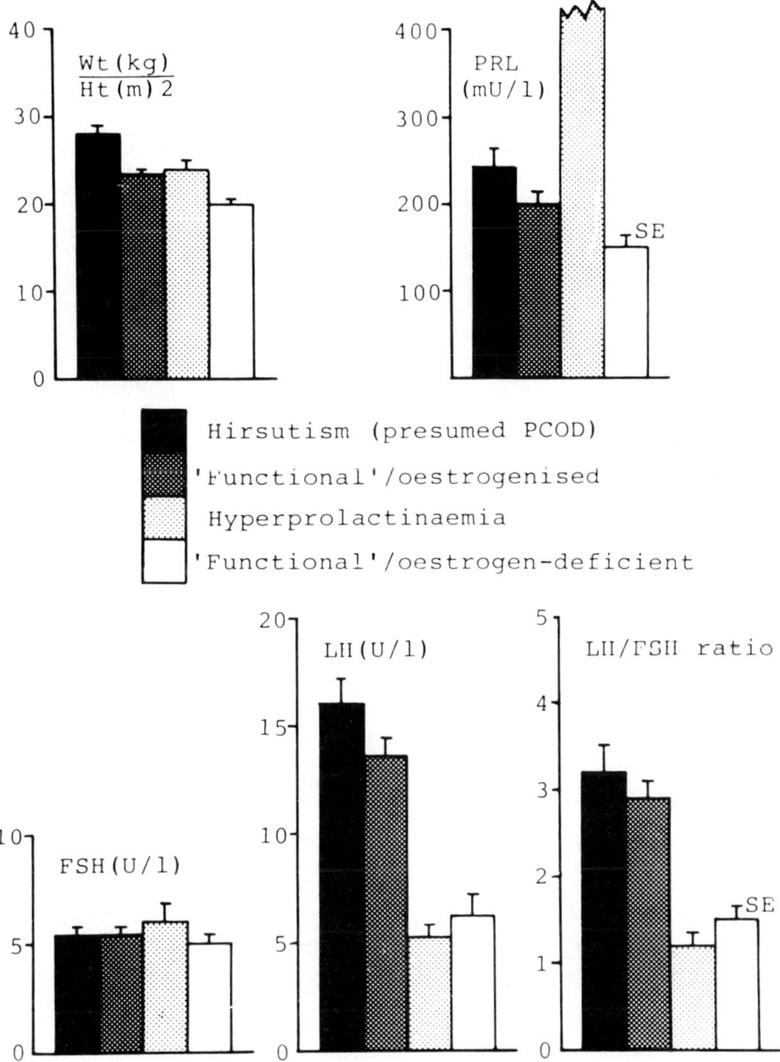

Figure 3-5

Mean body mass index and serum hormone values in four groups of infertile women with functional disorders of the hypothalamic-pituitary-ovarian axis presenting with oligo- or amenorrhea. (SE = standard error.)

Source: Reproduced with permission from Hull, 1987.

References

Aakvaag, A. Gjonnaess H. Hormonal response to electrocautery of the ovary in a patient with polycystic ovarian disease. *British Journal of Obstetrics and Gynaecology*, 1985; 92: 1258.

Abraham, G.E., Chalmajan Z.H., Buster J.E. Ovarian and adrenal contributions to peripheral androgens in hirsute women. *Obstetrics and Gynaecology*, 1965; 46: 169.

Adams, J., Polson D.W., Franks. Prevalence of polycystic ovaries in women with anovulation and idiopathic hirsutism. *British Medical Journal*, 1986; 293: 355.

Adams, J., Polson D.W., Abdulwahid, N., Morris D.V., Franks, S., Mason H.D., Tucker, M., Price, J. Multifollicular ovaries: Clinical and endocrine features and response to pulsatile gonadotrophin releasing hormone. *Lancet* 1985; i: 1375.

Adashi, E.Y. Clomiphene citrate: Mechanism(s) and site(s) of action — a hypothesis revisited. *Fertility and Sterility*, 1984; 42: 331.

Adashi, E.Y., Hsueh, A.J.W., Yen, S.S.C., Insulin enhancement of luteinising hormone and follicle-stimulating hormone release by cultured pituitary cells. *Endocrinology*, 1987; 108: 1441.

Adashi, E.Y., Resnick, C.E., D'Ercole A.J., Svoboda M.E., Van Wyk, J.J. Insulin-like growth factors as intraovarian regulators of granulosa cell growth and function. *Endocrine Reviews*, 1985; 6: 400.

Alberti, K.G.M.M., Christiansen S.E., Iversen, J. Inhibition of insulin secretion of somatostatin. *Lancet* 1973; i: 1299.

Aleem F.A., Eltabbakh G.H., Omar, R.A., Southern, A.L. Ovarian follicular fluid β-endorphin levels in normal and polycystic ovaries. *American Journal of Obstetrics and Gynecology*, 1987; 156: 1197.

Aleem F.A., McIntosh, T. Elevated plasma levels of β-endorphin in a group of women with polycystic ovarian disease. *Fertility and Sterility*, 1984; 42: 686.

Anderson, D.C., Yen, S.C.C. Effect of estrogens on adrenal 3 β ol hydroxysteroid-dehydrogenase in ovariectomised women. *Journal of Clinical Endocrinology & Metabolism*, 1976; 43: 561.

Aono, T., Miyazake M., Miyake A., Kinugasa, T., Kurachi K., Matsumoto K. Responses of serum gonadotrophins to LH-releasing hormone and oestrogens in Japanese women with polycystic ovaries. *Acta Endocrinologica*, 1977; 85: 840.

Baird, A., Walicke, P. Growth factors and the regulation of the neuroendocrine response. *Journal of Endocrinology*, 1987; 115 (suppl), abstract 4.

Baird, D.T., Corker, C.S., Davidson, D.W., Hunter, W.M., Michie, E.A., Van Look, P.F.A. Pituitary-ovarian relationships in polycystic ovary syndrome. *Journal of Clinical Endocrinology and Metabolism*, 1977; 45: 798.

Bar, R.S., Muggeo, M., Roth, J., Kahn, C.R., Havrankova, J., Imperato-McGinley, J. Insulin resistance, acanthosis nigricans and normal insulin receptors in a young woman: Evidence for a postreceptor defect. *Journal of Clinical Endocrinology and Metabolism*, 1978; 47: 620.

Barbieri, R.L., Makris, A., Ryan, K.J. Insulin stimulates androgen accumulation in incubations of human ovarian stroma and theca. *Obstetrics and Gynaecology*, 1984; 64: 743.

Barbieri, R.L., Ryan K.J. Hyperandrogenism, insulin resistance, and acanthosis nigricans syndrome: A common endocrinopathy with district pathophysiologic features. *American Journal of Obstetrics and Gynecology*, 1983; 147: 90.

Barlow, D., Bromwich, P., Wiley, M., Walker, A., Ross, C., Kennedy, S., Lopez Bernel, A. Transvaginal compared with transvesical ultrasonography for recovery of oocytes for in-vitro fertilisation. *British Medical Journal*, 1988; 296: 751.

Benjamin F., Deutsch, S., Saperskin, H., Seltzer, V. Prevalence of and markers for the attenuated form of congenital adrenal hyperplasia and hyperprolactinaemia masquerading as polycystic ovarian disease. *Fertility and Sterility*, 1986; 46: 215.

Berger, M.J., Taymor, M.L., Karam, K., Nudemberg F. The relative roles of exogenous and endogenous follicle stimulating hormone and luteinising hormone in human follicular maturation and ovulation induction. *Fertility and Sterility*, 1972; 23: 783.

Billiar R.B., Richardson, D., Anderson, E., Mahajan, D., Little, B. The effect of chronic and acyclic elevation of circulating androstenedione or estrone concentrations on ovarian function in the rhesus monkey. *Endocrinology*, 1985; 116: 2209.

Burghen, G.A., Givens, J.R., Kitabchi, A.E. Correlation of hyperandrogenism with hyperinsulinism in polycystic ovarian disease. *Fertility and Sterility*, 1980; 50: 113.

Buttram V.C., Vaquero C., Post-ovarian wedge resection adhesive disease. *Fertility and Sterility*, 1975, 26: 874.

Calogero, A.E., Macchi, M., Montanini, V., Mongioi, A., Maugeri, G., Vicari, E., Coniglione, F., Sipione, C., D'Agata R. Dynamics of plasma gonadotrophin and sex steroid release in polycystic ovarian disease after pituitary-ovarian inhibition with an analog of gonadotrophin-releasing hormone. *Journal of Clinical Endocrinology and Metabolism*, 1987; 64: 980.

Carmina, E., Rosato, F., Janni, A. Increased DHEAS levels in PCO syndrome: Evidence for the existence of two subgroups of patients. *Journal of Endocrinology Investigation*, 1986; 9: 5.

Chamlian, D.L., Taylor, H.B. Endometrial hyperplasia in young women. *Obstetrics and Gynaecology*, 1970; 36: 659.

Chang, R.J., Geffner, M.E. Insulin resistance in polycystic ovarian disease. *Clinics in Obstetrics and Gynaecology*, 1985; 12(3): 675.

Chang, R.J., Laufer, L.R., Meldrum, D.R., DeFazio, J., Lu, JKH, Vale, W.W., Rivier, J.E., Judd, H.L. Steroid secretion in polycystic ovarian disease after ovarian suppression by a long-acting gonadotrophin-releasing hormone agonist. *Journal of Clinical Endocrinology and Metabolism*, 1983a; 56: 897.

Chang, R.J., Mandel, F.P., Lu, J.K.H., Judd, H.L. Enhanced disparty of gonadotrophin secretion by estrone in women with polycystic ovarian disease. *Journal of Clinical Endocrinology and Metabolism*, 1982; 54: 490.

Chang, R.J., Mandel F.P., Wolfsen, A.R., Judd, H.L. Circulating levels of plasma adrenocorticotrophin in polycystic ovary disease. *Journal of Clinical Endocrinology and Metabolism*, 1982; 54: 1265.

Chang, R.J., Nakamura, R.M., Judd, H.L., Kaplan S.A. Insulin resistance in nonobese patients with polycystic ovarian disease. *Journal of Clinical Endocrinology and Metabolism*, 1983b; 57: 356.

Charbonnel, B., Krempf, M., Blanchard, P., Dano, F., Delage, C. Induction of ovulation in polycystic ovary syndrome with a combination of a luteinising hormone-releasing hormone analog and exogenous gonadotrohophins. *Fertility and Sterility*, 1987; 47: 920.

Chrousos, G.P., Loriaux, D.L., Mann, D.L., Cutler, G.B. Late-onset 21 hydroxylase deficiency mimicking idiopathic hirsutism or polycystic ovarian disease, an allelic variant of congenital virilizing adrenal hyperplasia with a milder enzymatic defect. *Annals of Internal Medicine*, 1982; 96: 143.

Cohen, M.B. Surgical management of infertility in the polycystic ovary syndrome. In Givens, J.R. (Ed), *Infertile Female*, Year-book Medical Publishers, Chicago, 1979; 273.

Cole, C., Kitabchi, A.E. Remission of insulin resistance with Orthonovum in a patient with polycystic ovarian disease and acanthosis nigricans. *Clinical Research*, 1978; 26: Abstract 412A.

Corenblum, B., Taylor, P.J. An investigation of the hyperprolactinaemia polycystic ovary (PCOD) syndrome. *Fertility and Sterility*, 1982; 37: 292 (abstract).

Coutts, J.R.T., Finnie, S., Conaghan, C., Black W.P., Fleming, R. Combined buserelin and exogenous gonadotrophin therapy for the treatment of infertility in women with polycystic ovarian disease. *Gynaecological Endocrinology,* 1988; 2 (suppl): Abstract 61.

Daly, D.C., Walter, C.A., Soto-Albors, C.E., Tohan, N., Riddick, D.H. A randomized study of dexamethasone in ovulation induction with clomiphene citrate. *Fertility and Sterility,* 1984; 41: 844.

Danisova, A., Sebokova, E., Kolena, J. Effect of corticosteroids on estradiol testosterone secretion by granulosa cells in culture. *Experimental and Clinical Endocrinology,* 1987; 89: 165.

Devesa, J., Perez-Fernandez, R., Lima, L., Cabezas-Cerrato, J. Adrenal cortex and type II polycystic ovary syndrome. *Gynaecological Endocrinology,* 1987; 1: 269.

Dewis, P., Newman M.C., Anderson, D.C. Does testosterone affect the normal menstrual cycle? *67th Annual Meeting of The Endocrine Society,* Baltimore, M.D., 1985; Abstract 223.

Dunaif, A., Scully, R.E., Anderson, R.A., Chapin, D.S., Crowley Jr, W.F. The effects of continuous androgen secretion on the hypothalamic-pituitary axis in woman: Evidence from a luteinized thecoma of the ovary. *Journal of Clinical Endocrinology and Metabolism,* 1984; 59: 389.

Eddy, C.A., Asch, R.H., Balmaceda, J.P. Pelvic adhesions following microsurgical and macrosurgical wedge resection of the ovaries. *Fertility and Sterility,* 1980; 33: 557.

Edman, C.D., MacDonald, P.C. Effect of obesity on conversion of plasma and rostenedione to estrone in ovulatory and anovulatory young women. *American Journal of Obstetrics and Gynecology,* 1978; 130: 456.

Erickson, G.F., Hsueh, A.J.W., Quigley, M.E., Rebar, R.W., Yen, S.S.C. Functional studies of aromatase activity in human granulosa cells from normal and polycystic ovaries. *Journal of Clinical Endocrinology and Metabolism,* 1979; 49: 514.

Evron, S., Navit, D., Laufer, N., Diamont, Y.Z. Induction of ovulation with combined human gonadotrophins and dexamethasone in women with polycystic ovarian disease. *Fertility and Sterility,* 1983; 40: 183.

Falaschi, P., Del Pozo, E., Rocco, A. Prolactin release in polycystic ovarian disease. *Obstetrics and Gynaecology,* 1980; 55: 579.

Feher, T., Halmy, L. Dehydroepiandrosterone and dehydroepiandrosterone sulfate dynamics in obesity. *Canadian Journal of Biochemistry,* 1975; 53: 215.

Fillicori, M., Michelacci, L., Ferrari P., Campaniello, E., Pareschi, A., Flamigni, C. Triplet pregnancy after low-dose pulsatile gonadotrophin-releasing hormone in polycystic ovarian disease. *American Journal of Obstetrics and Gynecology,* 1986; 155: 768.

Fleming, R., Haxton, M.J., Hamilton, M.R.P., McCune, G.S., Black, W.P., MacNaughton, M.C., Coutts, J.R.T. Successful treatment of infertile women with oligomenorrhoea using a combination of LHRH agonist and exogenous gonadotrophins. *British Journal of Obstetrics and Gynaecology,* 1985; 92: 369.

Fleming,R., Yates, R.W.S., Haxton, M.J., Coutts, J.R.T., Hamilton, M.P.R., Conaghan, C. Ovulation induction using the combination of buserelin and exogenous gonadotrophins in women with functional pituitaries. *British Journal of Clinical Practice,* 1987; 41 (suppl.): 34.

Flier, J.S., Young, J.B., Landsberg, L. Familial insulin resistance with acanthosis nigricans, acral hypertrophy and muscle cramps. *New England Journal of Medicine,* 1980; 303: 970.

Franks, S., Adams, J., Mason, H., Polson, D. Ovulatory disorders in women with polycystic ovary syndrome. *Clinics in Obstetrics and Gynaecology,* 1985; 12(3): 605.

Franks, S., Neagle, G., Leake, R., Mason, H., Harlow, C., Winston, R., Margara, R., Reed, M. Epidermal growth factor (EGF) concentrations in follicular fluid from normal or polycystic ovaries (PCO). *Journal of Endocrinology,* 1986; 112 (suppl.): Abstract 120.

Futterweit, W. *Polycystic Ovarian Disease*, Springer-Verlag, New York, 1984a; XI.
Futterweit, W. *Polycystic Ovarian Disease*, Springer-Verlag, New York, 1984b; 119.
Futterweit, W. *Polycystic Ovarian Disease*, Springer-Verlag, New York, 1984c; 58.
Futterweit, W. *Polycystic Ovarian Disease*, Springer-Verlag, New York, 1984d; 163.
Futterweit, W. *Polycystic Ovarian Disease*, Springer-Verlag, New York, 1984e; 118.
Futterweit, W. *Polycystic Ovarian Disease*, Springer-Verlag, New York, 1984f; 141.
Futterweit, W., Krieger, D.T. Pituitary tumours associated with hyperprolactinaemia and polycystic ovarian disease. *Fertility and Sterility*, 1979; 31: 608.
Garcea, N., Campo, S., Panetta, V., Vennen, M., Siccardi, P., Dargenio, R., De Tomasi, F. Induction of ovulation with purified follicle-stimulating hormone in patients with polycystic ovary syndrome. *American Journal of Obstetrics and Gynecology*, 1985; 151: 635.
Garcia, J.E., Jones, G.S., Wentz, A.C. The use of clomiphene citrate. *Fertility and Sterility*, 1977; 28: 707.
Geffner, M.E., Kaplan, S.A., Bersche, N., Golde, D.W., Landaw, E.M., Chang, R.J. Persistence of insulin resistance in polycystic ovarian disease after inhibition of ovarian steroid secretion. *Fertility and Sterililty*, 1986; 45: 327.
Gemzell, G.A., Kemman, E., Jones, J.R. Premature ovulation during administration of human menopausal gonadotrophins in non-ovulatory women. *Infertility*, 1978; 1: 1.
Giusti, G., Bassi, F., Borsi, L. Effects of prolactin on the human adrenal cortex: Plasma dehydro epiandrosterone sulphate in women affected by amenorrhoea with hyperprolactinaemia. In Crosignani, P.G. and Robyn, C. (Eds), *Prolactin and Human Reproduction*, Academic Press, New York, 1977; 239.
Givens, J.R., Kerber, L.J., Wiser, W.L., Anderson, R.N., Coleman, S.A., Fish, S.A. Remission of acanthosis nigricans associated with polycystic ovarian disease and a stromal luteoma. *Journal of Clinical Endocrinology and Metabolism*, 1974a; 38: 347.
Givens, J.R., Anderson, R.N., Wiser, W.L., Fish, S.A. Dynamics of suppression and recovery of plasma FSH, LH androstenedione and testosterone in polycystic ovarian disease using an oral contraceptive. *Journal of Clinical Endocrinology and Metabolism*, 1974b; 38: 727.
Givens, J.R., Anderson, R.N., Ragland, J.B., Wiser, W.L., Umstot, E.S. Adrenal function in hirsutism I. Diurnal change and response of plasma androstenedione, testosterone, 17-hydroxyprogesterone, Cortisol LH and FSH to dexamethasone and 1/2 unit of ACTH. *Journal of Clinical Endocrinology and Metabolism*, 1975a; 40: 988.
Givens, J.R., Anderson, R.N., Wiser, W.L., Donelson, A.J., Coleman, S.A. A testosterone-secreting, gonadotrophin-responsive pure thecoma and polycystic ovarian disease. *Journal of Clinical Endocrinology and Metabolism*, 1975b: 41: 845.
Givens, J.R., Anderson, R.N., Umstot, E.S., Wiser, W.L. Clinical findings and hormonal responses in patients with polycystic ovarian disease with normal versus elevated LH levels. *Obstetrics and Gynaecology*, 1976; 47: 388.
Gjonnaess, H. Polycystic ovarian syndrome treated by ovarian electrocautery through the laparoscope. *Fertility and Sterility*, 1984; 41: 20.
Goldzieher, J.W. Polycystic ovarian disease. *Fertility and Sterility*, 1981; 35: 371.
Goldzieher, J.W., Axelrod, L.R. Clinical and biochemical features of polycystic ovarian disease. *Fertility and Sterility*, 1963; 14: 631.
Goldzieher, J.W., Green, J.A. The polycystic ovary I. Clinical and histologic features. *Journal of Clinical Endocrinology and Metabolism*, 1962; 22: 325.
Goldzieher, J.W., Di Zerega, G.S. Polycystic ovarian disease. In Shearman, R.P. (Ed), *Clinical Reproductive Endocrinology*, Churchill-Livingston, Edinburgh, 1985; 406.

Green, J.A., Goldzieher, J.W. The polycystic ovary. IV. Light and electron microscopic studies. *American Journal of Obstetrics and Gynecology*, 1965; 91: 173.

Hague, W.M., Adams, J., Rodda, C., Brook, C.D.G., Dewhurst, C.J., Jacobs, H.S. Prevalence of ultrasonically detected polycystic ovaries in females with congenital adrenal hyperplasia. *Journal of Endocrinology*, 1986; III (suppl.): Abstract 46.

Haney, A.F., Maxson, W.S., Schomberg, D.W. Compartmental ovarian steroidogenesis in polycystic ovary syndrome. *Obstetrics and Gynaecology*, 1986; 68: 638.

Hann, L.E., Hall, D.A., McArdle, C.R., Seibel, M. Polycystic ovarian disease sonographic spectrum. *Radiology*, 1984; 150: 531.

Hartz, A.J., Barboriak, P.N., Wang, A., Katayama, K.P., Rimm A.A. The association of obesity with infertility and related menstrual abnormalities in women. *International Journal of Obesity*, 1979; 3: 57.

Hatch, R., Rosenfield, R.L., Kim, M.H. Hirsutism: Implications etiology and management. *American Journal of Obstetrics and Gynecology*, 1981; 140: 815.

Hill, D.J., Milner, R.D.G. Insulin as a growth factor. *Pediatric Research*, 1985; 19: 879.

Hoffman, D., Lobo, R.A. Serum dehydroepiandrosterone sulfate and the use of clomiphene citrate in anovulatory women. *Fertility and Sterility*, 1985; 43: 196.

Hoffman, D.I., Klove, K., Lobo, R.A. The prevalence and significance of elevated dehydroepiandrosterone sulfate levels in anovulatory women. *Fertility and Sterility*, 1984; 42: 76.

Homburg, R., Weissglas, L., Goldman, J. Improved treatment for anovulation in polycystic ovarian disease utilising the effect of progesterone on the inappropriate gonadotrophin release and clomiphene response. *Human Reproduction*, 1988; 3: 285.

Hosseinian, A.H., Kim, M.H., Rosenfield, R.L. Obesity and oligomenorrhoea are associated with hyperandrogenism independent of hirsutism. *Journal of Clinical Endocrinology and Metabolism*, 1976; 42: 765.

Hull, M.G.R., Knuth, U.A., Murray, M.A.F., Jacobs, H.S. The practical value of the progestogen challenge test, serum oestradiol estimation or clinical examination in assessment of the oestrogen state and response to clomiphene in amenorrhoea. *British Journal of Obstetrics and Gynaecology*, 1979; 86: 799.

Hull, M.G.R., Savage, P.E., Jacobs, H.S. Investigation and treatment of amenorrhoea resulting in normal fertility. *British Medical Journal*, 1979b; i: 1257.

Hull, M.G.R. Ovulation failure and induction. *Clinics in Obstetrics and Gynaecology*, 1981; 8: 753.

Hull, M.G.R. *Simplified Management of Anovulatory and Ovulatory Infertility*. MD Thesis, University of London, 1983; 263.

Hull, M.G.R., Glazener, C.M.A., Kelly, N.J., Conway, D.I., Foster, P.A., Hinton, R.A., Coulson, C., Lambert, P.A., Watt, E.M., Desair, K.M. Population study of causes, treatment and outcome of infertility. *British Medical Journal*, 1985; 291: 1693.

Hull, M.G.R. Epidemiology of infertility and polycystic ovarian disease: Endocrinological and demographic studies. *Gynaecological Endocrinology*, 1987; 1: 235.

Huppert, L.C. Induction of ovulation with clomiphene climate. *Fertility and Sterility*, 1979; 31: 1.

Jacobs, H.S. Polycystic ovaries and polycystic ovary syndrome. *Gynaecological Endocrinology*, 1987; 1: 113.

Jacobs, H.S. The use of GnRH analogues in the overall management of polycystic ovarian disease. *Gynaecological Endocrinology*, 1988; 2 (suppl.): Abstract 022.

James, V.H.T., Folkard, E.J., Bonney, R.C., Beranek, P.A., Reed, M.J. Factors influencing estrogen production and metabolism in postmenopausal women with endocrine cancer. *Journal of Endocrinological Investigation*, 1982; 5: 335.

Jeffcoate, S.L. Diagnosis of hyperprolactinaemia. *Lancet* 1978; ii: 1245.

Jialal, I, Naiter, K., Reddi, K., Moodley, J., Joubert, S.M. Evidence for insulin resistance in nonobese patients with polycystic ovarian disease. *Journal of Clinical Endocrinology and Metabolism*, 1987; 64: 1066.

Jones, G.S., Acosta, A.A., Garcia, J.E., Bernardus, R.E., Rosenwaks, Z. The effect of follicle-stimulating hormone without additional luteinising hormone on follicular stimulation and oocyte development in normal ovulatory women. *Fertility and Sterility*, 1985; 43: 696.

Judd, H.L., Rigg, L.A., Anderson, D.C., Yen S.S.C. The effects of ovarian wedge resection on circulating gonadotrophin and ovarian steroid levels in patients with polycystic ovary syndrome. *Journal of Clinical Endocrinology and Metabolism*, 1976; 13: 347.

Kahn, C.R., Flier, J.S., Bar, R.S., Archer, J.A., Gorden, P., Martin, M.M., Roth, J. The syndromes of insulin resistance and acanthosis nigricans. Insulin-receptor disorders in man. *New England Journal of Medicine*, 1976; 294: 739.

Kandeel, F., Butt, W.R., London, D.R. Regulation of serum prolactin levels by oestrone and oestrone sulphate in normally menstruating women. *Acta Endocrinologica*, 1977; 212: 42.

Kazer, R.R., Kessel, B., Yen, S.S.C. Circulating luteinising hormone pulse frequency in women with polycystic ovary syndrome. *Journal of Clinical Endocrinology and Metabolism*, 1987; 65: 233.

Kirschner, M.A., Bardin, C.W., Hembree, W.C., Ross, G.T. Effect of estrogen administration on androgen production and plasma luteinising hormone in hirsute women. *Journal of Clinical Endocrinology*, 1970; 30: 727.

Kirschner, M.A., Jacobs, J.B. Combined ovarian and adrenal vein catheterisation to determine the site of androgen over production in hirsute women. *Journal of Clinical Endocrinology and Metabolism*, 1971; 33: 199.

Kletsky, O.A., Davanjan, V., Nakamura, R.M., Mishell, D.R. Jr. Classification of secondary amenorrhoea based on distinct hormonal patterns. *Journal of Clinical Endocrinology and Metabolism*, 1975; 41: 660.

Kokko, E., Janne, O., Kaupila, A., Vinko, R. Cyclic clomiphene citrate treatment lowers cytosol estrogen and progestin receptor concentrations in the endometrium of postmenopausal women on estrogen replacement therapy. *Journal of Clinical Endocrinology and Metabolism*, 1981; 52: 345.

Korth-Schutz, S., Levine, L.S., Merkatz, I.R. An unusual case of Cushing's syndrome, hilus cell tumor and polycystic ovaries. *Journal of Clinical Endocrinology and Metabolism*, 1974; 38: 794.

Lachelin, G. The polycystic ovary syndrome. In Studd, J. (Ed), *Progress in Obstetrics and Gynaecology*, Vol 4, Churchill-Livingston, Edinburgh, 1984; 290.

Lachelin, G.C., Barnett, M., Hopper, B.R., Brink, G., Yen, S.S.C. Adrenal function in normal women and women with the polycystic ovary syndrome. *Journal of Clinical Endocrinology and Metabolism*, 1979; 49: 892.

Lachelin, G.C., Judd, H.L., Swanson, S.C., Hauck, M.E., Parker, D.C., Yen, S.S.C. Long term effects of nightly dexamethasone administration in patients with polycystic ovarian disease. *Journal of Clinical Endocrinology and Metabolism*, 1982; 55: 768.

Ladenheim, R.G., Tesone, M., Charreau, E.H. Insulin action and characterisation of insulin receptors in rat luteal cells. *Endocrinology*, 1984; 115: 752.

Lewis, J.T., Foglia, V.G., Rodriquez, R.R. The effect of steroids on the incidence of diabetes in rats after subtotal pancreatectomy. *Endocrinology*, 1950; 46: 111.

Lobo, R.A. The role of adrenal in polycystic ovary syndrome. *Seminars in Reproductive Endocrinology*, 1984; 2: 251.

Lobo, R.A. Disturbances of androgen secretion and metabolism in polycystic ovary syndrome. *Clinics in Obstetrics and Gynaecology*, 1985; 12 (3): 633.

Loba, R.A., Granger, L., Goebelsmann, U., Mishell, D.R. Elevation in unbound serum estradiol as a possible mechanism for inappropriate gonadotrophin secretion in women with polycystic ovaries. *Journal of Clinical Endocrinology and Metabolism*, 1981; 52: 156.

Lobo, R.A., Goebelsmann, U. Adult manifestation of congenital adrenal hyperplasia due to incomplete 21-hydroxylase deficiency mimicking polycystic ovarian disease.: *American Journal of Obstetrics and Gynecology*, 1980; 138: 120.

Lobo, R.A., Goebelsmann, U., Horton, R. Evidence for the importance of peripheral tissue events in the development of hirsutism in polycystic ovary syndrome. *Journal of Clinical Endocrinology and Metabolism*, 1983; 57: 383.

Lobo, R.A., Gysler, M., March, C.M. Goebelsmann, U., Mishell, D.R. Clinical and laboratory predictors of clomiphene response. *Fertility and Sterility*, 1982; 37: 168.

Luciano, A.A., Chapler, F.K., Sherman, B.M. Hyperprolactinaemia in polycystic ovary syndrome. *Fertility and Sterility*, 1984; 41: 719.

Lunenfeld, B., Insler, V. *Investigation, Diagnosis and Treatment of Functional Infertility*, Grosse Verlag, Berlin, 1978.

Macgregor, A.H., Johnson, J.E., Buride, C.A. Further clinical experience with clomiphene citrate. *Fertility and Sterility*, 1968; 19: 616.

MacLeod, A., Conaglen, J., Gordon, P., Richardson, P., Lowy, C., Sunksen, P., Wheeler, M. The effect of long term buserelin administration in the polycystic ovary syndrome. *Journal of Endocrinology*, 1986; 111 (suppl.): Abstract 228.

Mahesh, V.B. Current concepts of the pathophysiology of the polycystic ovary syndrome. In Tozzini, R.I., Reeves, G. and Pineda, R.L. (Eds), *Endocrine Physiopathology of the Ovary*, Elsevier/North Holland Biomedical Press, Amsterdam, 1980; 275.

Mason, H.D., Harlow, C.R., McNeill, J.M., Reed, M.J., Franks, S. Effects of epidermal growth factor and transforming growth factor in FSH-stimulated oestradiol production by rat grannulosa cells in culture. *Journal of Endocrinology*, 1986; III (suppl.): Abstract 100.

Meldrum, D.R., Abraham, G.E. Peripheral ovarian venous concentrations of various steroid hormones in virilizing ovarian tumors. *Obstetrics and Gynaecology*, 1979; 53: 36.

Melis, G.B., Mais, V., Gambacciani, M., Paoletti, A.M., Antinori, D., Fioretti, P. Dexamethasone reduces the post-castration gonadotrophin rise in women. *Journal of Clinical Endocrinology and Metabolism*, 1987; 65: 237.

Mennin, S.P., Gorski, R.A. Effects of ovarian steroids on plasma LH in normal and persistent oestrus adult female rats. *Endocrinology*, 1975; 96: 486.

Mortimer, H., Lev-Gur, M., Freeman, R., Fleischer, N. Pituitary response to bolus and continuous intravenous infusion of luteinising-hormone-releasing factor in normal women and women with polycystic ovarian syndrome. *American Journal of Obstetrics and Gynecology*, 1978; 130: 630.

Nagamani, M., Lingold, J.C., Gomez, L.G., Garza, J.R. Clinical and hormonal studies in hyperthecosis of the ovaries. *Fertility and Sterility*, 1981; 36: 326.

Nagamani, M., Van Dinh, T., and Kelver, M.E. Hyperinsulinaemia in hyperthecosis of the ovaries. *American Journal of Obstetrics and Gynecology*, 1986; 154: 384.

O'Herlihy, C., Pepperell, R.T., Robinson, H.P. Ultrasound timing of human chorionic gonadotrophin administration in clomiphene-stimulated cycles. *Obstetrics and Gynaecology*, 1982; 59: 40.

Orsini, L.F., Venturoli, S., Lorusso, R., Pluchinotta, V., Paraclisi, R., Bovicelli, L. Ultrasonic findings in polycystic ovarian disease. *Fertility and Sterility*, 1985; 43: 709.

Parisi, L., Tramonti M., Casciano, S., Zurli A, Gazzarrini, O. The role of ultrasound in the study of polycystic ovarian disease. *Journal of Clinical Ultrasound*, 1982; 10: 167.

Parker, L.N., Lifrak, E.T., Odell, W.D. A 60,000 molecular weight human pituitary glycopeptide stimulates adrenal androgen secretion. *Endocrinology*, 1983; 113: 2092.

Pasquali, R., Fabbri, R., Venturoli, S., Paradisi, R., Antenucci, D., Melchionda N. Effect of weight loss and antiandrogenic therapy on sex hormone blood levels in insulin resistance in obese patients with polycystic ovaries. *American Journal of Obstetrics and Gynecology*, 1986; 154: 139.

Pasquali, R., Venturoli, S., Paradisi, R., Capelli, M., Parenti, M., Melchionda, N. Insulin and C-peptide levels in obese patients polycystic ovaries. *Hormone and Metabolism Research*, 1982; 14: 284.

Paterson, M.E.L., Wade-Evans, T., Sturdee, D.W., Thorn, M.H., Studd, J.W.W. Endometrial disease after treatment with oestrogens and progestogens in the climacteric. *British Medical Journal*, 1980; i: 822.

Pehrson, J.J., Vaitukaitis, J., Longcope, C. Bromocriptine, sex steroid metabolism and menstrual patterns in the polycystic ovary syndrome. *Annals of Internal Medicine*, 1986; 105: 129.

Plymate, S.R., Fariss, B.L., Bassett, M.L. Obesity and its role in polycystic ovary syndrome. *Journal of Clinical Endocrinology and Metabolism*, 1981, 52: 1246.

Polan, M.L., Daniele, A., Russell, J.B., De Cherney, A.H. Ovulation induction with human menopausal gonadotrophin compared to human urinary follicle-stimulating hormone results in a significant shift in follicular fluid androgen levels without decernible differences in granulosa-luteal cell function. *Journal of Clinical Endocrinology and Metabolism*, 1986; 63: 1284.

Polson, D.W., Adams, J., Wadsworth, J., Franks, S. Polycystic ovaries — a normal variant? *Lancet* 1988; i: 870.

Polson, D.W., Sagle, M., Mason, H.D., Adams, J., Jacobs, H.S., Franks, S. Ovulation and normal luteal function during LHRH treatment of women with hyperprolactinaemic amenorrhoea. *Clinical Endocrinology*, 1986; 24: 531.

Poretsky, L., Kalin, M.F. The gonadotropic function of insulin. *Endocrine Reviews*, 1987; 8: 132.

Quigley, M.E., Rakoff, J.S., Yen, S.S.C. Increased luteinising hormone sensitivity to dopamine inhibition in polycystic ovary syndrome. *Journal of Clinical Endocrinology and Metabolism*, 1981; 52: 231.

Raj, S.G., Berger, M.J., Grimes, E.M., Taymor, M.L. The use of gonadotrophins for the induction of ovulation in women with polycystic ovarian disease. *Fertility and Sterility*, 1977; 28: 1280.

Rajaniemi, H.J., Ronnberg, L., Kauppila. Luteinising hormone receptors in ovarian follicles of patients with polycystic ovarian disease. *Journal of Clinical Endocrinology and Metabolism*, 1980; 52: 1054.

Randolph, J.F., Kipersztok, S., Ayers, J.W.T., Ansbacher, R., Peegal, H., Menon, K.M.J. The effect of insulin on aromatase activity in isolated human endometrial glands and stroma. *American Journal of Obstetrics and Gynecology*, 1987; 157: 1534.

Rebar, R., Judd, H.L., Yen, S.S.C, Rakoff, J., Vandenberg, G., Naftolin, F. Characterisation of the inappropriate gonadotrophin secretion in polycystic ovary syndrome. *Journal of Clinical Investigation*, 1976; 57: 1320.

Rogers, J., Mitchell, G.W. The relation of obesity to menstrual disturbances. *New England ournal of Medicine*, 1952; 247: 53.

Ruutiainen, K., Erkkola, R., Irjala, K. Endorphin basal levels in hirsute women. *European Journal of Obstetrics, Gynaecology and Reproductive Biology*, 1985; 20: 373.

Sarris, S., Swyer, G.I.M., Ward, R.H.T., Lawrence D.M., McGarrigle, H.H., Little, V. The treatment of mild adrenal hyperplasia and associated infertility with prednisone. *British Journal of Obstetrics and Gynaecology*, 1978; 85: 251.

Serio, M., Dell'Acqua, S., Calabresi, E. et al Androgen secretion by the human ovary: Measurement of androgens in ovarian venous blood. In James, V.H.T., Serio, M., and Giusti, G. (Eds), *The Endocrine Function of the Human Ovary*, Academic Press, London, 1976; 471.

Shaw, R.W., Duignan, N.M., Butt, W.R., Logan-Edwards, R., London, D.R. Hypothalamic-pituitary relationships in the polycystic ovary syndrome: Serum gonadotrophin levels following injection of oestradiol benzoate. *British Journal of Obstetrics and Gynaecology*, 1975; 82: 952.

Shaw, R.W., Ndukwe, G., Imueclemhe, D.A.G., Bernard, A., Burford, G., Bentick, B. Endocrine changes following pituitary desensitization with LHRH agonist and administration of purified FSH to induce follicular maturation. *British Journal of Obstetrics and Gynaecology*, 1987; 94: 682.

Sitteri, P.K., MacDonald, P.C. Role of extraglandular estrogen in human endocrinology, In Geep, R.O. and Astwood, E.B. (Eds), *Handbook of Physiology: Endocrinology*, Vol II, American Physiology Society, Washington, 1973; 615.

Smith, S., Ravnikar, V.A., Barbieri, R.L. Androgen and insulin response to an oral glucose challenge in hyperandrogenic women. *Fertility and Sterility*, 1987; 48: 72.

Sommers, S.C., Wadman, P.J. Prevalence of polycystic ovaries. *American Journal of Obstetrics and Gynecology*, 1956; 72: 160.

Stanger, J.D., Yovich, J.L. Reduced in-vitro fertilisation of human oocytes from patients with raised basal luteinising hormone levels during the follicular phase. *British Journal of Obstetrics and Gynaecology*, 1985; 92: 385.

Stanhope, R., Adams, J., Pringle, J.P., Jacobs, H.S., Brook, C.G.D. The evolution of polycystic ovaries in a girl with hypogonadotrophic hypogonadism before puberty and during puberty induced with pulsatile gonadotrophin-releasing hormone. *Fertility and Sterility*, 1987; 47: 872.

Stein, I.F., Cohen, M.R., Elson, R. Results of bilateral ovarian wedge resection in 47 cases of sterility. *American Journal of Obstetrics and Gynecology*, 1949; 58: 267.

Stein, W.F., Leventhal, M.L. Amenorrhoea associated with bilateral polycystic ovaries. *American Journal of Obstetrics and Gynecology*, 1935; 29: 181.

Stevens, V.C., Goldzieher, J.W. Urinary excretion of gonadotrophins in congenital adrenal hyperplasia. *Pediatrics*, 1968; 41: 421.

Stevens, C.A., Prince, M.J., Peters, E.J., Meyer, W.J. Hyperinsulinaemia and hyperandrogenaemia: In-vivo androgen response to insulin infusion. *Obstetrics and Gynaecology*, 1987; 69: 921.

Tan, S.L., Jacobs, H.S. Recent advances in the management of amenorrhea. *Clinics in Obstetrics and Gynaecology*, 1985; 12 (3): 725.

Thorner, M.O., Besser, G.M., Jones, A., Dacie, J., Jones, A.F. Bromocriptine treatment of female infertility: Report of 13 pregnancies. *British Medical Journal*, 1975; iv: 694.

de Vane, G.W., Czekala, N.M., Judd, H.L., Yen, S.S. Circulating gonadotrophins, estrogens and androgens in polycystic ovarian disease. *American Journal of Obstetrics and Gynecology*, 1975; 121: 496.

Vejlsted, H., Albrechsten,R. Biochemical and clinical effect of ovarian wedge resection in the polycystic ovary syndrome. *Obstetrics and Gynaecology*, 1976; 47: 575.

Wang, C.F., Gemzell, C. The use of human gonadotrophins for the induction of ovulation in women with polycystic ovarian disease. *Fertility and Sterility*, 1980; 33: 479.

Woodard, T.L., Burghen, G.A., Kitabhri A.E., Williams, J.A. Glucose intolerance and insulin resistance in aplastic anaema treated with oxymetholone. *Journal of Clinical Endocrinology and Metabolism*, 1981; 53: 905.

Wortsman, J., Singh, K.B., Murphy, J. Evidence for the hypothalamic origin of the polycystic ovary syndrome. *Obstetrics and Gynaecology*, 1981; 58: 137.

Wilson, E.A., Erickson, G.F., Zarutski, P., Finn, A.E., Tulchinsky, D., Ryan, K.J. Endocrine studies of normal and polycystic ovarian tissues in vitro. *American Journal of Obstetrics and Gynecology*, 1979; 134: 56.

Yen, S.S.C. Chronic anovulation due to inappropriate feedback systems. In Yen, S.S.C. and Jaffe, R. (Eds), *Reproductive Endocrinology*, Saunders, Philadelphia, 1978; 297.

Yen, S.S.C. The polycystic ovary syndrome. *Clinical Endocrinology*, 1980; 12: 177.

4

Induction of ovulation using pulsatile luteinizing hormone releasing hormone

S.L. Tan, P.W. Thong and C. Chen

Introduction

Ten to 15 per cent of the general population are subfertile, and 30 to 40 per cent of female subfertile patients have disorders of ovulation. By virtue of its efficacy, safety and ease of administration, clomiphene citrate remains today the first line of therapy for the treatment of anovulation except in cases of hyperprolactinaemia, where treatment with bromocriptine would be appropriate (Tan and Jacobs, 1985). Unfortunately, 25 per cent of anovulatory women do not respond to clomiphene (Rust et al, 1974) and, in the past, these women had to be treated with human menopausal gonadotrophin (hMG). However, while hMG is effective and successfully induces ovulation in 75 per cent of cases, the conception rate on hMG therapy is much lower. For instance, Thompson & Hansen (1970) reported the combined results of approximately 100 clinical investigators in the United States and Canada and out of a total of 1286 patients who were administered 3002 courses of therapy, 75 per cent of the patients ovulated but only 25 per cent became pregnant. Moreover, use of hMG requires intensive monitoring because the amount of hMG that corrects anovulation varies from patient to patient and from cycle to cycle even in the same patient. A slightly inadequate dose fails to achieve ovulation while a marginally excessive dose leads to multiple follicular development, ovarian hyperstimulation and multiple pregnancy. Most major series have reported a multiple pregnancy rate of 25 to 35 per cent (Schwartz et al, 1980; Wang and Gemzell, 1980; Oelsner et al, 1978; Healy et al,1980) and a risk of ovarian hyperstimulation of roughly 10 per cent (Wang and Gemzell, 1980; Lunenfeld and Insler, 1974). Since the unravelling of the structure of luteinizing hormone releasing hormone (LHRH) and its subsequent synthesis by Schally and his colleagues (1980), numerous attempts have been made to use LHRH for induction of ovulation. The initial studies were largely unsuccessful because high dose injections were administered at infrequent intervals (Huang, 1975). It was found that administration of LHRH led to an initial rise in serum luteinizing hormone (LH) and follicle stimulating hormone (FSH) concentrations, followed by a decline with continued LHRH infusion. This phenomenon has since been attributed to desensitisation of pituitary receptors (Clayton, 1982). It was Knobil and his co-workers (1980) who first demonstrated in Rhesus monkeys with experimental lesions in the hypothalamic area that administration of LHRH in a pulsatile fashion, rather than continuously, could restore ovulatory cycles. In recent years, this observation has led to a number of studies in humans where administration of pulsatile LHRH has been successfully used to induce ovulatory cycles that were endocrinologically normal (Leyendecker et al, 1980; Mason et al, 1984; Tan et al, 1987, 1988a). This chapter reviews our experience of the use of pulsatile LHRH for the treatment of chronic anovulatory infertility.

Patients and methods

Forty-four women with anovulatory infertility were studied. All had failed to ovulate in response to multiple courses of clomiphene citrate at a minimum dose of 100mg for five days. Several of the patients had not responded to hMG as well. In all patients, their husbands' semen analyses were normal while tubal patency had been confirmed by laparoscopy. The patients treated were essentially in two categories. The first group of patients are those with hypogonadotrophic hypogonadism. These patients present with primary or secondary amenorrhea, a negative progestogen challenge test and measurement of their circulating serum gonadotrophin levels reveal low LH and FSH levels. Pelvic ultrasonography reveal an unstimulated ovary with little follicular activity and a small uterus with thin endometrium (Figures 4-1 and 4-2). The second group of patients are those with polycystic ovarian disease (PCOD). These patients are often fatter than normal and their serum LH and testosterone concentrations and LH to FSH ratio are raised. Ultrasound examination of their pelvis reveal enlarged ovaries with multiple small cysts scattered around the periphery with highly echogenic stroma (Figure 4-3) and a uterus that is larger than normal with thickened endometrium (Figure 4-4) reflecting the stimulation produced by the high endogenous levels of oestrogen.

LHRH pump therapy

There are many miniaturised portable infusion pumps which are suitable for pulsatile LHRH therapy. Some are unnecessarily sophisticated and rather expensive. We have used the Autosyringe AS6H infusion pump in our programme. (Figure 4-5). The syringe containing the LHRH is connected to a microvolume infusion set (Travenol, Hooksett, USA) which is made of a biochemically inert non-kinkable material and has a dead space of 60μl. The length of the needle is 1.5cm (needle gauge 27) and the preferred tubing length is 107 cm. The pump is concealed underneath the patient's clothes while the needle is inserted into the lateral aspect of the upper arm distal to the humeral attachment of the deltoid muscle. The needle is placed in the subcutaneous fat and it is important to place the needle at the correct depth (Armar et al, 1987). If it is placed too superficially, a blister may form when the LHRH solution is administered, while an excessively deep insertion causes considerable discomfort when the arm is moved. With correct placement of the needle the patient is comfortable throughout the whole range of arm movements. All our patients are taught to change the needles themselves at home. Most of our patients are working and all have been able to carry on a normal working and social life. In over 230 treatment cycles we have not had a single patient give up treatment because of practical difficulty with pump therapy. The needle and tubing set is changed every four days when a new syringe of LHRH is used. The standard solution we use is 15μg of LHRH administered at a pulse interval of 90 minutes.

Route of administration

Initial studies of the use of pulsatile LHRH suggested that it was preferable to use the intravenous route of administration as the subcutaneous route resulted in disordered folliculogenesis (Reid et al, 1981). Long term intravenous therapy on an outpatient basis, however, is complex and carries a number of potential hazards, including septicaemia and subacute bacterial endocarditis. As a result, many groups (Armar et al, 1986; Hurley et al, 1987; Tan, 1987; Tan et al, 1988b) have employed the subcutaneous route and they have found that, provided that the dose of LHRH administered was sufficient, ovulatory cycles that were endocrinologically normal could be obtained.

Recently, Hurley and his colleagues (1987) have evaluated the suitability of the subcutaneous route for pulsatile administration of LHRH by determining the plasma LHRH and gonadotrophin profiles in a group of women with

LHRH responsive hypothalamic amenorrhea after subcutaneous LHRH administration, and comparing the results with those obtained after bolus intravenous LHRH administration. They found that the patterns of LH response to subcutaneous and intravenous LHRH were similar, with maximum levels reached between 20 and 30 minutes after injection, then declining to 50 to 69 per cent of the peak value by 90 minutes after subcutaneous injection and 61 per cent of the peak value 90 minutes after intraveous injection. There was no significant difference between peak LH response to 10μg intravenous and subcutaneous doses of LHRH (15.2 $\pm$2.5 ($\pm$SEM) versus 13.2 $\pm$ 2.2 iU/l). They concluded that subcutaneous LHRH administration results in pulsatile plasma LHRH and gonadotrophin responses, the latter resembling those seen after intravenous administration, thus confirming the suitability of the subcutaneous route for pulsatile LHRH delivery. When the subcutaneous route is chosen, however, the needle should preferably be inserted into the upper arm rather than the lower abdominal wall. Blunt and her colleagues (1986) have reported that subtaneous injection of LHRH into the upper arm produces a pulse of greater peak height and shorter duration that more closely resembles the profile obtained after intravenous injections. This may explain the excellent rates of ovulation reported by investigators who have employed the upper arm site (Armar et al, 1986; Blunt et al, 1986; Tan et al, 1988b) in contrast with the poor success rates achieved in studies using the lower abdominal wall as the site of administration (Menon et al, 1984). Figures 4-6a, b and c illustrate the endocrine pattern of three ovulatory cycles obtained in a patient with hypogonadotrophic hypogonadism using a constant dose of 15 μg per pulse administered every 90 minutes.

The place of ultrasound in the assessment and monitoring of patients on pulsatile LHRH therapy

The use of ultrasound to differentiate the patients who do not respond to induction of ovulation with clomiphene citrate has been referred to. In summary, pelvic ultrasonography allows these patients to be categorised into two large groups, namely, those with hypogonadotrophic hypogonadism and those with polycystic ovarian disease. This has important prognostic implications because, as we shall discuss later, the main determinant of successful treatment is proper selection of cases. Treatment with LHRH in patients with hypogonadotrophic hypogonadism is associated with a much higher ovulatory rate as compared with polycystic ovarian disease. Ultrasonography is also used to monitor treatment and in our programme, we have relied mainly on the Aloka abdominal sector scanner with a 3.5 mHz long focussed transducer for this purpose. A baseline ultrasound scan is performed at the commencement of pump therapy on day five of the menstrual cycle. The length and breadth of the uterus are measured as well as the endometrial thickness (Figures 4-7 and 4-8). Serial ultrasound scans are then performed from day 10 and growth of the uterus, endometrium and ovarian follicles documented. Ultrasound scans are performed three times a week once a dominant follicle is present and daily in the peri-ovulatory period. Ultrasound evidence of ovulation is provided by sudden collapse of the pre-ovulatory follicle, fluid in the pouch of Douglas and formation of a corpus luteum (Figures 4-9 and 4-10).

Although blood samples are taken at every visit, these are essentially for research, and day to day management of the patient is determined by ultrasound monitoring. Follicular activity has proved a reliable bioassay of gonadotrophin secretion and changes in uterine dimensions and endometrial thickness an effective bioassay of the rise in serum oestradiol concentrations as a result of follicular growth and maturation (Adams et al , 1988; Adams et al, 1989). More recently we have used vaginal ultrasonography to assess the growth in endometrial thickness and follicular numbers and sizes. The major advantage of this approach is the greater resolution of the ultrasound picture as well as avoiding the need for the patient to have a full bladder which is generally accepted by patients to be the most uncomfortable part of monitoring. Figures 4-11a and b show the evolution of a pre-ovulatory follicle on vaginal ultrasonography using the Aloka vaginal probe.

Results of LHRH therapy

Table 4-1 shows the overall results of our LHRH programme. In the patients with hypogonadotrophic hypogonadism, the rate of ovulation is close to 90 per cent. A striking illustration of the response in these patients is seen when detailed endocrine studies are undertaken. Figure 4-12 shows the serum LH and FSH profile of a patient with hypogonadotrophic hypogonadism taken at 15 minute intervals for 10 hours. It can be seen that initially the levels of serum LH and FSH are very low and there is an apulsatile pattern as would be expected in such a patient. When the infusion of LHRH was commenced at a dose of 15 μg per pulse every 90 minutes, the immediate response in terms of a pulsatile release of LH and FSH can be seen. Patients with pituitary tumours which have been surgically extirpated leading to HH may also respond to LHRH therapy provided there is sufficient pituitary reserve to respond to LHRH stimulation. An example of such a patient is illustrated in Figure 4-13.

Notwithstanding the above, patients with HH who have had pituitary surgery, especially if in conjunction with radiotherapy, do not as a group respond as well as other patients with HH (Morris et al, 1987). As can be expected, patients with panhypopituitarism do not respond to LHRH therapy (Figure 4-14). In the case of patients with polycystic ovarian disease we treated in our programme, we found that the rate of ovulation exceeds 60 per cent. A total of 29 clinical pregnancies have been achieved in these 44 patients treated. Interestingly, in the group of patients with polycystic ovarian disease 63.8 per cent of the patients became pregnant on LHRH therapy. We have analysed the length of the follicular phase of ovulatory cycles induced by LHRH and we have found that in patients with hypogonadotrophic hypogonadism the majority of cycles have a follicular phase length of 10–19 days (97.44 per cent of cases) and the mean follicular phase length was 15.25 ± 3.79 days. In contrast, when we look at ovulatory cycles in patients with polycystic ovarian disease, while the majority of cycles have a follicular phase length between 10–19 days, a significant proportion of cycles (29 per cent) have a follicular phase length of 20 days or more. In fact the mean follicular phase length in the patients with PCOD was 19.66 ± 7.59 days, which is significantly longer than that in HH. Based on these results, we believe that in patients with PCOD at least 30 days of LHRH therapy should be administered before anovulation is diagnosed. Failure to follow this rule will result in almost 29 per cent of cycles being mistakenly diagnosed as non-responsive to LHRH, and this may explain the results of some studies which show a poor response of PCOD to subcutaneous LHRH therapy.

We have also studied the luteal phase of patients on treatment with pulsatile LHRH and have found that in both categories of patients, that is, those with HH and PCOD, the luteal phase is essentially normal. With regard to the incidence of multiple pregnancy, we have only had one twin pregnancy among all the pregnancies that have been achieved when LHRH alone, or in combination with clomiphene citrate, was used to induce ovulation. A disturbing feature in some of the treatment cycles has been the development of follicular cysts. This was seen in about five per cent of the cycles and was often recurrent in the same patient. The cause of such cyst formation is unclear and these patients tend to form cysts even when clomiphene alone is used to induce ovulation. There is still no satisfactory treatment for these patients but since they do not form cysts in every treatment cycle it is still possible for pregnancy to occur in those cycles when normal folliculogenesis occurs.

Cost of treatment

The cost of treatment comprises the cost of the pump, LHRH and monitoring. When the cost of using LHRH is compared with that of hMG therapy, it has been found that LHRH therapy is in fact cheaper (Sueldo and Swanson, 1986). This is largely because the amount of monitoring that is required with LHRH therapy is significantly less than when hMG is used. In fact, in our programme, hormone tests have been dispensed with where day to day management of the patient is concerned. The gynaecologist, provided that he is able to perform ultrasound scans, is able to monitor patients on LHRH therapy himself without relying on the availability of a good endocrine laboratory for hormone assays.

Induction of ovulation in patients resistant to subcutaneous pulsatile LHRH therapy

It is now generally accepted that patients with hypogonadotrophic hypogonadism are the ideal group of patients for pulsatile LHRH therapy. The response to treatment is excellent, and the risk of ovarian hyperstimulation and multiple pregnancy low. The cumulative conception rate in these patients is almost 90 per cent at the end of six months (Armar et al, 1986). The problem arises in patients with PCOD, which remains today the most difficult group of patients to treat in terms of in vivo induction of ovulation. The large studies of the use of hMG therapy in these patients that have been published suggest that hMG therapy will successfully induce ovulation in 75 to 95 per cent of anovulatory patients but many of these studies include both patients with HH as well as those with PCOD. Moreover, because the use of clomiphene citrate was initiated at about the same time as hMG, many studies of the use of hMG were in all anovulatory patients and not confined to clomiphene resistant cases alone. When we review the results of studies using hMG only in patients with PCOD which did not ovulate in response to clomiphene citrate, the successful response in terms of ovulation is about 70 to 75 per cent. Another feature of hMG therapy is that there is a discrepancy between the apparent rate of ovulation and the pregnancy rate, and most studies have reported only a 30 per cent pregnancy rate (Blankstein and Quigley, 1988) when hMG is used for treating patients who do not ovulate in response to clomiphene. What is most disturbing about the use of hMG, however, is the high rate of multiple pregnancy and ovarian hyperstimulation. The major advantage of LHRH therapy is that when it is successful unifollicular ovulation generally obtains and the rate of multiple pregnancy and ovarian hyperstimulation is very low (Armar et al, 1989).

In fact we have never encountered a single cycle which resulted in clinical hyperstimulation when pulsatile LHRH therapy was used via the subcutaneous route, either alone, or in combination with clomiphene citrate (see below). Other large studies using subcutaneous pulsatile LHRH therapy have reported the same experience (Armar et al, 1986). Nevertheless, in the context of PCOD, the role of LHRH therapy remains debated. On the one hand, Burger and co-workers (1986) successfully induced ovulation in nine out of 11 PCOD patients treated with LHRH, which supported the favourable results reported earlier by Ory et al (1985). On the other hand, Loucopoulos et al (1984) and Saffan and Seibel (1986) had poor results and suggested that subcutaneous LHRH therapy produces a low response in patients with PCOD and is therefore not a suitable mode of therapy in this group of patients.

However, most of these studies have been small ones reporting the results of very few cycles of treatment. In the largest published series to date by Eshel et al (1988) they reported a 48 per cent ovulation rate (52 ovulatory cycles out of 108) when subcutaneous LHRH was used alone in clomiphene resistant cases of PCOD and 61 per cent ovulation rate (21 out of 34 cycles) when clomiphene citrate was added to the LHRH therapy. In our LHRH programme we have followed a similar approach. When we find that there is failure of response to pulsatile LHRH given by itself the patient is administered clomiphene citrate 100mg a day for five days (Tan et al, 1988c). Using this protocol we have found similar results in our programme as Eshel and his colleagues. We have had a 50 per cent ovulation rate when LHRH is used alone and a 66.7 per cent ovulation rate when clomiphene was added to LHRH therapy, giving a composite 63.6 per cent ovulation rate when both treatments are considered together (82 out of 129 cycles of treatment). The mechanism by which exogenous pulsatile LHRH successfully induces ovulation in PCOD is probably by overriding the underlying hypothalamic pituitary dysfunction as it has been found that in PCOD there is abnormal pulsatile gonadotrophin release with an increased LH pulse frequency as well as increased LH pulse amplitude (Filicori et al, 1988).

How clomiphene works to augment the response to pulsatile LHRH remains speculative. It has been shown that clomiphene acts at the hypothalamic level by increasing the pulse frequency but not amplitude of LHRH release (Kerin et al, 1985). There is however, also evidence that clomiphene has a pituitary site of action where it enhances LHRH mediated release of LH and FSH by exerting a direct oestrogenic effect (Adashi, 1984). Finally, clomiphene may have a direct action at the ovarian level by stimulating ovarian aromatase activity (Engels et al, 1968). Whatever the mechanism of action, our results support the notion that clomiphene citrate augments the response to induction of ovulation by pulsatile LHRH and combined pulsatile LHRH and clomiphene citrate is safe and effective in inducing ovulation in over 65 per cent of patients with PCOD who do not respond to either treatment alone.

What happens if LHRH and LHRH + clomiphene citrate in combination fails to induce ovulation? Recently, a few studies have reported the combined use of pulsatile LHRH and hMG for inducing ovulation in this very recalcitrant group of patients. Eckstein et al (1985) studied five patients with hypothalamic amenorrhea who did not have follicular maturation after nine to 32 days of LHRH therapy. When they administered two to four ampoules of hMG for two days, they obtained seven ovulatory cycles and four out of the five patients conceived.

There were no cases of clinical hyperstimulation. Corenblum and Taylor (1987) reported three women with hypothalamic amenorrhea who did not respond to LHRH alone. One ampoule of hMG was added for three days when the dominant follicle reached 7 to 8mm. They obtained five ovulatory cycles in three women and all three women conceived. These studies have been in small numbers of patients and are confined to patients with hypothalamic amenorrhea who are not the usual patients who would require such therapy since the overwhelming majority would respond to LHRH alone. We have therefore studied a group of 16 patients all of whom had not responded satisfactorily to induction of ovulation with clomiphene citrate, pulsatile LHRH and combined LHRH and clomiphene citrate. Many of these patients had failed to ovulate with hMG or pure FSH as well. 15 μg of LHRH was administered subcutaneously every 90 minutes while one to two ampoules of FSH was administered for five days starting from day two of the menstrual cycle. This resulted in 15 out of the 16 women ovulating and eight of the 16 women becoming pregnant. Seventy-four per cent of cycles in this very recalcitrant group of patients were ovulatory (Tan et al, 1989) and there was mild hyperstimulation in only one out of 54 cycles of treatment. No treatment was required and, in fact, the patient conceived in that same cycle. The basis of using pure FSH to augment the response to LHRH is that granulosa cells from polycystic ovaries have a low rate of oestrogen production which increases when FSH, but not LH, is added (Erickson et al, 1979). It has also been shown that the reduction in aromatase activity in PCOD is due to a low local concentration of FSH rather than an intrinsic abnormality of the granulosa cells. The advantage of combining a small dose of FSH with LHRH instead of using large doses of hMG or FSH by themselves is to seek the threshold of stimulation that would be sufficient to induce ovulation but not to produce clinical hyperstimulation or multiple pregnancy. Our initial results with this protocol has been very encouraging in this respect.

Recent developments

Recently there has been a number of novel approaches using LHRH. Kotsuji and his colleagues (1988) have investigated the efficacy of every other day administration of LHRH in women with hypothalamic amenorrhea and found that they could induce clomiphene responsiveness in 10 out of 11 women who were hypogonadotrophic and in four out of eight women who were normogonadotrophic. Filicori et al (1988) reported a small study of six women with PCOD in which they found that the use of LHRH analogue suppression rendered the patients more susceptible to ovulation induction with pulsatile LHRH. Both these approaches are interesting but as yet the data supporting their use are limited. One fundamental point is that while treatment of infertility is life-giving it is not life-saving. As clinicians, our goal should be to achieve successful pregnancy but by the safest means possible. While conventional therapy with hMG is successful, it carries a significant risk of ovarian hyperstimulation and multiple pregnancy. Moreover, there are some patients who do not respond to hMG but who will respond to LHRH. For instance, we recently treated a woman with PCOD who did not respond satisfactorily to hMG therapy although 105 ampoules of hMG were used in the treatment cycle. When we started her on pulsatile LHRH treatment she ovulated for three successive cycles on a standard 15μg dose and she became pregnant in her third cycle of treatment. As such, we feel that patients with PCOD should be treated with pulsatile LHRH if they do not respond to induction of ovulation with clomphene citrate.

If they do not respond during the first cycle of treatment, clomiphene citrate should be added and if this fails to induce ovulation, then in the following cycle a small dose of pure FSH should be administered to augment the response to the pulsatile LHRH. Using this regimen the majority of patients with PCOD will ovulate and, as our results suggest, with a much smaller risk of ovarian hyperstimulation (one cycle of mild hyperstimulation out of 232 treatment cycles) and multiple pregnancy. The only exceptions may be in patients with PCOD who have a high body mass index because these patients do not seem to respond as well to subcutaneous LHRH therapy (Armar et al, 1986; Thong et al, 1988). This group of patients should preferably be started on gonadotrophin therapy if they fail to respond to clomiphene citrate and are unable to reduce their weight.

In summary, the use of pulsatile LHRH therapy has allowed the successful correction of anovulatory infertility in patients who do not respond to clomiphene citrate. In comparison with hMG or FSH which directly stimulate the ovaries, the major advantage of pulsatile LHRH is that pituitary modulation of treatment remains intact and the message to the gonad represents the product of pituitary stimulation by the releasing hormones, and modification of that stimulation by the normal feedback to the pituitary by gonadal steroids (Jacobs, 1987). In clinical practice, this means that less monitoring is necesssary, the risk of ovarian hyperstimulation is minimal and the rate of multiple pregnancy close to that observed in spontaneous human conception. The use of clomiphene citrate and small doses of FSH to augment the response to induction by LHRH allows a greater percentage of patients, especially those with PCOD, to ovulate without any significant increase in the risk of multiple pregnancy and ovarian hyperstimulation.

Acknowledgements

We are grateful to Dr Chew Chin Hin, Dr Koh Thong Sam and Professor Y.M. Salmon for their support and to Shaw Foundation for their generous research grant. We wish to thank Drs Dixie Chua, L.C. Cheng, A. Adhha, R. Chong and S.W. Jen for their help with our LHRH programme. Nurses Margaret Lee, C.I. Phua, N.K. Gin and T.J. Yeo helped to look after the patients in the pump programme and we express our sincere gratitude. We are grateful to Mr Chua Ee Kwang, Dr Peter Raff and Dr W. Schaub of Hoechst for the generous supplies of Fertiral (LHRH) used in our studies and to Mr Robert Barzelay and Mr Tai Cheong Hui of Serono for the Metrodin (pure FSH) used.

Table 4-1
Results of treatment with LHRH

	Hypogonadotrophic hypogonadism	*Polycystic ovarian disease*	*Total*
No. of patients	8	36	44
No. of cycles of treatment	49	183	232
No. of ovulatory cycles	44	123	167
(% ovulatory cycles)	(89.80)	(67.20)	
No. of clinical pregnancies	6	23	29
No. of chemical pregnancies	2	—	2
No. of abortions	2	4	6

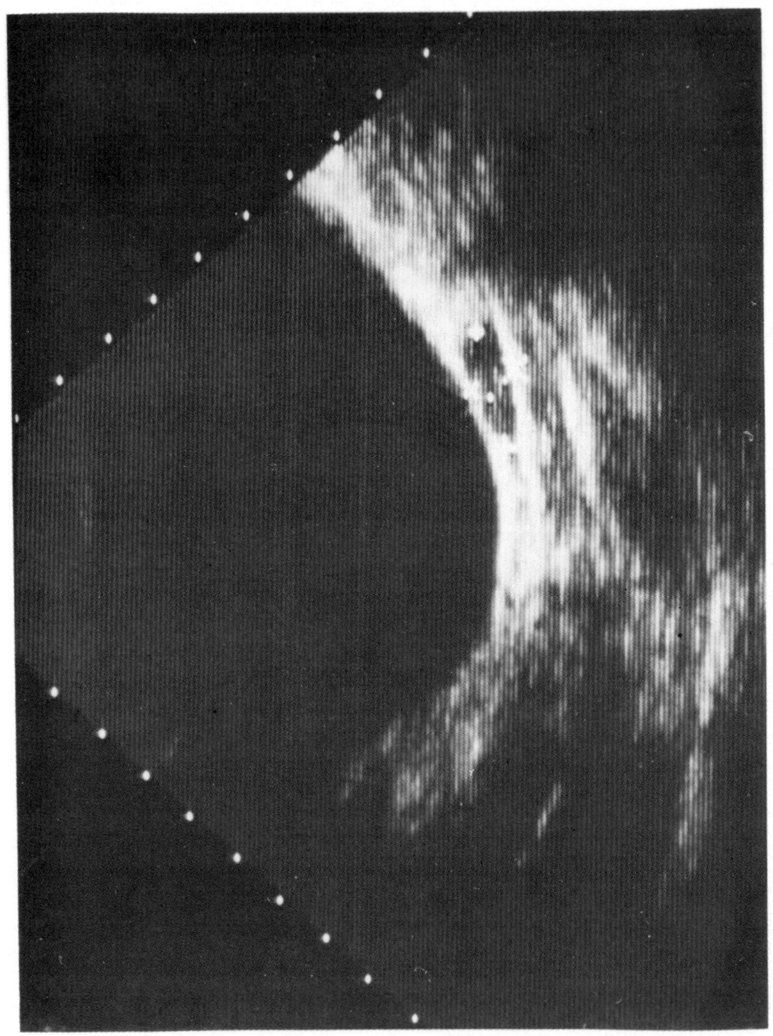

Figure 4-1
This shows a small unstimulated ovary in a patient with hypogonadotrophic hypogonadism.

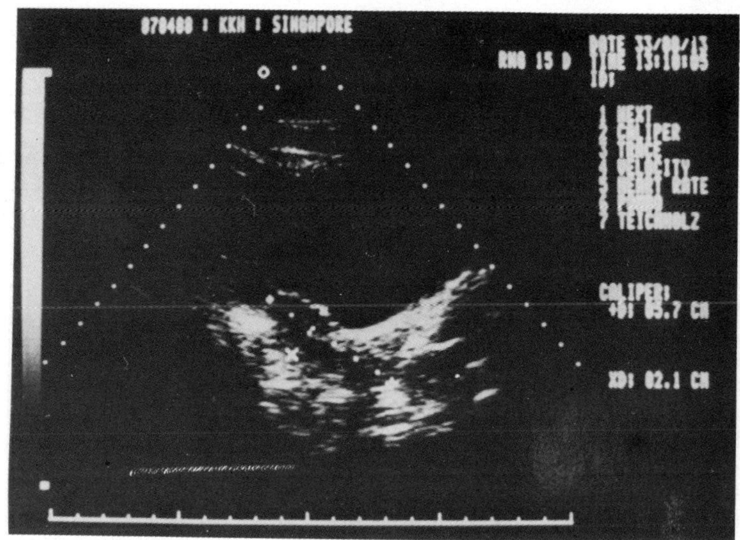

Figure 4-2
A small uterus with thin endometrium in a patient with hypogonadotrophic hypogonadism.

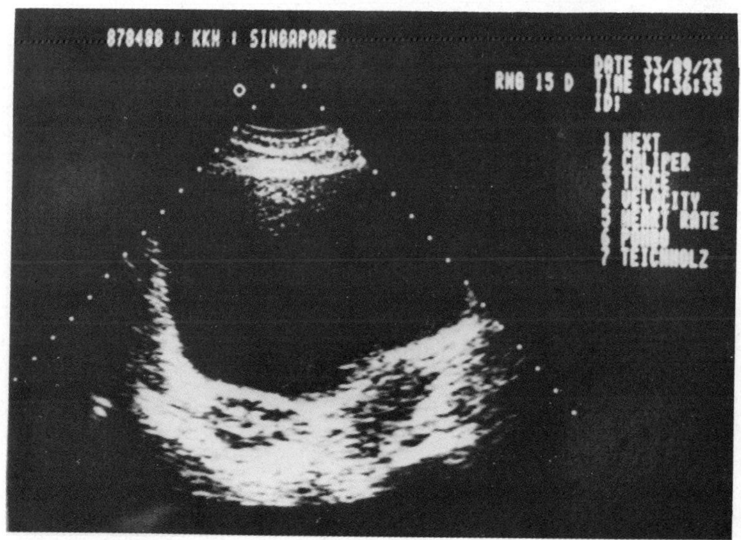

Figure 4-3
A picture of a polycystic ovary with multiple small cysts and highly echogenic stroma.

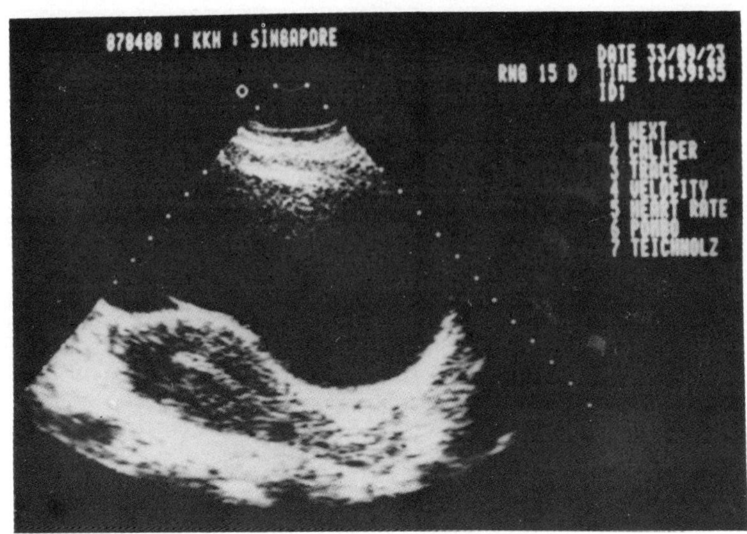

Figure 4-4
The uterus is large and the endometrium thick in this patient with polycystic ovarian disease reflecting stimulation by the high levels of endogenous oestrogen.

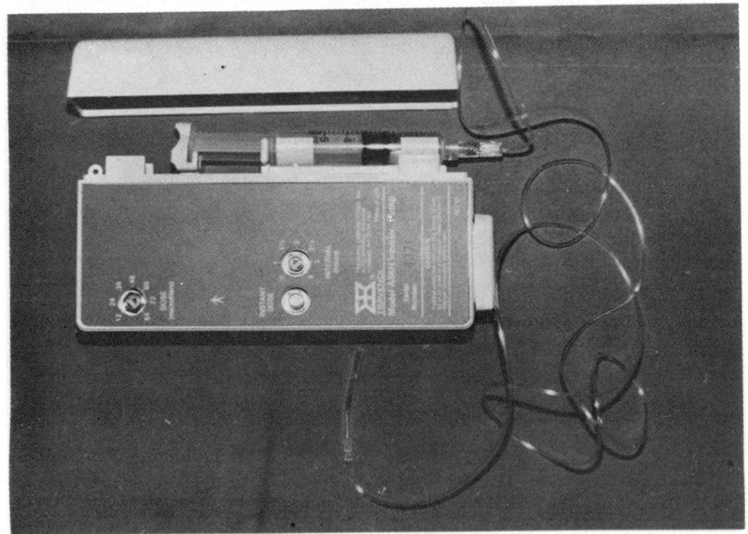

Figure 4-5
The Autosyringe AS6H infusion used in our studies.

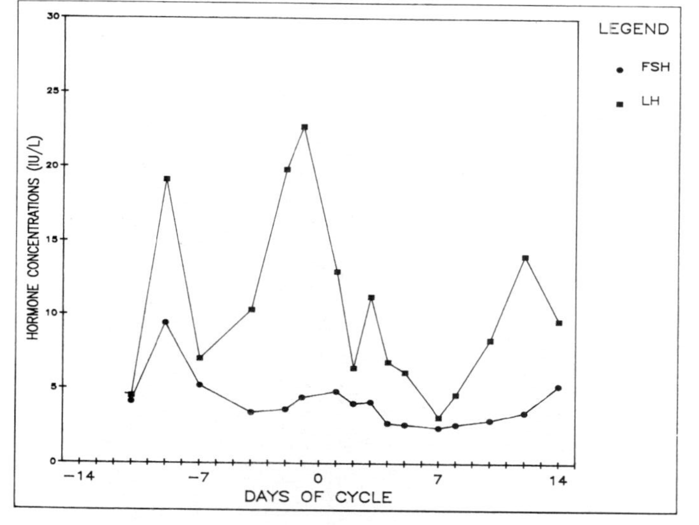

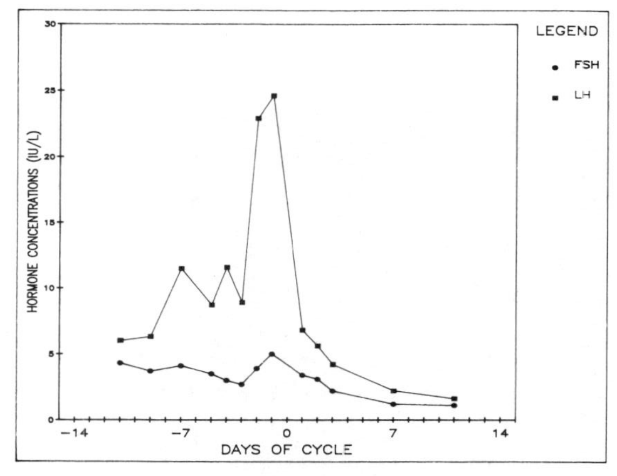

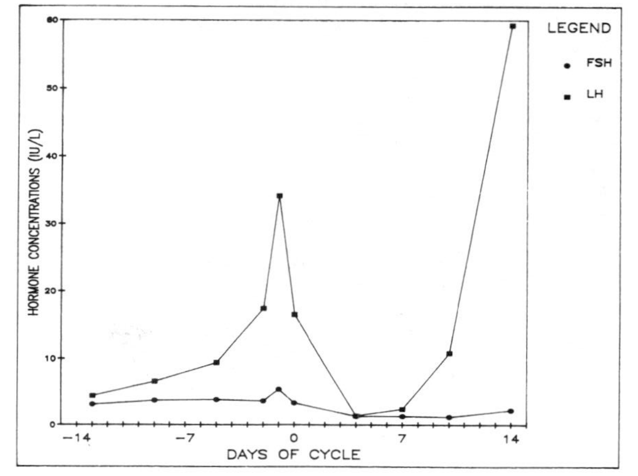

Figure 4-6a, b, c (clockwise from above)
The endocrine pattern of three ovulatory cycles (lst cycle a, 2nd cycle b, 3rd cycle c respectively) obtained in a patient with hypogonadotrophic hypogonadism treated with pulsatile LHRH at a constant dose of 15μg per pulse administered every 90 minutes. Day 0 is the day of presumed ovulation. Note in cycle three the apparent increase in LH concentration at the end of the cycle caused by chorionic gonadotrophin of pregnancy cross reacting with the LH assay.

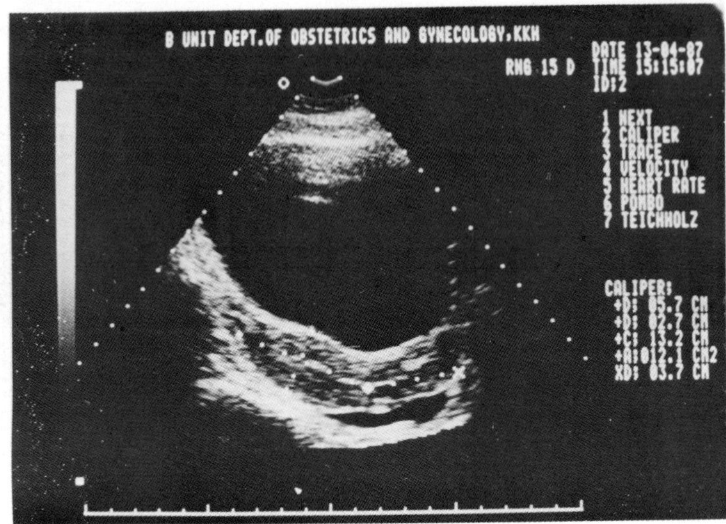

Figure 4-7
This shows how the length and breadth of the uterus is measured.

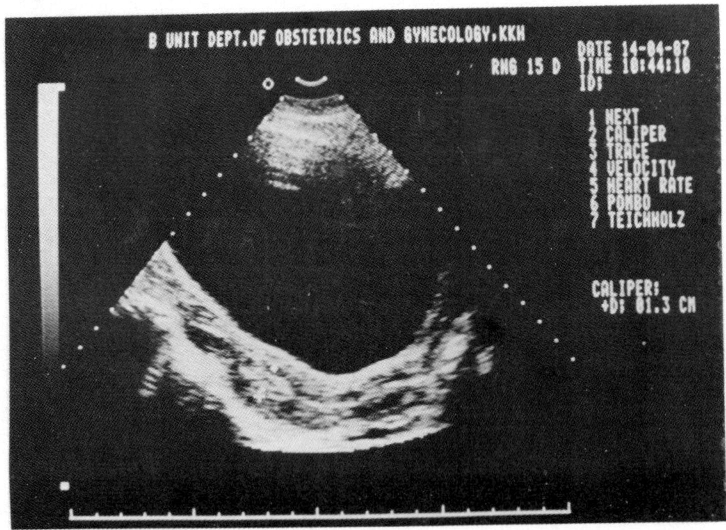

Figure 4-8
The endometrial thickness is shown between the two markings.

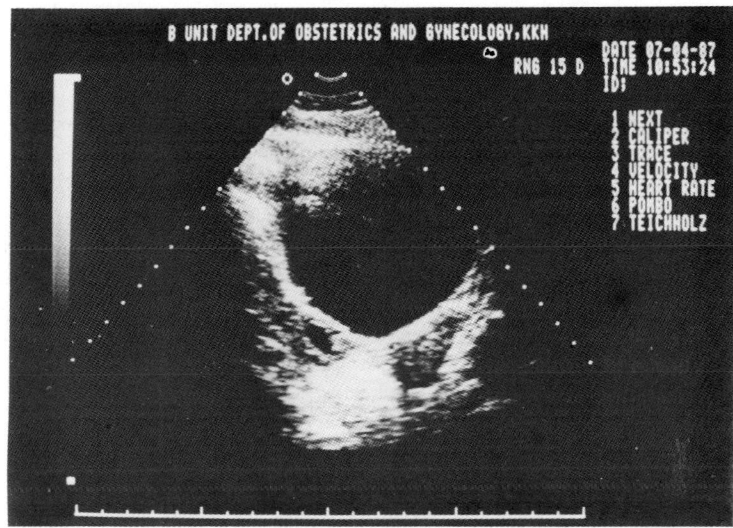

Figure 4-9
Fluid in the Pouch of Douglas as seen in the post ovulatory period.

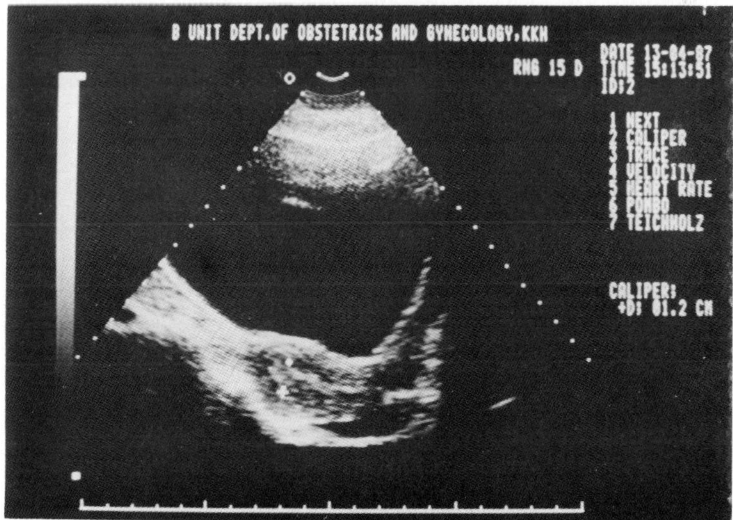

Figure 4-10
This shows the corpus lutuem in the ovary after ovulation has occurred.

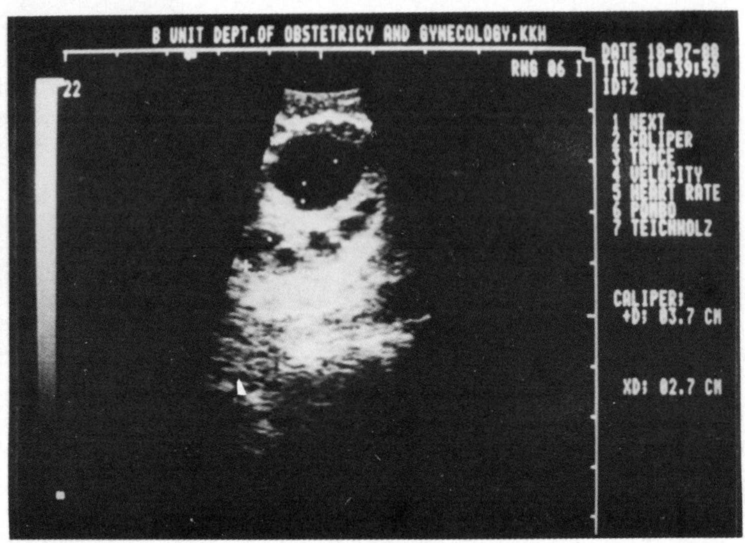

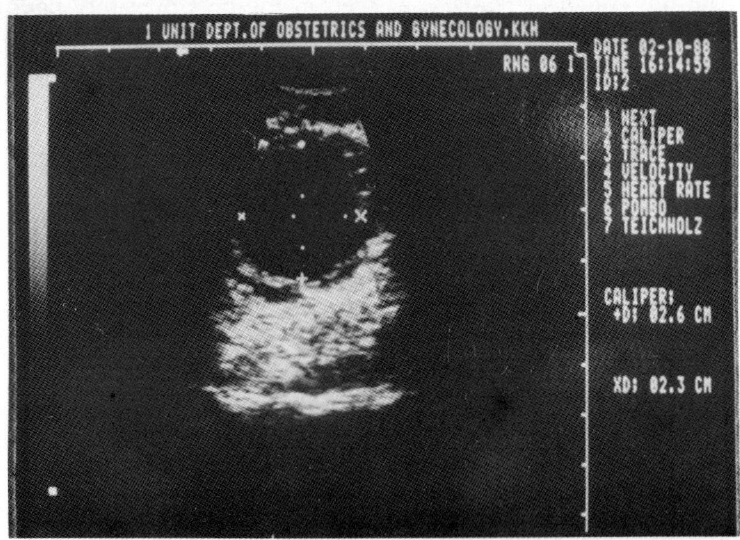

Figure 4-11a, b
This shows the evolution of a preovulatory ovarian follicle as seen on vaginal ultrasonography.

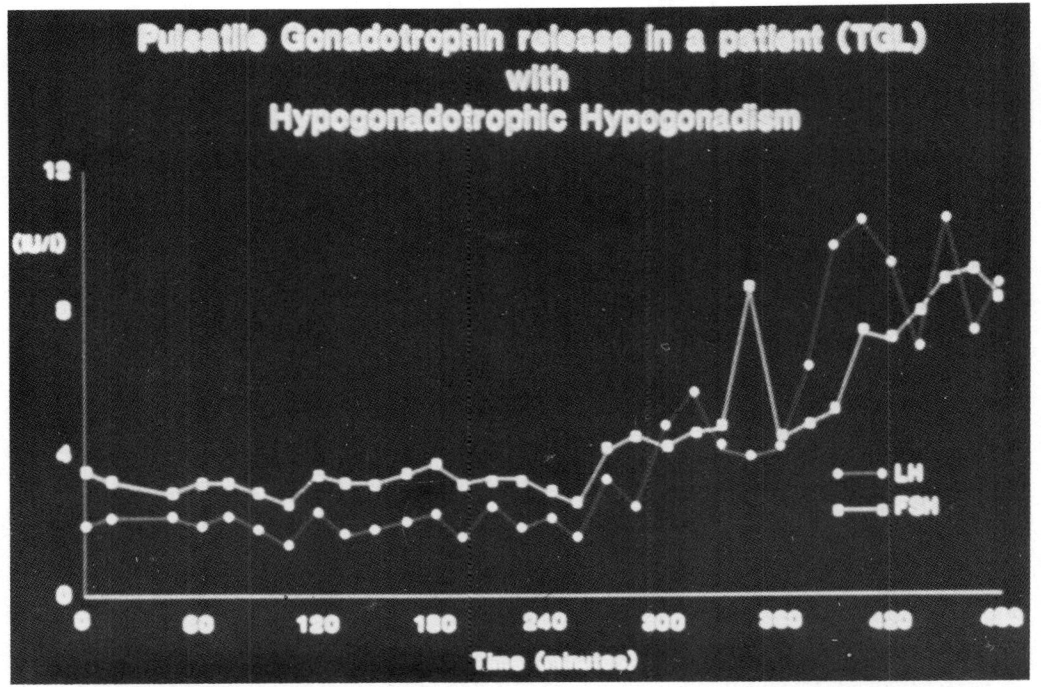

Figure 4-12
This illustrates the LH and FSH profile of a patient with hypogonadotrophic hypogonadism taken at 15 minute intervals. It can be seen that initially the levels of LH and FSH are very low but when LHRH infusion was commenced there was an immediate response in terms of a pulsatile release of LH and FSH.

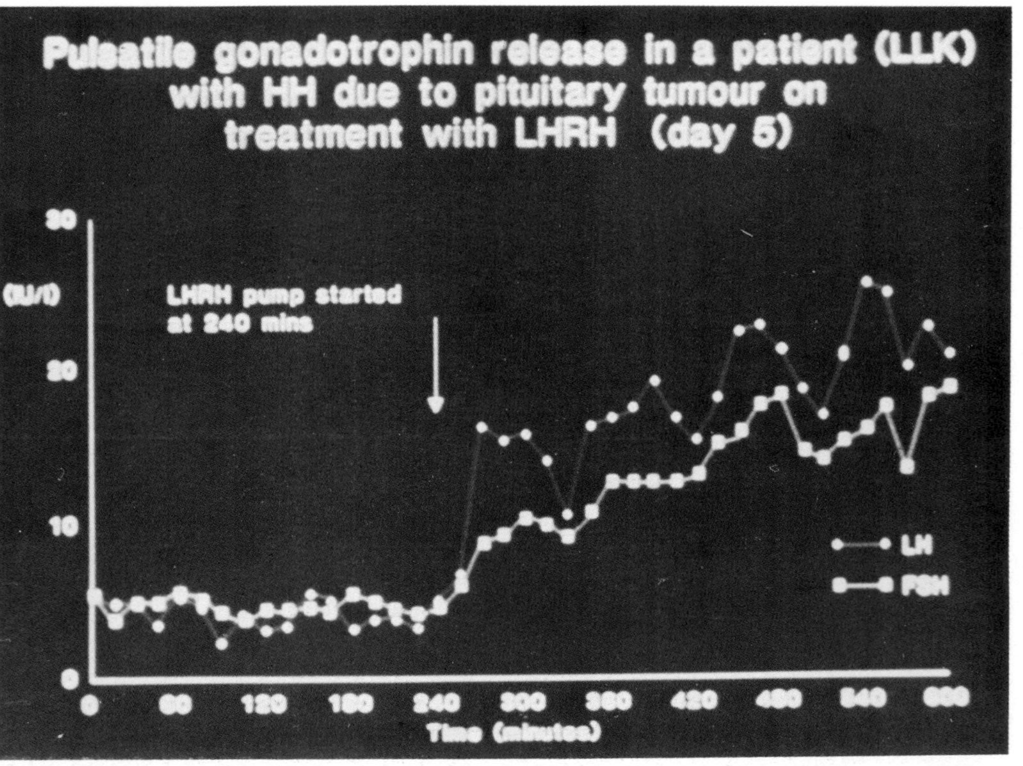

Figure 4-13
Patients who have pituitary tumours surgically removed leading to hypogonadotrophic hypogonadism may respond to LHRH therapy provided there is sufficient pituitary reserve. This shows the endocrine pattern in such a patient.

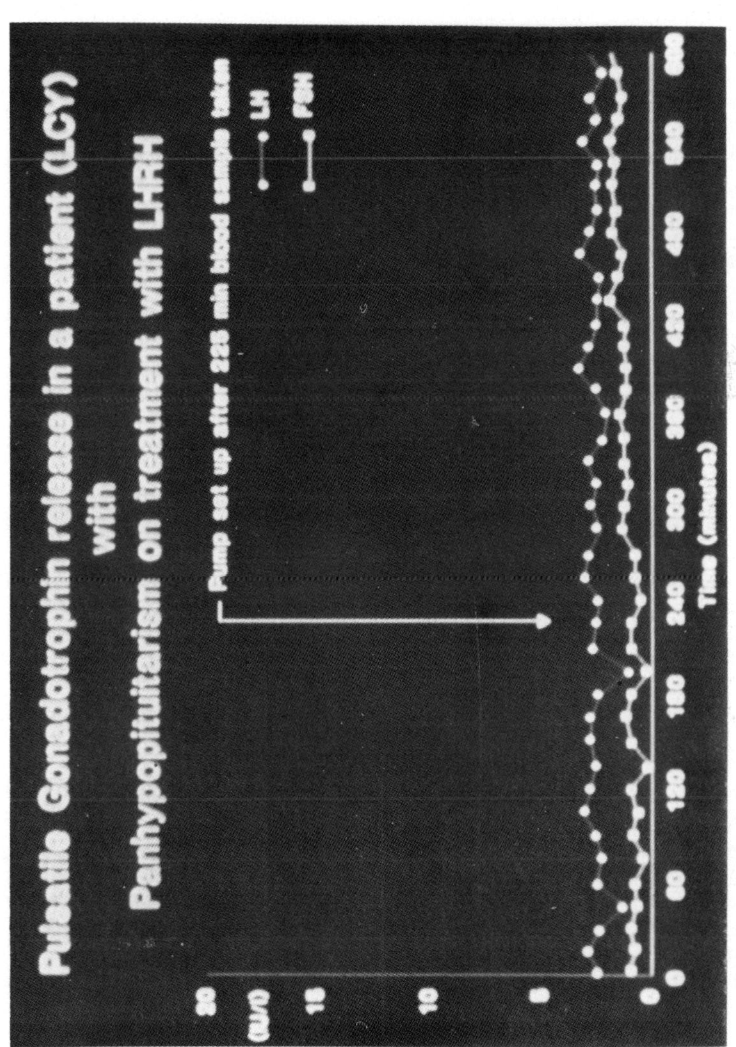

Figure 4-14
A patient with panhypopituitarism. There was no response to pulsatile LHRH infusion as would be expected.

References

Adams, J., Tan S.L., Wheeler, M., Morris, D., Jacobs, H.S. and Franks, S. Uterine growth in the follicular phase of spontaneous ovulatory cycles and during LHRH induced cycles in women with normal or polycystic ovaries. *Fertility and Sterility*, 1988; 49: 52.

Adams, J., Tan S.L., Jacobs, H.S. and Franks, S. Luteal phase correlation of ultrasonic and endocrinologic patterns during LHRH induction of ovulation. 1989 (Submitted for publication).

Adashi, E.Y. Clomiphene citrate: mechanism(s) and site(s) of action — a hypothesis revisited. *Fertility and Sterility*, 1984; 42: 331.

Armar, N.A., Adams, J. and Jacobs H.S. Induction of ovulation with gonadotrophin-releasing hormone. In Bonnar, J. (Ed), *Recent Advances in Obstetrics and Gynaecology*, 1986, 259.

Armar, N.A., Tan S.L., Adams J. and Jacobs, H.S. Practical aspects of pulsatile LHRH therapy *British Journal of Hospital Medicine*, 1987; 37: 429.

Armar, N.A., Tan S.L., Adams, J. and Jacobs H.S. Obstetric outcome of LHRH induced pregnancies. *Journal of Obstetrics and Gynaecology*, 1989 (in press).

Blankstein J. and Quigley M.M. Induction of ovulation in the patient with polycystic ovarian disease. *Endocrinology and Metabolism Clinics of North America*, 1988; 17: 733.

Blunt S.M., Clayton, R.N. and Butt, W.R. Effect of injection site on the pharmacokinetics and pharmacodynamics of subcutaneously administered luteinising hormone releasing hormone. *Clinical Endocrinology*, 1986; 25: 589.

Burger, C.W., Korsen, T.J.M and Hompes, P.G.A., et al. Ovulation induction with pulsatile luteinising hormone releasing hormone in women with clomiphene citrate resistant polycystic ovary-like disease. Clinical results. *Fertility and Sterility*, 1986; 46: 1045.

Clayton, R.N. Gonadotrophin releasing hormone modulation of its own pituitary receptors evidence for biphasic regulation. *Endocrinology*, 1982; 111: 152.

Corenblum, B. and Taylor, P. Augmentation of gonadotrophin-releasing hormone induced follicular growth with exogeneous gonadotrophins. *Fertility and Sterility*, 1987; 48: 954.

Eckstein, N., Vagman, I., Eshel, A., Naor, Z. and Ayalon, D. Induction of ovulation in amenorrhoeic patients with gonadotrophin-releasing hormone and human menopausal gonadotrophin. *Fertility and Sterility*, 1985; 44: 744.

Engels, J.A., Friedlander, R.L., Eik-Nes, K.B. An effect in vivo of clomiphene on the rate of conversion of androstenedione-C14 to estrone-C14 and estradiol-C14 by the canine ovary. *Metabolism*, 1968; 17: 189.

Erickson, G.F., Hsueh, A.J.W, Quigley. M.E., Rebar, R.W. and Yen S.S.C. Functional studies of aromatase activity in human granulosa cells from normal and polycystic ovaries. *Journal of Clinical Endocrinology and Metabolism*, 1979; 49: 514.

Eshel, A., Abdulwahid, N.A., Armar, N.A., Adams, J. and Jacob, H.S. Pulsatile luteinising hormone-releasing hormone therapy in women with polycystic ovary syndrome. *Fertility and Sterility*, 1988; 49: 956.

Filicori, M., Campaniello, E., Michelacci, L., Pareschi, A., Ferrari, P., Bolelli, G. and Flamign, C. Gonadotropin-releasing hormone (GNRH) analog suppression renders polycystic ovarian disease patients more susceptible to ovulation induction with pulsatile GnRH. *Journal of Clinical Endocrinology and Metabolism*, 1988; 66: 327.

Healy, D.L., Kovacs, G.T., Pepperell, R.J. and Burger, H.G. A normal cumulative conception rate after human pituitary gonadotropin. *Fertility and Sterility*, 1980; 34: 341.

Huang, K. Use of synthetic luteinising hormone releasing hormone in the induction of ovulation in amenorrhoeic patients. *Fertility and Sterility*, 1975; 26: 796.

Hurley, D.M., Clarke, I.J., Shelton, Rhonda and Burger, H.G. Subcutaneous administration of gonadotrophin-releasing hormone: absorption kinetics and gonadotrophin responses. *Journal of Clinical Endocrinology and Metabolism*, 1987; 65: 46.

Jacobs, H.S. Polycystic ovaries and polycystic ovary syndrome. *Gynaecological Endocrinology*, 1987; 1: 113.

Kerin, J.F., Liu J.H., Phillipou, G. and Yen S.S.C. Evidence for a hypothalamic site of action of clomiphene citrate in women. *Journal of Clinical Endocrinology and Metabolism*, 1985; 61: 265.

Knobil, E., Plant, T.M. and Wildt, L., et al. Control of the rhesus monkey menstrual cycle: permissive role of hypothalamic gonadotrophin releasing hormone. *Science*, 1980; 207: 1371.

Kotsuji, F., Aso, T., Kamitami, N., Tominaga, T., Kitaguchi M. and Okamura, Y. The efficacy of every other day administration of gonadotrophin-releasing hormone in women with hypothalamic amenorrhoea: gonadotrophin-releasing hormone treatment can induce clomiphene responsiveness. *Obstetrics and Gynecology*, 1988; 71: 615.

Leyendecker, G., Wildt, L. and Hansmann, M. Pregnancies following chronic intermittent (pulsatile) administration of GnRH by means of a portable pump (Zyclomat) — A new approach to the treatment of infertility in hypothalamic amenorrhoea. *Journal of Clinical Endocrinology and Metabolism*, 1980; 51: 1214.

Loucopoulos, A., Ferin, M., Vande Wiele, R.L., et al. Pulsatile administration of gonadotrophin-releasing hormone for ovulation. *American Journal of Obstetrics and Gynecology*, 1984; 148: 895.

Lunenfeld, B. and Insler, V. Classification of amenorrhoeic states and their treatment by ovulation induction. *Clinical Endocrinology* (Oxf), 1974; 3: 223.

Mason, P., Adams, J. and Morris, D., et al. Induction of ovulation with pulsatile luteinising hormone releasing hormone. *British Medical Journal*, 1984; 288: 181.

Menon, V., Butt, W.R., Clayton, R.N., Logan, Edwards R. and Lynch, S.S. Pulsatile administration of GnRH for the treatment of hypogonadotrophic hypogonadism. *Clinical Endocrinology*, 1984; 21: 223.

Morris, D.V., Abdulwahid, N.A., Armar, A. and Jacobs, H.S. The response of patients with organic hypothalamic pituitary disease to pulsatile gonadotrophin-releasing hormone therapy. *Fertility and Sterility*, 1987; 47: 54.

Oelsner, G., Serr, D.M., Mashiach, S., Blankstein, J., Snyder, M. and Lunenfeld, B. The study of induction of ovulation with menotrophins: Analysis of results of 1897 treatment cycles. *Fertility and Sterility*, 1978; 30: 538.

Ory, S.J., London, S.N. and Tyrey, L., et al. Ovulation induction with pulsatile gonadotrophin-releasing hormone administration in patients with polycystic ovarian syndrome. *Fertility and Sterility*, 1985; 43: 20.

Reid, R.L., Leopold, G.R. and Yen S.S.C. Induction of ovulation and pregnancy with pulsatile luteinising hormone releasing factor: dosage and mode of delivery. *Fertility and Sterility*, 1981; 36: 553.

Rust, L.A., Israel, R. and Mishell, D.R. An individualised therapeutic regimen for clomiphene citrate. *American Journal of Obstetrics and Gynecology*, 1974; 120: 785.

Saffan, D., Seibel, M.M. Ovulation induction with subcutaneous pulsatile gonadotrophin-releasing hormone in various ovulatory disorders. *Fertility and Sterility*, 1986; 45: 475.

Schally, A.V., Arimura, A. and Coy, D.H. Recent approaches to fertility control based on derivatives of LHRH. *Hormone Research*, 1980; 36: 53.

Schwartz, M., Jewelewicz, R., Dyrenfurth, I., Tropper, P. and Vande Wiele, R.L. The use of human menopausal and chorionic gonadotropins for induction of ovulation. *American Journal of Obstetrics and Gynecology*, 1980; 138: 801.

Sueldo, C.E. and Swanson, J.A. The economics of inducing ovulation with human menopausal gonadotropins versus pulsatile subcutaneous gonadotropin-releasing hormone. *Fertility and Sterility*, 1986; 45: 128.

Tan S.L. and Jacobs, H.S. Recent advances in the management of women with amenorrhoea. In Jacobs, H.S. (Ed), *Clinics in Obstetrics and Gynaecology*, W.B. Saunders, London, 1985, 725.

Tan S.L. The treatment of anovulatory infertility with pulsatile administration of luteinising hormone releasing hormone. *Singapore Journal of Obstetrics and Gynaecology*, 1987; 18: 11.

Tan S.L., Thong P.W., Jen S.W., Chong, R., Chua, D., Aw S.E., Salmon, Y.M. and Vengadasalam, D. Pregnancy after subcutaneous pulsatile administration of luteinising hormone releasing hormone in secondary amenorrhoea resistant to clomiphene therapy. *Singapore Journal of Obstetrics and Gynaecology*, 1987; 18: 97.

Tan S.L., Thong P.W., Jen S.W., Chong, R., Chua, D., Aw S.E., Salmon, Y.M. and Chen, C. Long term low dose pulsatile GnRH therapy for the treatment of anovulatory infertility. *Asia Oceania Journal of Obstetrics and Gynaecology*, 1988 (a); 14: 327.

Tan S.L., Chong, R., Thong P.W., Jen S.W., Salmon, Y.M. and Chen, C. Current concepts in the investigation and treatment of amenorrhoea in Cheng, W.C. and S.L. Tan (Eds), *Advances in Reproductive and Perinatal Medicine*, PG Publishing, Singapore, 1988, 1.

Tan S.L., Chong, R., Thong P.W., Jen S.W., Chua, D., Tay B.C., Aw S.E., Salmon, Y.M. and Chen, C. Clomiphene citrate augments the response to induction of ovulation with pulsatile luteinsing hormone releasing hormone. *Journal of Endocrinology*, 1988(c); 117 (supp): 274.

Tan S.L., Thong P.W., Chua, D., Tay B.C., Cheng L.C. and Chen, C. Combined gonadotrophin and pulsatile luteinising hormone releasing hormone is safe and effective therapy in polycystic ovarian disease resistant to conventional methods of induction of ovulation. *Journal of Endocrinology*, 1989 (in press).

Thompson, C.R. and Hansen, L.M. Pergonal (Menotropins): A summary of clinical experience in the induction of ovulation and pregnancy. *Fertility and Sterility*, 1970; 21: 844.

Thong P.W., Tan S.L., Chong, R., Chua, D., Tay B.C., Jen S.W., Aw S.E., Tan Y.O., Salmon, Y.M. and Chen. C. Pulsatile luteinsing hormone releasing hormone for induction of ovulation — endocrine and ultrasound determinants of response in 98 ovulatory cycles. *Proceedings of the XII World Congress of Gynaecology and Obstetrics*, Rio de Janeiro, Brazil, 1988.

Wang C.F. and Gemzell, C. The use of human gonadotrophins for the induction of ovulation in women with polycystic ovarian disease. *Fertility and Sterility*, 1980; 33: 479.

5
Clinical applications of LHRH agonist therapy

R.W. Shaw

Introduction

Although it was only in 1971 that the structure of the hypothalamic gonadotrophin releasing hormone (LHRH) was determined, this compound has already achieved an important role in clinical therapy. Indeed there are few sub-specialties in medicine which have remained untouched by the research advances associated with the use of LHRH and technological understanding in the production of releasing hormone analogues.

Within the field of gynaecology, many clinical applications for LHRH and its analogues have been investigated and therapeutic applications determined. However, for many conditions it may be still too early to determine the ultimate role of these compounds either as single entities or in combination with other agents. As new and more effective delivery systems for LHRH analogues are developed, other therapeutic applications will inevitably evolve.

The structure of native LHRH is shown in Figure 5-1. This compound is a decapeptide, and there are a number of sites at which enzymatic degradation occurs. Substitution, particularly of the amino acid in position 6, and an alteration or deletion of the amino acid in position 10, produce agonistic analogues of GnRH which are between 40 and 200 times more potent than the native hormone in terms of pituitary release of LH and FSH. Initial administration of these LHRH agonists result in increased gonadotrophin secretion with resultant steroid output from the gonads over a period of some days. Continued administration, however, induced desensitisation of the pituitary gonadotroph, down regulation of the pituitary gonadotroph receptors, reduced secretion of gonadotrophins and resultant reduced ovarian steroidogenesis and arrest of follicular maturation and growth. This continued action of inhibition of ovarian follicular steroidogenesis can be utilised in a number of gynaecological conditions which are oestrogen dependent.

Antagonistic analogues have also been synthesised. To achieve such activity, substitution of a larger number of the amino acid sequences is required than for agonistic analogues. The mode of action of such LHRH antagonists is immediate receptor blockade with rapid inhibition of gonadotrophin secretion. The majority of currently available LHRH antagonists however have induced local sensitivity reactions at the site of injection, thus delaying their introduction to clinical trials.

A wide range of clinical applications for LHRH analogues in the field of gynaecology can be suggested. To achieve optimal therapeutic effect in wide ranging different conditions, it is logical that a varying degree of suppression of the hypothalamic pituitary ovarian axis will be required. This is suggested in Table 5-1. Many of these applications are already being investigated in ongoing clinical studies and some of these will now be discussed.

Use of LHRH analogues in ovulation induction of multiple follicular growth for IVF

Induction of ovulation in women with hypogonadotrophic hypogonadism using human menopausal gonadotrophins has been performed successfully for many years. High pregnancy rates with low complication rates can be achieved with appropriate monitoring. With increasing functional pituitary capacity as a spectrum of disorder in the field of endocrinology, the use of hMG therapy has an increased incidence of complications and a decrease in pregnancy rate. Major complications are hyperstimulation and premature ovulation. The problem of hyperstimulation in response to hCG administration itself does not interfere with the process of ovulation but affects the chances of implantation. "Premature luteinization" is caused by a surge or rise of LH occurring as a response to increase in the levels of oestradiol 17B, and happening prior to the criteria for administration of the ovulatory dose of hCG being satisfied. Premature luteinization is usually evidenced by increasing serum LH and of rising levels of serum progesterone at a time when there is inadequate maturation of the lead follicle.

In several reported studies, 30 per cent of women with normal menstrual rhythms (Fleming & Coutts, 1986), and a similar percentage with polycystic ovary syndrome (Fleming et al, 1985) who were undergoing treatment with hMG for ovulation induction, showed evidence of premature (pre-hCG) luteinization.

Since the development of in-vitro fertilisation and gamete intrafallopian transfer techniques, many women with normal menstrual rhythms are now receiving high dose gonadotrophin therapy. Similar problems have been encountered during stimulation of multiple follicular growth for these procedures (Hillier et al, 1985). In many instances this premature luteinization will occur prior to the development of a lead follicle of 17mm in diameter.

Ovulation can occur in response to such LH surges but the released oocytes are likely to be immature. Indeed the onset of such surges usually leads to cancellation of planned oocyte collection, or unplanned pre-operative follicle rupture. Furthermore, elevated LH levels may also be associated with the occurrence of post-mature oocytes with poor fertilisation rates (Jamieson et al, 1987) and poor embryonic development (Stanger & Yovich, 1985). The effects of these inappropriate gonadotrophin surges are likely to reduce the chances of successful pregnancy being established in such cycles.

It has now been found possible to prevent premature luteinization occurring in patients undergoing ovulation induction therapy by the administration of LHRH analogues for a period of time to desensitise the pituitary. Once this situation has been achieved, then commence controlled ovulation induction using appropriate exogenous gonadotrophin administration.

A number of treatment regimes have been developed utilizing this approach, but what we have had extensive experience with is a regime in which LHRH analogue is commenced during the mid-luteal phase of the cycle — starting Day 22 of the cycle. Our own studies involve the administration of LHRH analogue, Buserelin, 100μg intranasally five times daily. Following the initial luteotrophic effects with the commencement of the analogue at this time in the cycle, patients experience menstrual bleeding from eight to 13 days after the commencement of treatment. This is a delay of their normal menstruation of between three to six days. Onset of menstruation indicates achievement of hypothalamic pituitary desensitisation.

Lowering and suppression of circulating LH and FSH and the induction of the hypogonadal state induced is confirmed by the absence of follicular growth and a low circulating plasma oestradiol 17B levels. The detailed hormonal changes seen in a group of patients so treated are shown in Figures 5-2a and b. The onset of withdrawal bleeding is an adequate indicator of the attainment of pituitary desensitisation and detailed hormonal investigations and monitoring are not necessary. Once the situation of hypogonadotrophic-hypogonadism has been established, the LHRH analogue therapy is continued but at the same time follicular growth is stimulated by the administration of exogenous gonadotrophin.

We have found that the administration of exogenous gonadotrophins of two to three ampoules daily of either human menopausal gonadotrophin (Pergonal) or purified FSH (Metrodin), usually takes between eight to 12 days before attainment of mature pre-ovulatory follicles with appropriate size (17mm or more) to allow administration of the ovulation dose of hCG.

The results of some 70 treatments cycles using the above regime are summarised in Table 5-2. In this table, results are compared with conventional gonadotrophin treatment with multiple follicular stimulation. With these combined regimes, a few patients failed to achieve adequate follicular growth patterns but the incidence of such problems is no greater than with hMG alone. What is particularly apparent is the lack of incidence of premature luteinization in patients receiving Buserelin and then hMG treatment in comparison with hMG alone. This meant that the combined Buserelin-hMG group were much more likely to achieve operative oocyte recovery and produce better quality oocytes with higher percentage for fertilisation and cleavage rates. This in turn meant that there were more pre-embyros available for possible transfer with improved pregnancy rates. (See Table 5-3).

These combined regimes of pituitary desensitisation with LHRH analogue followed by exogenous gonadotrophin therapy have positive advantages with certain difficult patients undergoing IVF with problems of premature luteinization and produced poor quality oocytes. It may also be useful for patients with polycystic ovary syndrome who are perhaps even more prone to the above complications than normal regularly ovulating patients.

Endometriosis

Endometriosis remains a disorder which is often difficult to diagnose, and if left untreated may progress (with implications for fertility impairment), and frequently reoccurs throughout the reproductive lifespan. Not uncommonly, patients presenting with infertility are found to have endometriosis and although this disease has been studied for decades the factors controlling its initiation and maintenance are still not fully understood. What has been established, however, is that ovarian steroids are needed for initial development and the continued presence of endometriotic deposits. Following the menopause with resultant lowering of circulating oestradiol levels, endometriotic deposits tend to resolve.

Currently one of the most effective treatment regimes has been the administration of Danazol, which has been shown to be highly effective in cases of mild to moderate endometriosis. Danazol, however, may induce androgenic type side effects, the incidence of which is related to the dose required to suppress ovulation/menstruation. For these reasons, new therapeutic approaches are being sought, and one such has been to evaluate the role of LHRH analogues in patients with endometriosis.

A number of studies have now reported symptomatic improvement and absorption of endometriotic deposits following LHRH against treatment (Shaw et al, 1983; Lemay et al, 1984; Shaw & Matta, 1986). These initial studies were open studies but more recently randomised prospective clinical trials comparing LHRH analogues and other established treatments, in particular, Danazol, have begun to appear.

The accompanying results present our preliminary data of a randomised, open label, prospective clinical trial comparing the LHRH analogue, Buserelin (D-Ser But)^{6}-des Gly^{10} LHRH), (administered intranasally) with Danazol in terms of endocrine effects. Clinical figures show patient tolerance and safety.

Patients and methods

Sixty patients were recruited into the study, aged between 21 and 40 years. Endometriosis was diagnosed and confirmed at laparoscopy, and scored according to the American Fertility Society classification. No patient entered into the study had received Danazol or other sex steroid hormones within six months of entry. Following laparoscopy, patients were randomised by open label to receive either Buserelin (N=40) or Danazol (N=20). Both treatments were commenced in the early follicular phase of the cycle and continued for six months, at the end of which a second laparoscopy was performed with repeat evaluation and scoring of endometriosis. Subjects were followed up for a further six months after ceasing therapy.

Patients allocated to receive Buserelin received a fixed dose of 400μg three times daily intranasally, whilst those randomised to Danazol received between 400–800 mg total daily dose, depending upon the severity of the endometriosis and the patient's response. Throughout the treatment and follow up period, patients were reviewed from both clinical, endocrine and various other safety laboratory assessment viewpoints at monthly intervals.

Results and conclusions

Two of the 40 patients receiving Buserelin and two of 20 patients receiving Danazol were withdrawn during the treatment period for reasons unrelated to drug tolerance. It was found that consistent suppression of serum oestradiol 17B concentrations to below early follicular phase levels were achieved in all patients receiving Buserelin, mean circulating levels of oestradiol being 87 $\pm$ 14 pmols/1 at the end of six months' treatment. The patients receiving Danazol achieved less consistent and dose related hypo-oestrogenism, levels of oestradiol 17B at the end of six months' treatment being 115 $\pm$ 31 pmols/1.

Laparoscopic comparisons are shown in Table 5-4. At the post treatment laparoscopy, mean AFS score for endometriotic lesions alone was reduced from the mean score pre-treatment by 86 per cent in the Buserelin group (38 patients) and by 67 per cent in the Danazol group (18 patients). These reductions in score were comparable in patients with mild endometriosis in both groups. In patients with moderate to severe disease, reduction in scores were more marked in patients who received Buserelin, although we appreciate that the numbers of patients in these groups were small.

Both drugs appeared comparable in their figures for improvement in subjective symptoms of pelvic pain, deep dyspareunia, and dysmenorrhea. The major side effects of both drugs are shown in Table 5-5. In general, the side effects caused by Danazol tended to be more troublesome although 18 per cent of patients on Buserelin experienced severe hot flushes (a mixed total of 74 per cent experienced some form of hot flushes). None of the patients dropped out from either form of treatment because of side effects alone.

Following completion of treatment, the first menstrual period returned within a mean of 44 days (range 24–79) in patients who had received Buserelin, with a mean of 35 days (range 22–95) in patients who had received Danazol. Twelve months after discontinuing treatment, there had been seven patients who conceived out of 11 patients presenting with infertility in the Buserelin treated group, and five patients who conceived out of 10 patients in the Danazol treated group. Recurrence of endometriosis diagnosed by laparoscopy, within 12 months after completion of treatment, had been observed in six patients out of 38 receiving Buserelin, and in three of the 18 patients receiving Danazol.

Both Buserelin and Danazol were effective in inducing a reversible state of hypooestrogenism and would be a suitable mode of therapy for treatment of endometriosis. Both treatments were highly effective in inducing complete or partial resolution of the endometriotic lesions. Buserelin seemed more effective in patients with more severe disease. Associated with the objective regression of endometriotic implants, as observed laparoscopically, was a marked improvement in the subjective symptoms of the endometriosis which was comparable with both treatments. Where the two drugs differed largely was in the incidence and nature of side effects. These were primarily anabolic, psychological and androgenic in patients receiving Danazol, while the more tolerable vasomotor side effects predominated in the Buserelin treated group.

Pregnancy and recurrence rates appear similar following both treatments in this group of patients studied. We therefore conclude that Buserelin administered by the intranasal route offers an alternative effective treatment for patients with endometriosis to the current other best option of Danazol. LHRH analogues may have some positive advantages in terms of less severe side effect profiles. Whether in the long term they are more effective in preventing recurrence of the disease awaits further larger comparative trials and longer term follow up studies.

Uterine Fibroids

It has been estimated that approximately 20 per cent of women over the age of 30 years will be found to have uterine fibroids (Dewhurst, 1981). Fibroids may be associated with a number of gynaecological symptoms: eg. menorrhagia, dysmenorrhea, infertility; or may present simply as asymptomatic pelvic abdominal masses. Management of patients with uterine fibroids has traditionally been surgical — either myomectomy for patients wishing to preserve fertility, or hysterectomy as the preferred choice in patients whose families are complete.

Pathogenesis of uterine fibroids

Each of the cells within a single myoma contain the same glucose-6-dehydrogenase enzyme, suggesting that the residual fibroid develops from a unicellular origin (Townsend et al, 1970). It remains unclear why neoplastic transformation occurs in some smooth muscle cells within the uterus, but it has been established that several hormones may influence the rate of growth of fibroid tumours.

Oestradiol

Unopposed oestrogen action is thought to be the strongest factor in the pathogenesis of uterine fibroids. Evidence to substantiate this has arisen from the findings that fibroids tend to reduce in size and fibrose following the menopause, when endogenous oestrogen levels are reduced, but when oestrogen levels increase they may rapidly increase in size, eg. during pregnancy. The risk of developing fibroids seems to be decreased consistently with an increasing number of term pregnancies (Ross et al, 1986) and this may be related to the reduced growth in nascent fibroid tumours during the puerperium. The risk is also lower with increasing duration of oral contraceptive use, lower body weight and in women who smoke cigarettes.

However, in many studies in which serum oestradiol concentrations have been measured there appear to be no differences in the concentrations in women with uterine fibroids or of those in control groups (Spellacy et al, 1972).

Progesterone

Progesterone receptors have also been reported in uterine fibroids. Unlike oestrogen receptors, no clear increase in the amount of specific binding sites in fibroids has been found (Soules & McCarty, 1982).

Local growth factors

A number of putative growth factors have been measured in the circulation of patients with uterine fibroids but no consistent changes have been found in concentrations of growth hormone, human placental lactogen, or insulin. Recently, the demonstration of local secretion of insulin-like growth factor 1 (IGF-1) or epidermal growth factor within the ovary and the identification of receptors suggest the possibility of local stimulators which may well effect fibroid growth (Adashi et al, 1985).

Attempts at medical treatment of uterine fibroids

Goldzieher and colleagues (1966) administered large doses of the progestogen, Medrogestone, 25mg per day, given three weeks prior to hysterectomy, and induced degenerative changes in fibroids. More recently, Gestrinone, an oestrogen-progesterone receptor antagonist, at doses of 5mg twice weekly, induced reduction in uterine fibroid size with treatment extending between four and 13 months (Coutinho et al, 1986). Administration of Danazol has also been attempted but with variable results (Maheux et al, 1983).

Ideally, since fibroids appear to be oestrogen sensitive, a therapy which induces hypooestrogenism is more logical approach in the medical treatment of uterine fibroids. LHRH analogues do just this and are currently being investigated as possible medical treatments for uterine fibroids.

Effect of LHRH analogues on fibroid size

Recent reports on the use of LHRH agonists in patients with uterine fibroids have been encouraging (Healey et al, 1986; Coddington et al, 1986; Rolland et al, 1986; Maheux et al, 1987). These reports lack data on controls and on the long term follow up changes following discontinuation of therapy.

We have recently evaluated the effects of LHRH agonist, Buserelin, [D-Ser $(tBU)^6$-des Gly^{10} LHRH] Hoechst Pharmaceuticals. A group of patients with large uterine fibroids were treated for a period of six months and have been followed up for at least 12 months post-treatment.

Detailed results of the study are currently in press.

Patients and methods

Ten women, five Caucasian, three Negroid, two Asian, aged 28–45 years, were entered into the study. All had abdominally palpable fibroid uteri. The presenting symptoms of the patients were menorrhagia, seven; dysmenorrhea and/or pelvic pain, eight; infertility, two. Two patients had previously undergone myomectomy seven years prior to entry into the study. None of the patients had received any steroid hormone therapy during the 12 months prior to the study or during the 18 months after the study.

To exclude other pelvic pathology prior to entering into the study, all subjects underwent examination under anaesthesia and diagnostic curettage. Examination of the overall clinical size of the uterus was established and assessed by at least two clinicians, and ranged between 12–18 weeks pregnancy size. Two patients appeared to have single large fibroids but the remainder had multiple fibroid uteri. These findings were confirmed by ultrasound assessment.

The patients were then commenced on Buserelin at a dose of 300 μg eight-hourly, intranasally, and treatment continued for a period of six months. The first day of treatment was between days two to four of a menstrual period following the diagnostic curettage.

During treatment and follow up assessments by clinical examination, ultrasound measurement and full haematological biochemical evaluation was carried out every second month during treatment and the first six months of follow up and then at nine and 12 months post-treatment. Endocrine evaluation was performed at similar intervals.

The total uterine volume measurements performed by one observer (NM) provided the formula for use for studying therapeutic effects on ellipsoid tumours — $D1 \times D2 \times D3 \times 0.5233$. Measurements were taken by a linear secter scan (Diasonics 100).

A group of four patients with clinical findings who did not receive Buserelin treatment acted as controls and had monthly endocrine and ultrasound measurements for uterine volume. All 10 patients who received Buserelin completed six months' treatment. Four weeks after commencing therapy, a marked degree of hypooestrogenism was achieved and sustained throughout treatment at or below levels consistent with early follicular phase levels. During the first three weeks following commencement of therapy with Buserelin, patients experienced some light withdrawal bleeding. Following this no further true menstrual periods occurred during treatment in any patients. However, irregular, infrequent episodes of bleeding without the usual menstrual symptons were reported by five patients and these episodes continued throughout treatment in two patients. The expected symptoms of hot flushes were experienced by seven of the 10 patients and two of these patients found the hot flushes quite severe and moderately inconvenient, particularly when occurring at night.

Five patients had haemoglobin levels below 11 g/dl before commencing treatment, due to increased menstrual blood losses. In all subjects after six months' treatment, haemoglobin levels increased to within the normal range with a mean of 12.4 g/dl.

The uterine volumes of patients prior to commencing treatment had a mean of 620.8 $cm^3 \pm 85.75$, although there was a wide variation in the total uterine volume with a range between 300 cm^3 and 1032 cm^3.

Although there was a wide variation in hypooestrogenism and speed at which suppression was achieved, there was an overall general trend in the effect of treatment of fibroid size. It demonstrated a very consistent rate of reduction in total uterine volume during the first four months of Buserelin administration with a much slower rate of change in the subsequent fifth and sixth months of therapy. Clinical size at the commencement of treatment was 14.7 weeks pregnancy size and this was reduced to a mean of 10.6 weeks by the end of six months' treatment. There was a tendency for patients with the largest pretreatment volumes to have the most marked percentage reduction in size on the therapy (Table 5-6).

Effects from discontinuation of LHRH analogue

The first menstrual period after the cessation of treatment occurred at a mean of 41 days. Because of prolonged uterine bleeding and associated pain, one patient underwent hysterectomy three months following discontinuation of treatment. Two others underwent myomectomy within four months of ceasing therapy. In the remaining seven who were followed up for a period of 12 months post treatment, uterine volume had returned to, or slightly exceeded, pretreatment values by the end of six months' post treatment in five of the seven patients and their symptoms had gradually returned towards pretreatment problems. The other two patients demonstrated a slower increase in uterine volume but in both patients volumes had returned to pretreatment size by 12 months' follow up (See Table 5-6).

Discussion

This study demonstrated that administration with LHRH analogue induced a sustained and reversible hypooestrogen state with resultant marked reduction in uterine fibroid volumes and good relief of associated symptoms. Reduction in total uterine volume was comparable to that reported in other studies who often administered LHRH analogues either by subcutaneous injections or subcutaneous continuous infusion.

The treatment was well tolerated by patients and accompanied by a sense of wellbeing, partly because of induced amenorrhea and reduction of uterine blood loss and correction of anaemia. There was quite a marked variation in response. Reduction in uterine volume ranged between 23 per cent and 62 per cent pretreatment volumes at the end of six months' therapy. This measure of reduction in volume associated with hypooestrogenism with LHRH agonist treatment is much more rapid than that observed in the immediate post-menopausal period. The group of control patients showed no significant change in uterine volumes during the six months' close monitoring period. This is of relevance when one considers the rapid rate of regrowth of the fibroids in our LHRH analogue treated group when cyclical ovarian function recommenced.

The re-enlargement of fibroid volumes found in these patients after six months' post treatment appears to indicate that the use of these agents will not replace surgery in the long term management of uterine fibroids, as had been hoped. The major indication for use of these drugs with fibroids appears to be administration for a pre-operative period of three to four months prior to myomectomy or hysterectomy. This appears to be adequate since the maximum effects in most patients of reduction in size were achieved after that period of time. Further, little reduction occurred with continuing treatment.

Our recent studies also reported a significant increase in the impedence to blood flow from both the uterine and fibroid vasculature when measured by Doppler ultrasound in patients undergoing analogue therapy for uterine fibroids (Matta et al, 1988). This increase of impedence to blood flow and reduction in blood flow can also be beneficial at the time of surgery in reducing the amount of perioperative blood loss. This would have beneficial effects in reducing the incidence of postoperative infection, adhesion formation, and anaemia problems. Studies on randomised control trials to assess these aspects of treatment are underway and the results are awaited with interest.

Summary

There is a wide range of applications for LHRH analogues in the field of benign gynaecological disorders. When greater understanding of the physiology and mechanism of LHRH agonists has accrued, and perhaps as more varied and efficient delivery systems become available, it may be possible to develop new applications. This would certainly be so if a variable degree of suppression of the hypothalamic pituitary axis could be achieved. The true potential of these potent agents has yet to be fully realised but there can be no doubt that they are going to influence clinical practice dramatically over the next decade.

Table 5-1
Degree of suppression of hypothalamic-pituitary-ovarian axis to achieve therapeutic effect from LHRH analogue administration in various gynaecological conditions

Partial:	Contraception.
Moderate:	Fibroids Endometriosis Menorrhagia Premenstrual syndrome.
Complete:	Precocious puberty Polycystic ovary syndrome Ovulation induction.

Table 5-2
Stimulation of multiple follicular growth for IVF. Comparison of hMG therapy alone, with combined LHRH analogue (Buserelin) and hMG sequential treatment

	Cycle starts	*Inadequate follicular growth*	*Premature luteinization*	*No. achieving oocyte recovery*	*(% of cycle starts)*
hMG alone	68	6	9	53	77.9
Buserelin + hMG	68	4	Nil	64	94.1

Table 5-3
Outcome of IVF cycles — Comparison of hMG alone and Buserelin and hMG sequential treatments

	Oocytes/OR (mean %)	*Cleaving embryos (mean %)*	*Embryo transfer (% of patients)*	*Pregnancies (% cycle starts)*
hMG alone	6.3	57.3	84.3	9.4
Buserelin + hMG	5.8	52.4	97.1	17.3

Table 5-4
Results of treatment of endometriosis — Comparison of Buserelin and Danazol treated patients

	Buserelin treated	*Danazol treated*
Number completing	38	18
Initial AFS Staging		
Mild	21	13
Moderate	10	3
Severe	7	2
Resolution of Endometriotic deposits		
Complete	31 (82%)	11 (61%)
Partial	7 (18%)	5 (28%)
No change	—	2 (11%)
Worsened	—	—

Table 5-5
Most common side effects experienced whilst receiving Buserelin or Danazol for six months in the treatment of endometriosis

Buserelin (n = 38)			*Danazol (n = 18)*		
Hot flushes	—	29	Fluid retention symptoms	—	17
Recurrent bleeding	—	9	Irritability/mood swings	—	15
Vaginal dryness	—	9	Weight gain (> 3 kg)	—	13
Headaches	—	8	Acne/oily skin	—	10
			Headaches	—	7

Table 5-6
Mean serum oestradiol-17B and mean percentage of original uterine volume in 10 patients receiving Buserelin 300μg + d.s. intranasally as medical therapy for uterine fibroids

	Serum oestradiol 17B pmol/1 (mean ± SEM) n = 10	*Percentage (%) original volume (mean ± SEM) n = 10*
Pretreatment	356 ± 49	100
Treatment		
2 months	156 ± 39	74.6 ± 4.3
4 months	131 ± 24	51.5 ± 8.4
6 months	109 ± 12	49.6 ± 9.6
Post-treatment		
2 months	319 ± 57	64.3 ± 6.7
4 months	407 ± 64	71.6 ± 9.8
6 months	384 ± 39*	90.3 ± 9.4*
9 months	451 ± 60*	98.5 ± 10.5*
12 months	389 ± 63*	108.4 ± 11.6*

* *Results from remaining seven patients in study.*

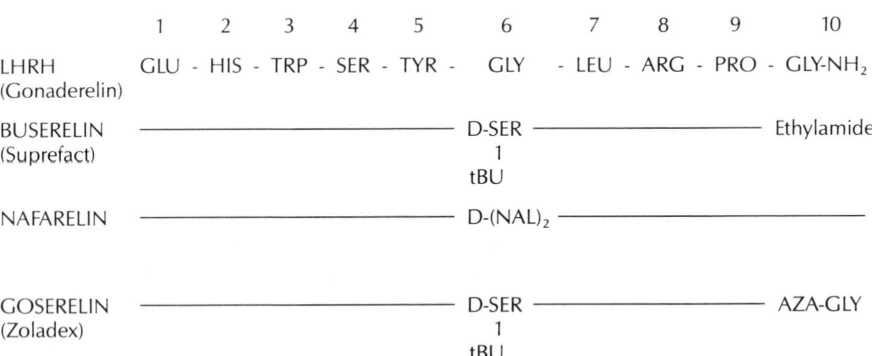

Figure 5-1
Structure of LHRH and three currently investigated agonistic analogues

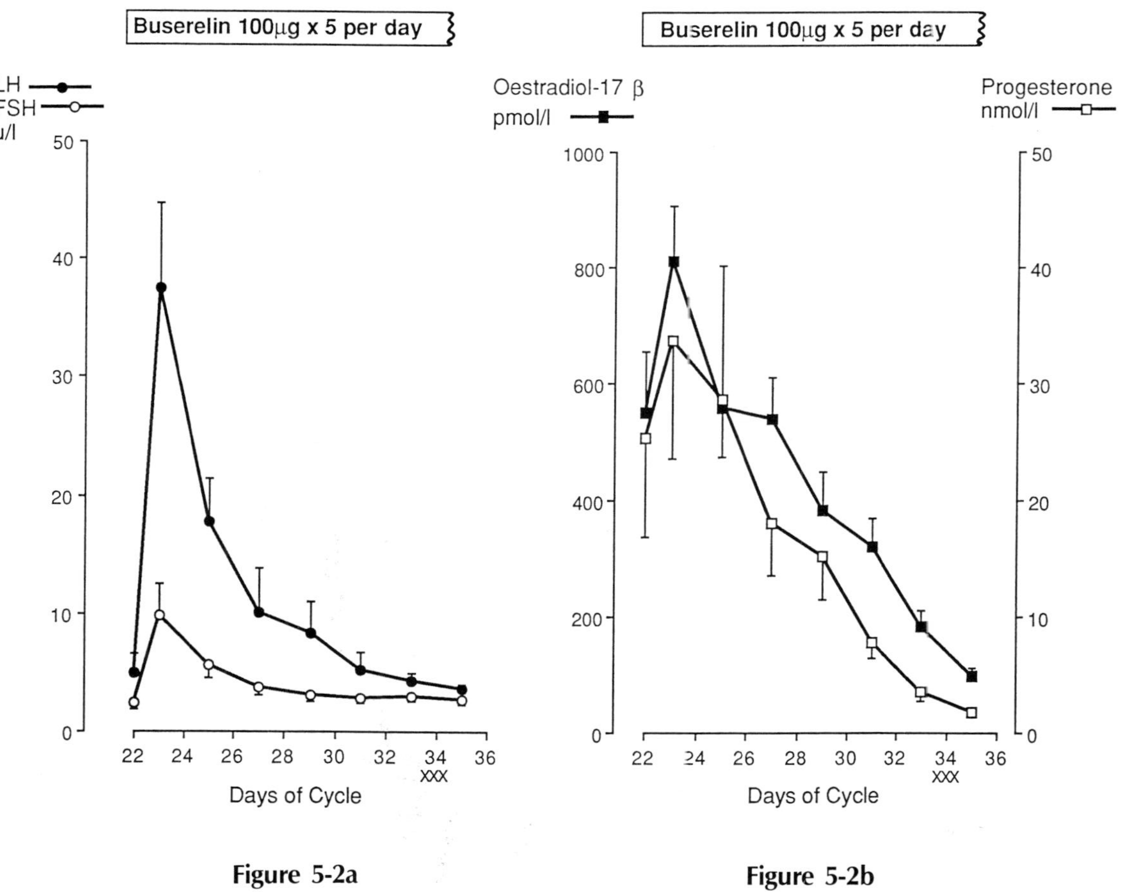

Figure 5-2a

Figure 5-2b

References

Adashi, E.Y., Resnick, C.E., D'Ercole, A.J., Szerboda, M.E. and Van Wyk, J.J. Insulin-like growth factors as intraovarian regulators of granulosa cell growth and function. *Endocrine Reviews*, 1985; 6: 400.

Coddington, C.C., Collins, R.L., Shwker, T.H., Anderson, R., Loriaux D.L. and Winkel, C.A. Long-acting gonadotrophin hormone-releasing hormone analog used to treat uteri. *Fertility and Sterility*, 1986; 45: 624.

Coutinho, E.M., Baulanger, G.A. and Goncalvas, M.T. Regression of uterine leiomyomas after treatment with gestrinone, and antiestrogen, antiprogesterone. *American Journal of Obstetrics and Gynecology*, 1986; 155: 761.

Dewhurst, C.J. (Editor), *Integrated Obstetrics and Gynaecology for Postgraduates*, 3rd Edition, Blackwell Scientific Publications, London, 1981.

Fleming, R. and Coutts, J.R.T. Induction of multiple follicular growth in normally menstruating women with endogenous gonadotrophin suppression. *Fertility and Sterility*, 1986; 45: 226.

Fleming, R., Haxton, M.J., Hamilton, M.P.R., McCune, G.S., Black, W.P., MacNaughton, M.C. and Coutts, J.R.T. Successful treatment of infertile women with oligomenorrhea using a combination of LHRH agonist and exogenous gonadotrophins. *British Journal of Obstetrics and Gynaecology*, 1985; 92: 369.

Goldzieher, J.W., Maqueo, M., Ricaud, L., Aquilar, A.J. and Canale, S.E. Induction of degenerative changes in uterine myomas by high dose progestin therapy. *American Journal of Obstetrics and Gynecology*, 1966; 96: 1078.

Healy, D.L., Lawson, S.R., Abbott, M., Baird, D.T. and Fraser, H.M. Towards removing uterine fibroids without surgery: Subcutaneous infusion of a luteinising hormone-releasing hormone agonist commencing in the luteal phase. *Journal of Clinical Endocrinology and Metabolism*, 1986; 63: 619.

Hillier, S.G., Afnan, A.M., Marara, R.A. and Winston, R.M. Superovulation strategy before in-vitro fertilisation. *Journal of Obstetrics and Gynaecology*, 1985; 12: 687.

Jamieson, M.E., Yates, R.W.S., Fleming, R. and Coutts, J.R.T. Induction of follicular growth for IVF-comparison of oocytes and hormone profiles in cycles treated with hMG alone or in combination with a GnRH analog. *Human Reproduction*, 1987; Abstracts 3rd Meeting ESHRE. 30 Abstract 107.

Lemay, A., Maheux, R., Faure, N., Jean, C. and Fazekas, A.T.A. Reversible hypogonadism induced by a luteinising hormone-releasing hormone (LHRH) agonist (Buserelin) as a new therapeutic approach for endometriosis. *Fertility and Sterility*, 1984; 41: 863.

Maheux, R., Lemay, A. and Merat, P. Use of intranasal luteinising hormone-releasing hormone agonist in uterine leiomyomas. *Fertility and Sterility*, 1987; 47: 229.

Matta, W.H.M., Stabile, I., Shaw, R.W. and Campbell, S. Doppler assessment of uterine blood flow changes in patients with fibroids receiving the gonadotrophin releasing hormone agonist Buserelin. *Fertility and Sterility*, 1988; in press.

Matta, W.H.M., Shaw, R.W. and Nye, M. Long-term follow up of patients with uterine fibroids after treatment with the LHRH agonist Buserelin. *British Journal of Obstetrics and Gynaecology*, 1988; in press.

Rolland, R., Franssen, A.M.H.W., Willemsen, W.N.P. and Corbey, R.S. Uterine leiomyomas and LHRH agonist treatment — A preliminary report. In Rolland, R., Chadha, D.R. and Willemsen, W.N.P. (Eds), *Gonadotrophin Down-Regulation in Gynaecological Practice*, Alan R. Liss, New York, 1986; 313.

Ross, R.K., Pike, N.C., Vessey, N.P., Bull, D., Yates, D. and Casagrande, J.T. Risk factors for uterine fibroids: Reduced risk associated with oral contraceptives. *British Medical Journal*, 1986; 293: 359.

Shaw, R.W., Fraser, H.M. and Boyle, H. Intranasal treatment with luteinising hormone-releasing hormone agonist in women with endometriosis. *British Medical Journal*, 1983; 287: 167.

Shaw, R.W. and Matta, W. Reversible pituitary ovarian suppression induced by an LHRH agonist in the treatment of endometriosis — comparison of two dose regimens. *Clinical Reproduction and Fertility*, 1986; 4: 329.

Soules, M.R. and McCarty, K.S. Leiomyomas: Steroid receptor content. *American Journal of Obstetrics and Gynecology*, 1982; 143: 6.

Spellacy, W.N., Lemaire, W.J., Buhl, W.C., Birk, S.A. and Bradley, B.A. Plasma growth hormone and estradiol levels in women with uterine myomas. *Obstetrics and Gynecology*, 1972; 40: 829.

Stanger, J.D. and Yovich, J.L. Reduced in-vitro fertilisation of human oocytes from patients with raised basal luteinising hormone levels during the follicular phase. *British Journal of Obstetrics and Gynaecology*, 1985; 92: 385.

Townsend, D.E., Sparkes, R.S., Baluda, M.C. and McClelland, G. Unicellular histogenesis of uterine leiomyomas as determined by electrophoresis of glucose-6-phosphate dehydrogenase. *American Journal of Obstetrics and Gynecology*, 1970; 107: 1168.

6

Advances in the management of endometriosis

I. Johnston

Introduction

It is now nearly 130 years since Von Rokitansky first reported this condition and despite the hundreds of papers that have addressed the subject, there is still no uniformity of opinion regarding its etiology and there is considerable debate about the roles of medical and surgical management of endometriosis. Its reported incidence depends largely on the population that has been examined. In gynaecological laparotomies, this varies from 20 to 50 per cent and in infertility patients between 30 and 50 per cent. That any disease should have such a high incidence would suggest that it has either become much more common than previously described or that our methods of diagnosis have improved very considerably.

There is no doubt that endometriosis and infertility are closely related, but it is difficult to understand how the most minor of endometriotic lesions can lead to a continuing problem of infertility. In the absence of our understanding of the evolution of this disease, one can speculate as to whether they do have a clear cause and effect relationship or whether there is some other factor which is producing both conditions.

I do not intend here to address the problem of the pathogenesis of endometriosis, but rather to examine the more clinically oriented problems of diagnosis and treatment. Practically every paper that appears on the subject of endometriosis highlights the "enigmatic" nature of the disease and perhaps that is the only thing on which everyone is agreed.

Diagnosis

While the etiology remains unclear, there is no doubt that the classic triad of dysmenorrhea, dyspareunia and infertility is highly suggestive of the condition. However, it is evident that each symptom may exist on its own. In particular, infertility may have its genesis in quite advanced endometriosis without the patient having experienced any pain at all. While even recent gynaecological texts still persist with the classification of primary and secondary dysmenorrhea, the usefulness of this separation in the diagnosis of endometriosis is debatable. Endometriosis is found in adolescent women who have classic primary dysmenorrhea and, unless the pain is completely relieved by anti-prostaglandins, it should generate a high order of suspicion. Deep dyspareunia is highly suggestive of the condition but can equally be produced by other pelvic pathology or even a prolapsed normal ovary. Palpable masses in the adnexae and uterine fixity can also be highly suggestive.

The one sign that is almost pathognomonic of endometriosis is the finding of tender nodularity in the uterosacral ligaments. Visible endometriotic lesions can be seen in the posterior fornix of the vagina. The final diagnosis must always rest on pelvic inspection either by laparotomy, where this is indicated by significant cyst formation, but more frequently by laparoscopy.

There is absolutely no place in modern gynaecology of initiating therapy for endometriosis on the basis of a presumptive diagnosis. Once the diagnosis is confirmed, a charted record should be made of the lesions such as is recommended by the American Fertility Society (1979). Such charting enables satisfactory comparisons to be made when different treatments are compared, particularly from different centres. If these charts are not immediately available, a simple line drawing suffices equally well. Because of the progressive and recurrent nature of the disease, it is an extremely useful guide in long term patient management.

Treatment decisions

Expectant treatment

A number of authors (including Decker and Lafery et al, 1979; Skenken and Malinak, 1982) have published pregnancy rates similar to those achieved following medical or surgical treatment. However, some of these papers have suffered from problems related to retrospective study and others have inadequately randomised their patients or controlled for other factors. There is, therefore, inadequate information at this stage to definitely say that expectant treatment has a role in mild endometriosis. Despite this possibility there are a number of publications (Naples et al, 1981; Wheeler et al, 1983) showing a much higher rate of spontaneous abortion in those patients with untreated disease. Rates varying between 34 per cent and 46 per cent in patients with untreated endometriosis decreased to eight or nine per cent following conservative treatment. The rate is particularly high in mild endometriosis (Decker and Lafery, 1979) although the specific relationship between pregnancy loss and endometriosis is unknown. It appears, therefore, that even mild disease may be associated with a high incidence of abortion and I, therefore, believe that there exists little evidence at the moment to justify expectant therapy. These concepts are still undergoing debate (Metzger et al, 1986).

Laparoscopic fulguration

In those patients with one or two spots of endometriosis there is a temptation to treat this by unipolar diathermy or laser therapy at the time of diagnosis. This approach, however, ignores the fact that for every macroscopic area of endometriosis, microscopic endometriosis is also almost certainly present. This has been confirmed when peritoneal biopsies have been taken from apparently normal areas of peritoneum at the time of conservative surgery for endometriosis and one would certainly expect this to be true when the genesis of endometriosis is considered. Almost without exception the reports of such treatment include only patients who have been treated with laparoscopic fulguration followed by some form of medication for several months (Daniell and Christianson, 1981; Sulewski et al, 1980). The more sophisticated approach using the new generation argon lasers suffers from the same problems. As these mild lesions respond well to medical treatment, there seems little justification for adopting an approach which carries a significant risk of damage to either underlying tissues or to other intraperitoneal structures. In highly skilled hands and with the most modern sophisticated equipment, the argon laser is probably the safest (Keye and Dixon, 1983) as the wavelength is such that is is selectively absorbed by the endometriotic lesion, but one cannot escape from the fact that the disease is almost certainly more widespread than the individual macroscopic lesions found at the original examination. The same argument could be applied to the new Excimer laser technology. Excimer laser uses kinetic energy rather than thermal energy but its role in this condition is unproven.

The decision for treatment, therefore, really revolves around the choice of a satisfactory medical approach to the problem or to open surgery or some combination of both. It is probably appropriate at this stage to say that as far as subsequent pregnancy rates are concerned there is really little to pick between these two modalities of treatment. Pregnancy rates vary between 50 per cent and 75 per cent depending on the length of follow up and other associated infertility factors (Dmowski and Cohen, 1978; Malinak, 1980). One of the more convincing papers written on this subject was presented by Gurzick and Rock (1983) from the Johns Hopkin Hospital in Maryland who studied 224 infertile women with mild or moderate endometriosis. They were given either Danazol or conservative surgical treatment and the cumulative pregnancy rates were then assessed on a life table analysis. The two are almost identical as were the pregnancy outcome of the two treatments. If there is a bias at all it is probably slightly in favour of conservative surgery. If combination therapy is chosen it is probably better to use medical treatment prior to surgery (Buttram and Reiter, 1984) rather than after it but even this is debatable.

The choice of treatment, therefore, tends to be made primarily on the extent of the disease. Where the lesions are superficial and there has been little or no distortion of the pelvic anatomy, the trend is to adopt a conservative approach and use medical treatment. Once cyst formation has occurred within the cortex of the ovary, and certainly if the cyst exceeds 1cm in size then conservative surgery is the treatment of choice. Experience with progestins and Danazol have certainly shown that they are not effective when significant cyst formation has occurred. Whether the same rule will apply to GnRH analogues is yet to be proven although these do result in shrinkage of the cyst but it is very likely that the cyst will "reactivate" once the analogue is stopped. If surgery is to be the treatment of choice then one has the choice between conserving reproductive function as far as one can or of a complete surgical excision of the disease. This conventionally means a total abdominal hysterectomy and bilateral salpingo-oophorectomy. Obviously the patient's age, her previous reproductive performance, her previous history of surgery and the severity of her symptoms will all have to be considered in making this decision.

Medical treatment

I wish to confine my remarks to four preparations which are currently available — Duphaston (Rx) (dydrogesterone), Danazol (Isoxazole) derivitive of 17-ethinyl testosterone), Provera (Rx) (medroxyprogesterone) and GnRH analogues. I do not believe that testosterone has any place in the treatment of endometriosis in modern gynaecology and I do not intend to discuss it further.

In the early 1970s, a trial of treatment with Duphaston was conducted at The Royal Women's Hospital (Johnston, 1976). Forty-nine patients were diagnosed as having mild endometriosis endoscopically and each received

Duphaston 5mg b.d. continuously for nine months, the length of the treatment based on the original Kistner concepts. After nine months, 32 of these patients were re-examined endoscopically to assess the progress of the disease, the remainder declining re-examination. Eighty-four percent were assessed as being clear of the disease and of the 19 who were attempting pregnancy, 10 (52.6 per cent) were successful over a period of follow up averaging 18 months. The relatively low dose used in that trial was chosen because of the expense of the medication. As Duphaston is pure progesterone with no oestrogenic or androgenic potential, there was an absolute minimum of side effects and compliance was very high. Interestingly, although medication was given continuously, the patients continued to menstruate regularly and, in a separate study, the majority of patients given Duphaston at this dose level also continued to ovulate. However, none of the patients conceived during the course of the trial and our subsequent experience with Duphaston confirms this. It is presumed that this is probably due to the effect of Duphaston on the cervical mucus, which effect is now being used formally in the progesterone-only pills.

Danazol then became available and a study was carried out comparing the use of Danazol (200mg t.d.s. for six months) with Duphaston (5mg t.d.s. for six months). One hundred infertile patients were included in this trial and the patients were randomised on the toss of a coin. All patients were assessed before and after treatment by laparoscopy. Any patient who had previously received treatment for endometriosis was excluded from the trial. The anatomic distribution of the disease is shown in Table 6-1 and is remarkably similar for both groups, as were age distribution and duration of infertility. All the couples were assessed for associated infertility factors and these are shown in Table 6-2. These are also very similar and, as far as pregnancy outcome is concerned, it is unlikely that any bias could be introduced via other infertility factors due to this distribution.

Response to treatment is shown in Table 6-3 and it is clear that Danazol is significantly better than Duphaston as far as the immediate resolution of the lesions is concerned. It is interesting to compare this degree of response with the original Duphaston trial where the same total dose of Duphaston was given, but over a nine month period as opposed to six months. Here the results are identical, which would suggest that progestogen treatment is both dose and time related. The mean follow up period was 17 months and in most it exceeded 12 months. Forty-one per cent of those patients who had received Danazol became pregnant in this time, compared with 33 per cent of those who had received Duphaston. There is no significant difference between these two rates and it is of interest to note that 85 per cent of the pregnancies were achieved within six months of completing the therapy and all occurred within 12 months. Again a comparison of the numbers achieving pregnancy in the previous Duphaston trial shows no significant difference, but because that analysis lacked a formal assessment of associated infertility factors, no direct comparison can be made. The structure of the latter trial allowed for crossover treatment if the second laparoscopy showed any residual disease.

Of the 36 patients who had further treatment, 47 per cent became pregnant within the follow up period, giving an overall pregnancy rate of the whole trial of 40 per cent. A comparison of the side effects from these drugs is shown in Table 6-4. Weight gain, troublesome androgenic side effects and muscular cramps were certainly more common with Danazol, which is known to be both androgenic and anabolic. These can be troublesome unless the patient has the high level of committment to her medication that one finds in an infertile population. The one potentially serious side effect that must be watched for is a deepening of the voice, which on occasions can be permanent, demanding immediate cessation of treatment if it occurs.

As a result of these two trials, it would appear that Danazol has a more immediate impact on the lessions in mild forms of endometriosis than does Duphaston, but there is no difference when Duphaston is used for the longer time period. Danazol has a higher incidence of significant side effects which can affect patient compliance unless the motivation is strong. There is no difference in the pregnancy rates following treatment. Of the two, Duphaston is still the drug of choice for mild endometriosis as it is certainly better tolerated than Danazol and is much cheaper (one-sixth the price) but treatment needs to be extended for nine months for best results. However, if the patient is anxious to complete her treatment as quickly as possible and if the condition tends to be more extensive, then Danazol is probably the drug of choice.

Although medroxprogesterone has been available for some years, there have been no formal trials reported with this drug as yet. At this stage, one can only assume that the appropriate dose to use would be in a menstrual suppressive range, probably of the order of 30–60mg per day, as it suppresses pituitary gonadotrophins and thereby causes ovulatory suppression; any lesser dose would cause very troublesome bleeding. One could perhaps reasonably assume that its effect would be similar to other progestational agents and its sporadic use with satisfactory results has been reported. I believe it may well have a more significant place in a drug armamentarium.

More recently, GnRH analogues have been used in the treatment of endometriosis with good results. All the analogues currently available for treatment are, in fact, GnRH agonists. These are a group of substances which are produced by modifying the normal GnRH decapeptide usually at the sixth or tenth position of the natural sequence. Such analogues have a markedly enhanced effect when compared with the parent substance and induce a profound and selective desensitisation of the pituitary gonadotrophin secretion. Examples are Buserelin Rx, Nafarelin Rx and Lucren Rx. When administered on their own, they can be used either subcutaneously or by intranasal spray. When incorporated in microspheres, the depot preparation is administered by monthly injections as the spheres produce a slow release mechanism. There are currently two such preparations available but more are appearing and the ease of their clinical application is such that they have an obvious place in the treatment of endometriosis.

The agonists must be differentiated from antagonists which, while having a more immediate impact, have until recently been plagued with marked oedoematogenic and anaphylactoid properties that have made their application in the human unacceptable. However, the peptide chemists have made the inevitable breakthrough and early trials with antagonists free of these problems have now been reported in the human.

At a recent symposium on GnRH analogues held in Geneva in February 1988, a large number of papers appeared detailing the use of these analogues in the treatment of endometriosis. Without exception the same response that can be achieved with other medical treatments can also be achieved with these preparations. There is a satisfactory resolution of the endometriotic lesions and an associated relief of symptoms while post-treatment pregnancy rates in those patients suffering from infertility again approach 50 per cent. Because of the profound suppression of oestrogen excretion in patients receiving analogue therapy, the principal side effects are the same as severe oestrogen deprivation from any cause, but it is reported that the concommitant administration of small doses of Norethisterone can significantly alleviate the symptoms of hot flushes and dryness in the vagina which inevitably occur on this therapy. Because the treatment for endometriosis must be continued for six to nine months, there is potential for development of osteoporotic changes. It would seem in the time frame mentioned that there can be some trabecular bone loss during this time but very little loss can be demonstrated in cortical bone. It would appear, however, that once the ovarian suppression is stopped, the trabecular bone loss is recovered reasonably quickly (Waibel, 1988).

What is lacking is any long term study of recurrence rates of endometriosis following completion of GnRH treatment. At this stage one can only assume that a similar recurrence rate that follows other medical treatments can be expected. At this stage of the evolution of the analogues, it would seem that they are effective but they do not have any major advantage over current medical therapy. If this is true, then one has to take into consideration the cost structure. At present these preparations are expensive and, unless their cost can be made comparable to the more conventional medication, then their use may be somewhat limited. As previously mentioned, that may have a singular place in those patients with small endometriomas who would otherwise require surgery.

I have not discussed the contraceptive pill in this section as there is, I believe, no place for such medication in the treatment of endometriosis today. To be effective, they must be given continuously in high doses to induce complete amenorrhea. This results in a high dose of oestrogen, which produces unacceptable side effects and a corresponding low compliance. The standard contraceptive dose of "the pill" does not control the disease and its only use may be diagnostic, as continuing dysmenorrhea experienced by patients taking the pill is strongly suggestive of active endometriosis and demands investigation.

Surgical treatment

Conservative treatment

As the ultimate aim of this surgery is to both enhance and preserve the patient's reproductive potential, everything that can be done to foster this must be done. It is, therefore, important to adopt all the detail that is inherent in a microsurgical approach to these patients. Irritant powder must be washed from the surgeon's, the assistant's and the scrub sister's gloves prior to the start of the operation. Peritoneal and serosal surfaces should be protected from dehydration by both packing and covering all the peritoneal and serosal surfaces that are not immediately being worked on with moist packs using a physiologic solution such as Hartmanns. Exposed peritoneal and serosal surfaces should be continually irrigated to prevent dessication. Tissue should be handled gently and preferably with teflon coated or glass rods. Surgical trauma should be minimal and all surfaces should be repaired accurately with fine non-reactive suture material. All raw areas should be re-peritonealized accurately and the final anatomy should be restored as near as possible to normal. The use of adjuvants to prevent post-operative adhesions is still debated but I personally use Rheomacrodex (6 per cent Dextran) leaving between 400–500mls in the peritoneal cavity. Where extensive disease exists, it is impossible to follow each of these tenets absolutely because of the extensive nature of the surgery involved but the principles remain the same. As a result of the work presented from Houston, either pre or post operative treatment with Danazol appears to produce some improvement in results (Malinak, 1980; Buttram and Reiter, 1984).

Occasionally, extensive associated scarring in the region of the uterosacral ligaments necessitates excision of these fibrous areas so that relief of severe deep dyspareunia can be achieved even though the disease process may have been arrested by chemotherapy. If such a resection is being done, preliminary dissection of the lower portion of the ureter is required, to avoid inadvertent damage to this structure as it lies very close to the uterosacral ligament on each side. This dissection is difficult as in such patients the very fibrosis that one is excising prevents any significant elevation of the uterus prior to its excision but the symptomatic relief that this procedure produces makes the effort worthwhile. Occasionally, endometriotic involvement of the cornu of the tube produces either the picture of salpingitis isthmica nodosa or complete cornual obstruction. Such tubal involvement requires resection and reanastomosis of the tube.

Relocation of the ovaries

Relocation of the ovaries can be and is occasionally a useful form of conservative management in patients with severe disease, particularly where the disease is recurrent and previous surgery has failed to control the condition. It is applicable to patients who are suffering from severe intractable deep dyspareunia brought about by either recurrent endometriosis or extensive adhesions which weld the ovary into the ovarian fossa and completely destroy the interface between the ovarian serosa and the peritoneal lining of the ovarian fossa.

In such patients merely remobilising the ovary will not be an effective treatment as the extent of the disease almost guarantees that the ovary will readhese into the lower reaches of the pelvis behind the uterus and the patient's dyspareunia will persist. The relocation procedure consists of firstly mobilising the ureter by extraperitoneal dissection, thus avoiding damage to this structure. The suspensory ligament of the ovary and its attendant blood vessels are divided and the pelvic peritoneum is opened longitudinally both superior to and inferior to the infundibula pelvic vessels up as far as the brim of the pelvis. This leaves the ovary freely mobile on a pedicle containing its superior blood supply. The ovary is then sewn to the peritoneal surface anterior to the round ligament to a point near the internal inguinal ring. During this procedure, great care must be taken to preserve the blood supply to and from the ovary passing through the infundibular pelvic ligament. Once the ovary has been located in this position, the peritoneum covering the blood vessels is then sewn to the adjacent peritoneal surface to avoid any bowel slipping through the space between the ovarian pedicle and the lateral pelvic wall.

This procedure can almost guarantee complete relief from dyspareunia but because of the disruption of the normal relationships between the tube and the ovary, it makes it almost impossible for the patient to achieve a pregnancy naturally. However, it does enable conservation of both ovarian tissue and the uterus and pregnancies are still possible through the process of IVF.

Radical surgery

Because of the hormone dependent nature of endometriosis, there is no point in leaving any ovarian tissue if extirpation of the disease is intended. Patients must, therefore, be prepared psychologically for this pre-operatively, as it is now possible to completely replace both oestrogen and androgens post-operatively at satisfactory therapeutic levels. They must be reassured that a bilateral oophorectomy is not going to produce the drastic effects of a surgical menopause and both their sex life and their femininity will be retained intact following the procedure. If hormone replacement post-operatively does reactivate any endometriotic deposits, which rarely occurs, these can readily be treated with appropriate chemotherapy.

Surgical removal of the uterus and ovaries in a case of severe endometriosis can be one of the most difficult gynaecological surgical procedures undertaken. The disease can penetrate through the peritoneum, completely obliterating normal planes and can surround the ureter and involve other adjacent structures. It is, therefore, wise as a preliminary step to open the peritoneum lateral to the line of the infundibular pelvic ligament and identify and free the ureter from the medial structures prior to their removal.

It the disease has spread anteriorally into the base of the bladder, it may be necessary to open through the fundus of the bladder so that the base of the bladder can be safely dissected from the cervic. Similarly, significant difficulty may be experienced in freeing the rectosigmoid from the back of the cervix. As it is obviously undesirable to open the bowel it may be necessary to shave through the outer layers of the cervix, thereby leaving a small amount of tissue attached to the front of the rectosigmoid. Once the hysterectomy has been completed, this tissue can be dissected free from the anterior wall of the rectosigmoid and the serosal layer repaired.

Many people advocate the use of appropriate chemotherapy for two to three months prior to surgery as it can make the surgical dissection easier and safer. This may be another role for GnRH analogues, particularly the new antagonists, because of their speed of action.

Conclusion

These then are the more conventional methods of treatment that have been applied to endometriosis, and either individually or in combination will provide adequate relief of the symptoms and control of the disease. However, some 20 to 40 per cent of the patients will still fail to achieve their desired pregnancy and IVF and GIFT have now emerged as significant modalities of treatment in this condition. In our own IVF Unit we have been able to achieve pregnancy rates almost equal to those of patients with tubal disease on an IVF programme, providing the endometriosis has been effectively controlled with appropriate treatment (Johnston et al, 1985). There may even be a case to withhold conventional treatment to expedite a patient's re-entry to an IVF programme, but because of the known increased incidence of miscarriage in the presence of active endometriosis following spontaneous pregnancy, this may ultimately prove to be the wrong approach.

Despite the fact that endometriosis can be an extraordinarily extensive disease process, the tubes are rarely involved and the majority of patients are therefore appropriate for gamete intra fallopian transfer (GIFT). Our experience with this so far has produced a pregnancy rate of 20 per cent which exceeds that produced by more conventional IVF. More recently PROST has emerged as an alternative method of treatment to GIFT but no major study is available yet. These newer modalities have already been established as definitive extensions of the more conventional treatments as far as the correction of infertility is concerned and we have, therefore, reached the stage where they must be included in the overall treatment protocols. However, because of the respective success rates of the medical and surgical approaches to this condition, there is no doubt that these remain the most appropriate primary treatments while IVF, GIFT and PROST should be reserved for those who have failed to respond appropriately.

It should always be remembered that endometriosis has a recurrence rate which probably approaches 50 per cent regardless of the treatment used. As the majority of pregnancies occur within 12 months of either medical or surgical treatment, review laparoscopy to assess any recurrence is probably best deferred for that period of time following the completion of a treatment programme. As significant pregnancy rates can be obtained following repeat medical treatment and, to a lesser extent, following repeat surgical treatment, both are justified. However, in the more severe cases, crippling pain can force both the patient and the surgeon to the conclusion that radical surgery is the best course.

One can only hope that the GnRH analogues may have a more major role to play in the long term management of endometriosis. They may allow for a reduction in the need for open surgery while the new laser therapies applied via laparoscope may well be used effectively to the same end.

Encouraging results have recently been reported indicating that preliminary suppression of pituitary function using GnRH analogues can increase the pregnancy rate prior to hyperstimulation for IVF. It may even be possible to immediately initiate a course of IVF treatment towards the end of, or even during, the period of suppression with GnRH analogues. We are now embarking on a whole new era of treatment of this perplexing condition. We certainly have a number of new tools at our disposal but how best they may be applied have still to be determined.

Table 6-1
Distribution of the lesions

	Danazol	*Duphaston*
Peritoneal only	59.2%	59.8%
Ovarian only	8.2%	5.9%
Both	32.7%	35.8%

This represents the classic distribution of lesions seen in early endometriosis.

Table 6-2
Associated infertility factors

	Danazol	*Duphaston*
Ovulating disturbances	32.7%	22.0%
Male factors	53.1%	50.0%
Mucous factors	8.1%	10.0%
Tubal factors	6.1%	2.0%

These are remarkably evenly distributed between the two groups. The multifactorial nature of infertility is well demonstrated.

Table 6-3
Result of treatment

	Danazol	*Duphaston*	*Significance*
Complete resolution	65.3%	39.2%	.02
Improvement	89.8%	54.9%	.001

Danazol is clearly superior when treatments with each drug is given for six months.

Table 6-4
Side effects of the drugs

	Danazol	*Duphaston*
Weight gain	63.4%	41.2%
Amenorrhea	83.7%	0
Androgenic effects	12.2%	2%
Irregular bleeding	14.3%	13.7%
Depression	6.1%	0
Cramps	12.2%	2%

Duphaston is clearly superior, which can affect patient compliance.

References

Buttram, V.C. Jnr. and Reiter, C. Treatment of endometriosis with danazol — Second interim report. *Fertility and Sterility*, 1984; 41: 365.

Daniell, J.F. and Christianson, C. Combined laparoscopic surgery and danazol therapy for pelvic endometriosis. *Fertility and Sterility*, 1981; 35: 521.

Decker H.W. and Lafery, H. Conservative surgical treatment of endometriosis and infertility. *Infertility*, 1979; 2: 155.

Dmowski, W.P. and Cohen, M.R. Antigonadotrophin (danazol) in the treatment of endometriosis: Evaluation of post treatment fertilization and three-year follow-up data. *American Journal of Obstetrics and Gynecology*, 1978; 130: 41.

Gurzick, D.S. and Rock, J.A. A comparison of danazol and conservative surgery for the treatment of infertility due to mild or moderate endometriosis.*Fertility and Sterility*, 1983; 40: 580.

Johnston, W.I.H. Dydrogesterone and endometriosis. *British Journal of Obstetrics and Gynaecology*, 1976; 83: 77.

Johnston, W.I.H., Oke, K., Speirs, A., Clarke, G., McBain, J., Bayly, C. and Hunt, J. Patient selections for in vitro fertilisation — Physical and psychological aspects. *Annals. New York Academy of Sciences*, 1985; 442: 490.

Keye, W.R. Jnr. and Dixon, J. Photocoagulation of endometriosis by the argon laser through the laparoscope. *Obstetrics and Gynecology*, 1983; 62: 383.

Malinak, L.R. Infertility and endometriosis: Operative techniques clinical staging and prognosis *Clinical Obstetrics and Gynaecology*, 1980; 23: 92.

Metzger, D.A., Olive, D.L. and Stohs, G.F. Franklin Association of endometriosis and spontaneous abortion: Effect of control group selection. *Fertility and Sterility*, 1986; 45: 19.

Naples, J.D., Batt, R.E. and Sadigh, H. Spontaneous abortion rate in patients with endometriosis. *Obstetrics and Gynecology*, 1981; 57: 509.

Shenken, R.S. and Malinak, L.R. Conservative surgery versus expectant management for and infertile patient with mild endometriosis. *Fertility and Sterility*, 1982; 37: 183.

Sulewski, J.M., Curcio, F.D., Bronitsky, C. and Stenger, V.G. The treatment of endometriosis at laparoscopy for infertility. *American Journal of Obstetrics and Gynecology*, 1980; 138: 128.

Waibel, S. et al. Bone density in patients treated with GnRH agonists for myomata and endometriosis: Abst.96 Internal symptoms on GnRH analogues in cancer and human reproduction. *Gynaecological Endocrinology*, 1988; 2: Supp. No.1: 106.

Wheeler, J.M., Johnston, B.M. and Malinak, L.R. The relationship of endometriosis to spontaneous abortion. *Fertility and Sterility*, 1983; 39: 656.

7
Ultrasound directed follicle aspiration in IVF

M. Wren and J. Parsons

Introduction

The technique of in vitro fertilisation and embryo transfer (IVF-ET) was first described by Steptoe el al (1980), who performed oocyte collections under direct vision using a laparoscope. Although IVF-ET was originally developed for the treatment of infertility due to tubal damage, infertility due to other indications can also be treated successfully with this technique. These include unexplained infertility (Wood et al, 1984), oligozoospermia (Cohen et al, 1984), endometriosis, and immunological factors (Trounson and Conti, 1982). Since its introduction, the indications for IVF-ET have increased; hence patient demand exceeds still further the facilities available for treatment. In order to meet this increase in demand, particularly as funds are largely limited, it is found necessary to develop other ways of performing the treatment procedure that is less expensive.

One such technique is ultrasound directed follicle aspiration (UDFA) for oocyte collection. It is less costly than that of laparoscopic follicle aspiration because patients do not require a general anaesthetic or hospitalisation. Full theatre facilities are not necessary, and the number of staff required to perform the procedure is also reduced. In addition, UDFA may be performed on patients with extensive pelvic adhesions, for whom laparoscopy may be inappropriate or where laparoscopic oocyte retrieval may be impossible because of ovarian inaccessibility. Unlike UDFA, laparoscopy and general anaesthesia are both associated with a significant morbidity and mortality (Chamberlain and Brown, 1978). Furthermore, the insufflation of gases required during laparoscopy may also have an adverse effect on the oocyte.

UDFA was first described by Lenz et al (1981), who performed the procedure under general anaesthesia. The bladder was filled with saline, the aspirating needle passed through the anterior abdominal wall into the bladder, and then through the posterior bladder wall before entering the ovary, all under transabdominal ultrasound control. The procedure of transcutaneous transvesical UDFA was later performed under local anaesthesia (Wikland et al, 1983; Riddle et al, 1987). As a further development, the aspiration needle was either passed through a guide attached to the transducer, or manipulated freehand through the abdominal wall. Transvaginal UDFA was first described by Dellenbach et al (1984). A speculum was passed into the vagina and an aspiration needle penetrated through the vaginal fornix into the ovary under transabdominal ultrasound guidance. Perurethral UDFA was introduced by Parsons et al (1985). The technique involved passing the aspiration needle through the urethra into the bladder and out of the posterior bladder wall into the ovary. The most recent development of the UDFA technique is the direct transvaginal approach (Wikland et al, 1985; Feichtinger et al, 1986). The needle is introduced through the vaginal fornix into the ovary under vaginal ultrasound control using a vaginal ultrasound transducer and needle guide.

When IVF-ET first started at King's College Hospital (KCH), severe limitations were encountered with funding, and the absence of theatre facilities for laparoscopic oocyte collection. It was therefore necessary to develop an outpatient ultrasound based programme. Initially, oocyte collections were performed by the transcutaneous transvesical route. This was followed by the perurethral approach, and later by the direct transvaginal route. All the procedures were performed under intravenous sedation and the patients allowed home one to two hours later.

This chapter describes our two years' experience of UDFA at KCH. During the study period, January 1986 to December 1987, the most significant development in our IVF-ET programme was the introduction of transvaginal ultrasonography. This is presently our method of approach for both follicular monitoring and oocyte recovery.

Patients

A total of 562 patients underwent 1154 cycles of stimulation in preparation for IVF-ET during the study period. Table 7-1 shows the reasons for referral for IVF treatment. Patients were accepted who had failed laparoscopic retrieval or were considered risky by other IVF units. The use of UDFA circumvented the need for a preliminary laparoscopic pelvic assessment. The mean age of the patients was 33.4 years (range, 24 to 41 years).

Ovarian stimulation

The standard regimen for ovarian stimulation was a combination of clomiphene citrate (Clomid; Merrel, Hounslow, UK) 100mg given daily between days two and six of the menstrual cycle, and Human Menopausal Gonadotrophin (hMG; Pergonal; Serono, Welyn Garden City, UK) two to six ampoules daily. The day of commencement and the dosage of hMG was individualised according to the length of the patient's menstrual cycle, her age, and her response to previous treatment.

All our patients attended the Assisted Conception Unit on the second day of their cycle for an ultrasound scan to check for normal ovarian morphology prior to commencing stimulation. During the first year of the study, the majority of ultrasound scans were performed abdominally, using a mechanical sector scanner (DRF 100; diasonics, Bedford, UK) with an abdominal 3.5 MHz transducer. In the second year, vaginal ultrasound was introduced and became routine, with abdominal ultrasound being reserved for those patients whose ovaries could not be visualised vaginally or who specifically requested it. We used a mechanical sector scanner (Bruel and Kjaer, Copenhagen, Denmark) with a 7MHz vaginal transducer.

Patients received their second ultrasound examination on day six or day seven, to determine the number and size of the developing follicles. At the same time, blood was taken for baseline serum oestradiol estimation. Thereafter, follicular scans and oestradiol measurements were performed daily. Human Chorionic Gonadotrophin (hCG; Profasi; Serono, UK) 5000 IU, was given when the leading follicle had a mean diameter of 17mm, provided there was a satisfactory rise in serum oestradiol (corresponding to approximately 1,000 pmol/L per follicle with a mean diameter greater than 14mm). UDFA was performed 34–36 hours post hCG.

Treatment was abandoned when less than three follicles developed or where the rise in the serum oestradiol level was inadequate.

Ultrasound directed follicle aspiration

Patient preparation

Patients received lorazepam (Ativan; Wyeth, Maidenhead, UK) 1mg orally the evening before oocyte retrieval and again one hour pre-operatively. They were fasted for six hours prior to UDFA and were instructed to arrive at the hospital 30 minutes before the procedure with their bladder empty. Their partners were asked to produce a semen sample by masturbation either before or after the egg collection, which they were encouraged to attend.

UDFA was performed under intravenous sedation with diazepam and pethidine given through a 21G butterfly needle (Abbot, Queenborough, Kent, UK) sited on the back of the hand. The dose given varied depending on the patient's tolerance and the time taken to complete the procedure. Thus pethidine ranged from 25–150 mg IV and diazepam 2.5–15mg IV, in the proportion pethidine 25 mg and diazepam 2.5 mg. All the patients went home within two hours of completing the procedure.

Procedure room

UDFA was performed in a minor operating theatre with a laboratory adjacent. Theatre clothes and sterile rubber gloves were worn by the operator and assistant. Sterile gowns and face masks were not required.

Equipment

A 27.2cm long double channel needle (Figure 7-1) was used for UDFA (Casmed, Cheam, UK). the outer disposable channel was sharp ended and had an outer diameter of 1.7mm. the inner re-usable channel was blunt ended and had an inner diameter of 0.93 mm. The latter was connected by PTFE tubing to a 15ml test-tube (Falcon; Becton and Dickinson, London, UK) (Figure 7-2), to which suction was applied from a foot operated pump (Craft; Rocket, Watford, UK). When the needle was assembled, the two concentric channels were joined by a Luer lock fitting. Two cms of the outer needle, next to the sharpened tip, were roughened to enhance ultrasound visualisation (Figure 7-3). When the needle was inside a follicle and suction was applied, the follicular contents were aspirated into the test tube. If an oocyte was not found in the aspirate, then the follicle was flushed with medium (Earle's balanced salt solution; EBS; Gibco, Paisley, Scotland). For this purpose, a syringe containing EBS was connected to the side arm of the needle by PTFE tubing. The medium passed down the space between the two channels, refilling the follicle and was then reaspirated.

Techniques

Perurethral UDFA

The patient was placed in the lithotomy position, with the operator standing on her right, the ultrasound machine opposite on her left, and the assistant sitting between her legs. Vulval toilet was performed with a solution of cetrimide and chlorhexidine (Savlodil, ICI, Macclesfield, UK) as for routine urinary catheterisation, but this is followed by washing with EBS, to remove traces of the antiseptic.

The double channel needle, primed with flushing medium, was then inserted into the urethra, within the tip of a 12 French Foley catheter (Figure 7-4). Hartman's solution was introduced into the bladder through the catheter, until the follicles could be seen clearly by transabdominal ultrasonography. As the bladder was being filled, the catheter balloon was inflated and the needle tip disconnected from the end of the catheter. In order to visualise the maximum length of the needle within the bladder, the needle was kept at right angles to the ultrasound beam (Figure 7-5).

The needle was aimed at a suitable follicle and then advanced with a single, rapid thrust through the posterior bladder wall into the centre of the follicle. The follicular fluid was aspirated into a test-tube (Figure 7-6) and then examined in the adjacent laboratory. If an oocyte was not identified, the follicle was flushed with EBS. Once the oocyte was identified, or granulosa cells were no longer present in follicular flushes, the needle was redirected into another follicle. The procedure was repeated until all the follicles with a diameter of 10mm or greater in that ovary were aspirated. The needle was then withdrawn into the bladder and flushed with EBS before the procedure was repeated on the other side. Sometimes it was necessary to puncture the posterior bladder wall on more than one occasion for each ovary, in order to reach all the follicles. In each case, the needle was flushed with EBS before re-entering the ovary, to avoid urinary contamination of the next aspirate. When all the follicles were aspirated, the needle was removed, the bladder emptied, and the catheter withdrawn. The patient was then moved to the recovery area where she stayed until she felt well enough to go home.

Transvaginal UDFA

The patient was placed in the lithotomy position, with the operator and assistant sitting between her legs, and the vaginal ultrasound machine to her left (Figure 7-7). The vagina was cleansed with a solution of Savlodil, followed by flushing medium to remove traces of the antiseptic. The vaginal transducer was covered with a sterile condom containing ultrasound jelly in the tip. The sterile needle guide was then attached over the sheathed transducer (Figure 7-8).

The prepared vaginal transducer was then inserted into the vagina. The ovaries were scanned and the transducer rotated until the target follicle was on the monitor screen's biopsy guide line. The distance from the tip of the transducer to the centre of the follicle was estimated, the needle then passed down the needle guide and with a rapid movement thrust through the vaginal vault into the follicle. When the needle tip was visible inside the follicle (Figure 7-9) suction was applied and the follicular fluid aspirated.

The aspirate was examined in the adjacent laboratory and if an oocyte was not identified the follicle was flushed with medium, as for perurethral UDFA. The needle was then either advanced through the follicle wall into the adjacent follicle, or withdrawn into the ovarian stroma and redirected into another follicle. The procedure was repeated until all the follicles greater than 10mm MFD in that ovary were aspirated. It was usually possible to aspirate all the follicles from both ovaries by two punctures, one on each side of the vaginal vault. At the end of the procedure, the vaginal vault was inspected and, if necessary, pressure was applied to bleeding points.

Transabdominal transvesical UDFA

The patient was placed in the lithotomy position and catheterised with a 12 French gauge Foley catheter. The bladder was filled with Hartmans solution until the follicles could be seen clearly by transabdominal ultrasonography (Figure 7-10). A small area on the anterior abdominal wall was infiltrated with 10ml 1 per cent Lignocaine (Figure 7-11), through which the needle was passed into the bladder, under transabdominal ultrasound guidance (Figure 7-12). The follicles were needled, aspirated and flushed using a technique similar to that described for the perurethral approach.

Combined routes

In some patients, it was not possible to aspirate all the follicles using a single route and therefore a combination of approaches was required. For example, if an ovary was behind the uterus, it was impossible to aspirate the follicles transvaginally, without passing the needle through the uterus. Occasionally, an ovary would be situated subcutaneously beyond the reach of the vaginal transducer and above the level of the distended bladder. Such ovaries were approached directly through the lower abdominal wall, under transabdominal ultrasound guidance, following infiltration with local anaesthetic.

In vitro fertilisation and embryo culture

The oocytes were transferred into 1 ml drops of EBS supplement with 10 per cent (v/v) heat-inactivated patient's serum, under liquid paraffin, equilibrated in 5 per cent carbon dioxide (CO_2) in air at 37°C, to give a pH of 7.4. The semen sample was prepared by a simple wash and "swim-up" technique (Lopata et al, 1976). Insemination was performed four to six hours after egg collection, using an appropriate volume of prepared sperm suspension, to give a final concentration of 50,000–100,000 motile spermatozoa per ml. The oocytes were examined for the presence of two pronuclei, 17 to 19 hours after insemination, and a maximum of three embryos, usually at the two to four cell stage, were transferred 24 to 48 hours later.

Results

Between January 1986 and December 1987, 562 patients received treatment in our IVF-ET programme. In the first year, ovarian stimulation was commenced in 529 cycles, of which 385 (72.8 per cent) resulted in UDFA, and 304 (57.5 per cent) in ET. The majority of UDFAs were performed using the perurethral route (291; 75 per cent) but in a small number of patients (60; 15.6 per cent) transvaginal UDFA was performed. The following year, 625 stimulated cycles were commenced, of which 418 (66.9 per cent) resulted in egg collection, and 343 (54.8 per cent) in ET. That year, 338 collections (80.9 per cent) were performed using the transvaginal route and only 57 (13.6 per cent) were performed per urethrally (Table 7-2).

Complications

Perurethral UDFA

On two occasions, patients were unable to tolerate bladder filling during perurethral UDFA and were therefore changed to the direct transabdominal route. In one patient the procedure was abandoned due to pain, following the aspiration of six oocytes from one ovary.

In 11 cases, significant extravasation of Hartman's solution occurred. The patients were unaware of this event, but deterioration of the ultrasound picture made further follicle aspiration difficult and the procedure was abandoned.

Two patients developed respiratory depression after administration of pethidine. In both cases this was easily reversed with intravenous naloxone (Narcan; Du Pont, Stevenage, UK). Four more patients became confused during the procedure, but all were fit to go home within two hours.

There were four cases of gross haematuria following perurethral UDFA, requiring catheterisation and admission to hospital for bladder irrigation.

When the urine was no longer bloodstained, the patients were discharged. None of them had any long term complication.

Transvaginal UDFA

Amongst those patients receiving transvaginal UDFA, there was no immediate complication requiring hospital admission. Although the patients usually experienced some discomfort during the procedure, only one case was abandoned because of pain before all the follicles were aspirated.

Pelvic vessel puncture occurred on 17 occasions, without sequelae. Following the procedure, a small amount of bleeding from the vaginal puncture sites was common and a light bloodstained vaginal loss often occurred for one to two days after UDFA.

Two patients developed severe pelvic sepsis after transvaginal UDFA. Both patients had a past history of chronic pelvic inflammatory disease prior to commencing IVF and both had cystic structures in the pelvis, which were drained at the time of UDFA. In the first case, the patient presented five weeks after UDFA with a large pelvic abcess, which was successfully treated by surgical drainage through the posterior vaginal fornix. She has since had two further treatment cycles, and on both occasions perurethral UDFA was performed without complication. The second patient presented one week after transvaginal UDFA, with a tender adnexal mass. At laparotomy a tubo-ovarian abcess was identified. The abcess was drained and a salpingectomy and partial oophorectomy performed. Post operative intravenous antibiotics were given, and the patient recovered completely. She has returned for further IVF treatment.

Discussion

The data presented is retrospective. The patients were not matched and in the majority of the cases where a transvaginal approach was used, the procedure were performed later on in the series than those cases where a perurethral approach was used. Direct comparisons are therefore not appropriate. In view of the improvement in the quality of the image produced with the vaginal ultrasound transducer, it is reasonable to conclude that the transvaginal route for egg collection contributed to the improved results.

During the study period, the mean number of follicles aspirated by the perurethral route and the mean number of oocytes collected was 8.6 and 5.8 respectively. Transvaginally, the mean number of follicles aspirated and oocytes collected was 9.2 and 7.5. The mean yield of oocytes per follicle aspirated was 67 per cent for the perurethral collections and 81 per cent for the transvaginal collections.

The other major advantage of the transvaginal route for UDFA is that the technique is relatively easy and can be learnt quickly. In our unit, where we perform 12 to 15 collections per week, a new operator is usually able to perform a collection competently within four to five weeks. In contrast the full bladder techniques usually require more training and most new operators will need to be trained for two to three months before they can regularly perform perurethral or transabdominal transvesical UDFA without supervision. Although the transvaginal route is easier to learn and to perform, the full bladder techniques should also be learnt by all operators performing UDFA, since the ovaries of some patients will be inaccessible transvaginally.

The advantage of all the UDFA techniques is that they can be performed without general anaesthesia and therefore the patients may go home within two hours. Although the risks of general anaesthesia are avoided, great care must be taken to avoid the complications of intravenous pethidine and diazepam. Excessive use of these drugs, particularly in small patients, may easily cause respiratory depression.

Patients should be informed before IVF of possible complications that may occur following UDFA. Urinary extravasation and haematuria were the most frequent complications occurring after perurethral UDFA in the study. Although there is a potential risk of introducing infection into the bladder when performing catheterisation for perurethral UDFA, no post operative urinary tract infection was reported and no patient developed pelvic sepsis.

The potential disadvantage of transvaginal UDFA is the introduction of pathogenic organisms from the vagina into the pelvis. However, in our series only two of the 398 patients who had transvaginal UDFA developed pelvic sepsis. Both these patients already had irreparable tubal damage with encysted fluid around the ovaries, resulting from previous episodes of pelvic infection. Since the risk of sepsis following transvaginal UDFA is small, prophylactic antibiotic cover is unnecessary. However, in patients with a history of severe pelvic sepsis the risk of developing infection may be less following transabdominal, transvesical, or perurethral rather than transvaginal UDFA.

Table 7-1
Indications for inclusion in the IVF programme (1986–1987)

Indication	*No. of patients*	*Per cent*
Tubal damage	356	63.3
Unexplained infertility	91	16.2
Male factor	51	9.1
Endometriosis	31	5.5
Multiple factors	33	5.9

Table 7-2
Results for 1986 and 1987

Description	*Year* 1986	*Year* 1987
Stimulated cycles	529	625
Cycles abandoned prior to UDFA (%)	144 (27.2%)	207 (33.1%)
UFDA	385	418
Perurethral UDFA	291 (75.6%)	57 (13.6%)
Transvaginal UDFA	60 (15.6%)	338 (80.9%)
Transcutaneous/transvesical UDFA	4 (1.0%)	0
Combined route UDFA	30 (7.8%)	23 (5.5%)
Embryo transfer	304	343
Clinical pregnancies	60	90
Pregnancy rate/cycle	11%	14%
Pregnancy rate/UDFA	16%	22%
Pregnancy rate/ET	20%	26%

Clinical pregnancy is defined as amenorrhea of at least five weeks, with raised serum beta hCG, and a gestation sac demonstrable by ultrasound.

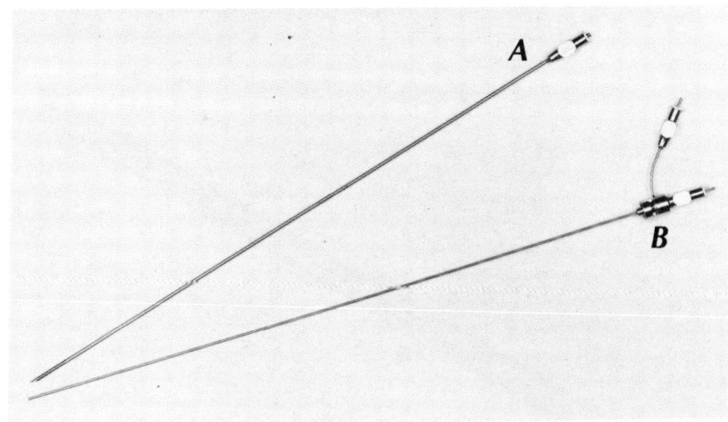

Figure 7-1
The King's College Hospital follicle aspiration needle.
A: the sharp ended, disposable outer needle;
B: the blunt ended, reuseable inner channel.

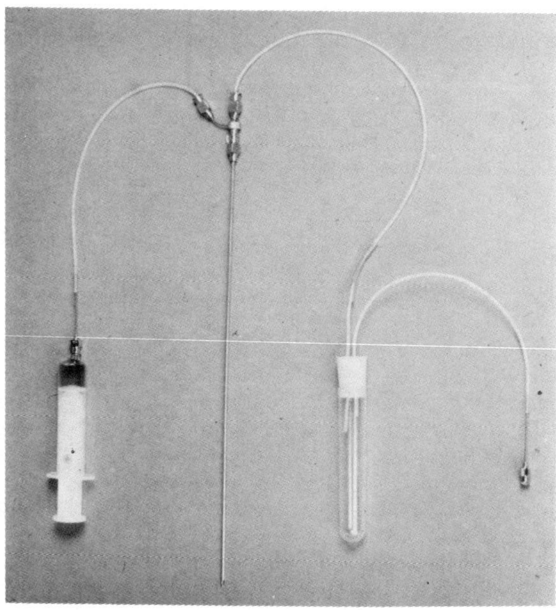

Figure 7-2
The King's College Hospital follicle aspiration needle assembled, and connected to the syringe and test tube with PTFE tubing.

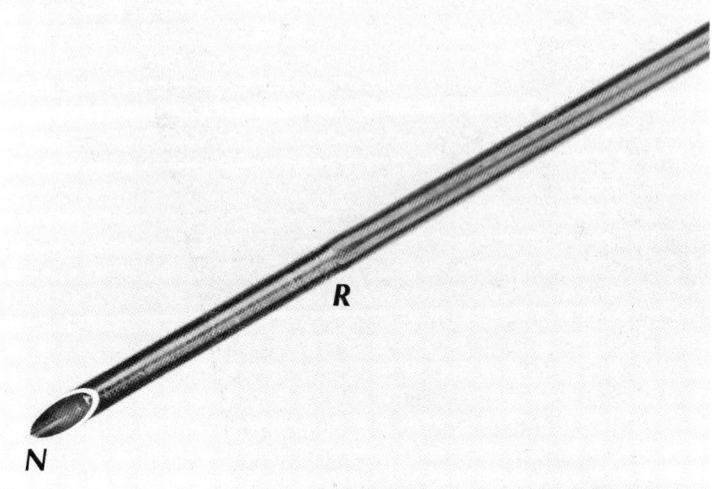

Figure 7-3
Magnified view of the King's College Hospital follicle aspiration needle showing the tip (*N*) and the roughened segment (***R***).

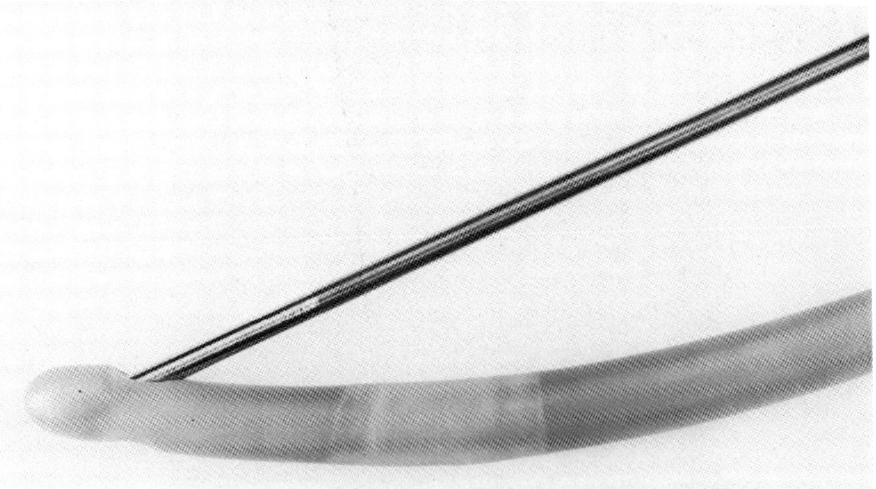

Figure 7-4
The King's College Hospital follicle aspiration needle inside the tip of a Foley catheter.

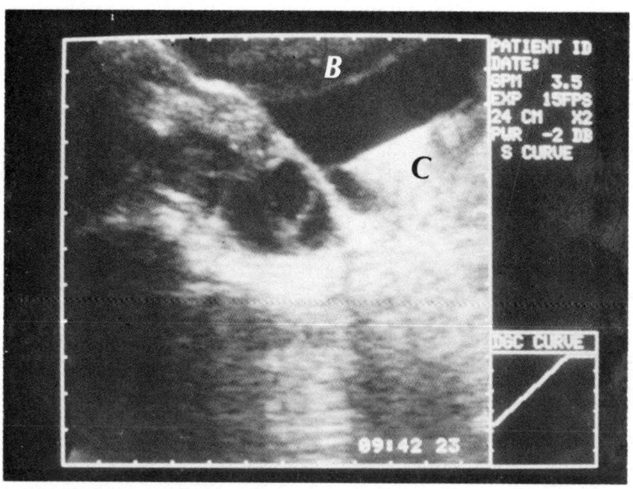

Figure 7-5
Perurethral UDFA: ultrasound image of the King's College follicle aspiration needle within the bladder (*B*), demonstrating the "curtain" of reverberation (*C*) beneath the needle.

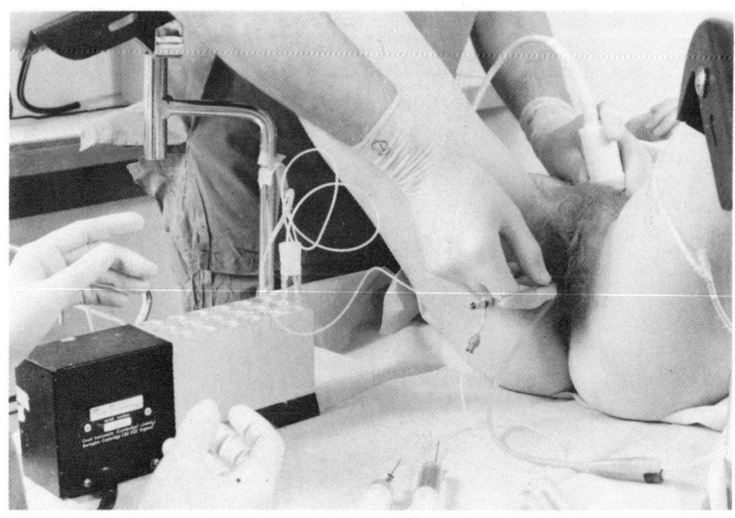

Figure 7-6
Perurethral UDFA: picture showing the needle and catheter *in situ*; follicular fluid is aspirated into the test tube in the metal block maintained at 37°C.

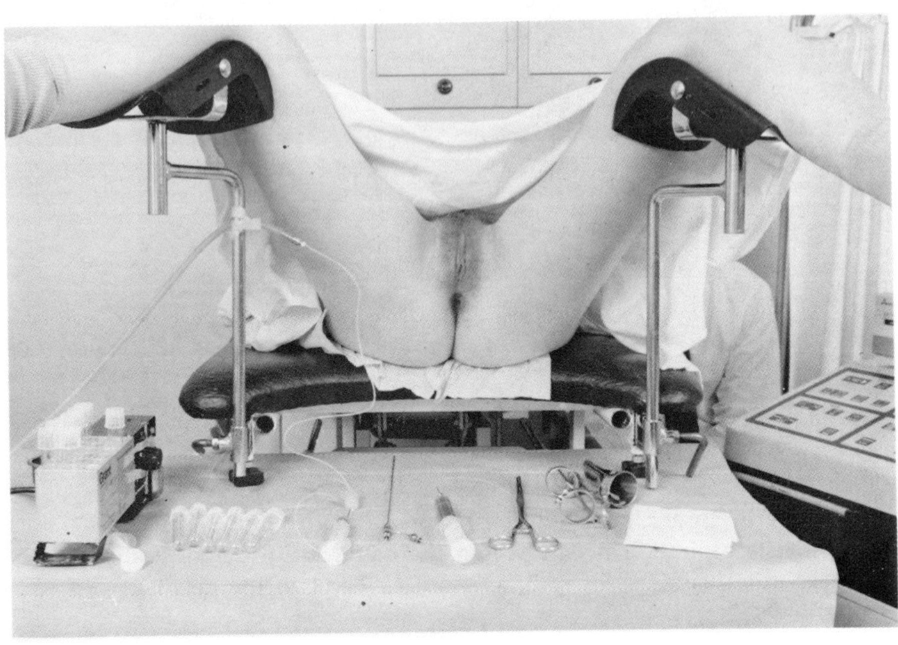

Figure 7-7
Transvaginal UDFA: picture showing the patient and equipment ready for egg collection.

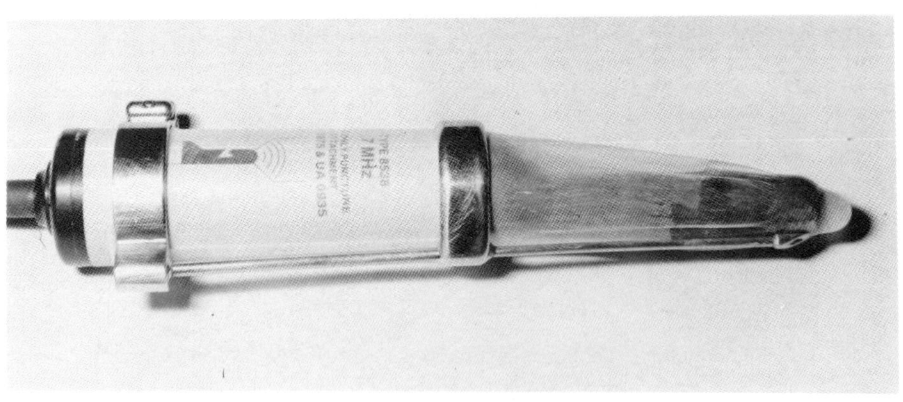

Figure 7-8
Transvaginal UDFA: the Bruel and Kjaer needle guide over the sheathed Bruel and Kjaer vaginal ultrasound transducer.

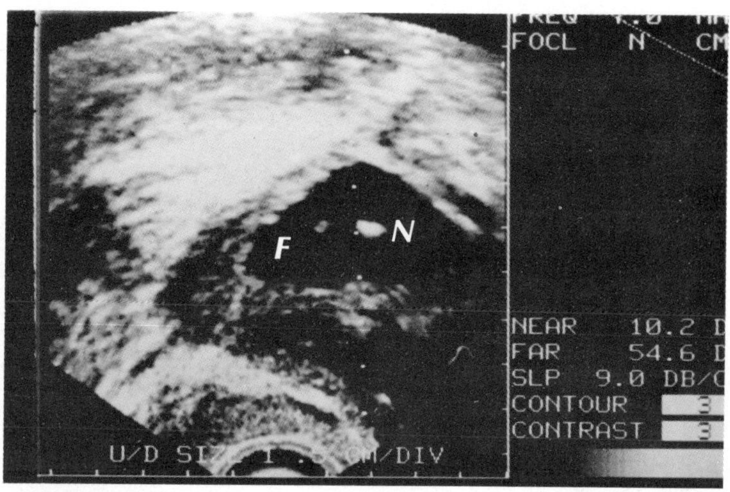

Figure 7-9
Transvaginal UDFA: ultrasound image of the needle tip (*N*) within the follicle (*F*).

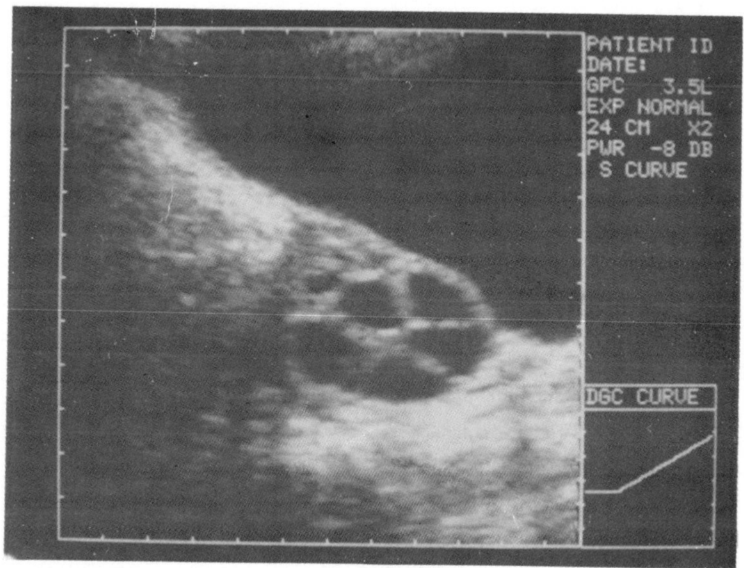

Figure 7-10
Transabdominal UDFA: ultrasound image of a hyperstimulated ovary prior to egg collection.

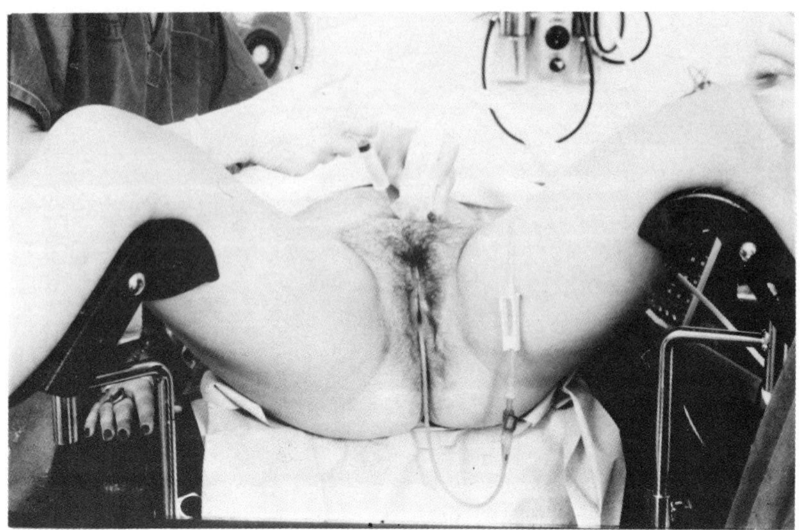

Figure 7-11
Transabdominal UDFA: picture showing the patient's position and infiltration of the anterior abdominal wall with local anaesthetic.

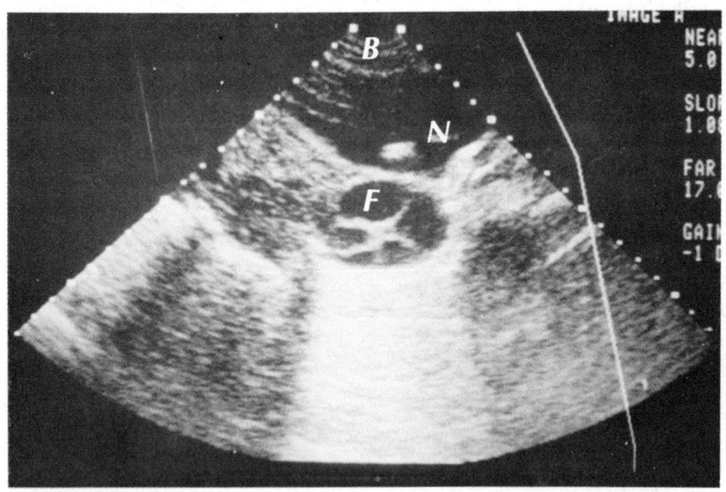

Figure 7-12
Transabdominal UDFA: ultrasound image of the needle tip (*N*) inside the bladder (*B*), before entering an ovarian follicle (*F*).

Picture by courtesy of Dr. V. Sharma.

References

Chamberlain, G.V.P. and Brown, J.C. *Report of the working party of the confidential enquiry into gynaecological laparoscopy.* London Royal College of Obstetricians and Gynaecologists, 1978, 105.

Cohen, J., Fehilly, C.B., Fishel, S.B., Edwards, R.G., Hewitt, J., Rowland, G.F., Steptoe, P.C. and Webster, J. Male infertility successfully treated by in vitro fertilization. *Lancet,* 1984; ii: 1239.

Dellenbach, P., Nisand, I., Moreau, L., Feger, B., Plumere, C., Gerlinger, P., Brun, B. and Rumpler, Y. Transvaginal, sonographically controlled ovarian follicle puncture for oocyte retrieval. *Lancet,* 1984; i: 1467.

Feichtinger, W. and Kemeter, P. Transvaginal sector sonography for needle guided transvaginal follicle aspiration and other applications in gynaecologic routine and research. *Fertility and Sterility,* 1986; 45: 722.

Lenz, S., Lauristen, J.G. and Kjellow, M. Collection of human oocytes for in vitro fertilisation by ultrasonically guided follicular puncture. *Lancet,* 1981; i: 1163.

Lopata, A., Patullo, M.J., Chang, A. and James, B. A method for collecting motile spermatozoa from human semen. *Fertility and Sterility,* 1976; 27: 677.

Parsons, J., Riddle, A., Booker, M., Sharma, V., Goswami, R., Wilson, L., Akkermans, J., Whitehead, M. and Campbell, S. Oocyte retrieval for in vitro fertilisation by ultrasonically guided needle aspiration via the urethra. *Lancet,* 1985; i: 1076.

Riddle, A.F., Sharma, V., Mason, B., Ford, N.T., Pampiglione, J.S. and Parsons, J. and Campbell, S. Two years' experience of ultrasound-directed oocyte retrieval. *Fertility and Sterility,* 1987; 48: 454.

Steptoe, P.C., Edwards, R.G. and Purdy, J.M. Clinical aspects of pregnancies established with cleaving embryos grown in vitro. *British Journal of Obstetrics and Gynaecology,* 1980; 87: 757.

Trounson, A. and Conti, A. Research in human in vitro fertilisation and embryo transfer. *British Medical Journal,* 1982; 285: 244.

Wikland, M., Nilsson, L., Hansson, R., Hamberger, L. and Janson, P.O. Collection of human oocytes by the use of sonography. *Fertility and Sterility,* 1983; 39: 603.

Wikland, M., Lennart, E. and Hamberger, L. Transvesical and transvaginal approaches for the aspiration of follicles by the use of ultrasound. *Annals of New York Academy of Science,* 1985; 442: 182.

Wood, C., Downing, B., Trounson, A. and Rogers, P. Clinical implications of developments in in vitro fertilisation. *British Medical Journal,* 1984; 289: 987.

8
GIFT: Current status in infertility management

P.C. Wong, C.L.K. Chan, A. Bongsu, S.C. Ng, Y.C. Wong, C. Anandakumar, V.H.H. Goh and S.S. Ratnam

Introduction

Five years ago, Asch and colleagues (1984, 1985) reported the first pregnancy following translaparoscopic gamete intrafallopian transfer (GIFT), followed by the subsequent delivery of the patient of a pair of twins. Since then the GIFT technique has found wide application in many infertility clinics around the world (Borrero, 1988; Confino et al, 1986; Corson et al, 1986; Guastella et al, 1985; Jansen et al, 1987; Lim-Howe et al, 1987; Madden et al, 1986; Molley et al, 1987; Matson et al, 1987; Wong et al, 1988; Yovich et al, 1988). This chapter will discuss the clinical results from the GIFT programme at the National University of Singapore. It will also show some data from the International Multicentric Study and finally discuss the future development of the technique.

Materials and methods

Between August 1985 to March 1987, 138 treatment cycles of GIFT were carried out on couples whose infertility ranged from 3 to 20 years, with a mean of 8.1 years. The female partners were aged between 27 and 42 years, with a mean $\pm$ SD of 34.5 $\pm$ 7.5 and a median of 34.5 years. The male partners on the other hand were aged 27–60 years with a mean $\pm$2SD of 37.6 $\pm$ 9.5 and a median of 37.0 years.

Induction of multiple follicular development

Four stimulation regimens were used. Patients on clomiphene, human menopausal gonadotrophin (hMG), received clomiphene citrate 50 mg twice a day between days two and six of the menstrual cycle. From days four to eight, hMG, (Pergonal®, Serono, Switzerland and Humegon®, Organon, Netherlands) two ampoules were given intra-muscularly. From cycle day nine onwards, the dose of hMG was individualised, based on the oestradiol response and follicular growth on ovarian ultrasonography. The second regimen used was a pure FSH-hMG combination. From day two to six of the menstrual cycle, the patients received pure FSH (Metrodin®, Serono, Switzerland) two ampoules (150 iu) daily from day two to six; the dose being individualised from day seven. The third stimulation regimen was a combination of gonadotrophin releasing hormone agonist — hMG. In this regimen, the patient self-administered intranasal Buserelin® (Hoechst, Frankfurt FRG) 400 μg eight-hourly for 15 days beginning on day 22 of the menstrual cycle. Day 16 was re-designated day one of the treatment cycle when the patient commenced daily hMG two ampoules till day five. The dose was individualised from day six. The fourth stimulation regimen was hMG alone. Patients received two ampoules hMG from day two to six. The dose was individualised from day seven.

Monitoring of follicular development

All the patients were monitored by serial ovarian ultrasonography and plasma oestradiol assays. The ultrasound scans were carried out on days six and eight of the cycle, and thereafter daily when the follicles reached 14mm in diameter. Plasma oestradiol assays were carried out daily beginning on day six.

Human chorionic gonadotrophin (hCG) administration

hCG (Pregnyl®, Organon, Netherlands or Profasi®, Serono, Switzerland) 5000 iu was given when the ultrasound scan showed at least two follicles with diameters $\geq$ 16mm and plasma oestradiol of about 300 pg/ml per large follicle. The hCG is usually administered 30–36 hours after the last dose of hMG.

Semen preparation

Semen from the husbands were obtained in split ejaculates two to two-and-a-half hours before oocyte recovery. The better fraction was used for semen processing. The sample was divided into 1ml aliquots and each washed with 2ml of T6 medium and centrifuged at 1000rpm, with the procedure being repeated once. The resulting sperm pellet was then layered with 0.3ml of medium and incubated at 37°C for 60 minutes after which the supernatant was removed. The final sperm concentration was adjusted to 10 million sperm/ml (100,000 per 10ul).

Oocyte recovery and identification

Oocyte recovery was carried out by laparoscopy under general anaesthesia 34 to 36 hours after hCG injection. Follicular fluid were aspirated in 5ml Falcon tubes. If oocytes were not found in the follicular fluid, the follicles were then flushed with T6 medium supplemented with 10 per cent heat inactivated serum. The oocytes were kept in a 37°C incubator in an atmosphere of 5 per cent CO_2, 5 per cent 0_2 and 90 per cent N2 until transferred.

Gamete loading and GIFT

After oocyte recovery was completed, the oocytes (usually two) were selected and loaded into a catheter (Mets 2020 or Teflon Reproductive Transfer Catheter, Cook, Melbourne, Australia) together with 100,000 motile sperm. The catheter was then introduced into the fimbrial ostium of the fallopian tube and its contents expelled into the ampulla. The same procedure was repeated on the other tube. No more than four oocytes were transferred to each patient.

Luteal phase support

Five days after the GIFT procedure, all patients except those on the clomiphene-hMG stimulation regimen received an intramuscular injection of 25mg progesterone-in-oil for luteal support.

Confirmation of pregnancy

β-hCG was measured at 14 and 16 days after GIFT. Two positive hCG tests were required to confirm pregnancy. This was followed by an ultrasound scan four weeks after the GIFT procedure. The demonstration of foetal heart activity was necessary to confirm the presence of a clinical pregnancy.

Results

The 138 GIFT treatment cycles resulted in 34 clinical pregnancies (24.6 per cent), seven of whom miscarried (29.2 per cent) (Table 8-1).

The mean number of oocytes recovered from each of the four stimulation regimens and their respective pregnancy rates are summarised in Table 8-2.

The pregnancy rates among the various etiological groups are summarised in Table 8-3. Patients with a male factor problem had relatively poorer outcomes.

Among the 34 clinical pregnancies were six twins and one triplet, giving a multiple pregnancy rate of 20.6 per cent (Table 8-4).

The relationship between pregnancy rates and number of oocytes transferred are given in Table 8-5. There was no pregnancy with only one oocyte transferred. The chances of pregnancy when two, three and four oocytes were transferred were 8.3, 25.0 and 28.0 per cent respectively. No multiple pregnancy occurred when two oocytes were transferred. Multiple pregnancies were obtained when three oocytes (20.0 per cent) and four (21.4 per cent) were transferred.

Five or more oocytes were recovered in 63 patients. Four were transferred and the excess inseminated. Excess eggs from 24 patients did not show fertilisation, yet five of the patients conceived (20.8 per cent). In the remaining 39 patients where their excess eggs fertilised, 16 (41.0 per cent) conceived. This difference was not statistically significant (Table 8-6).

International multicentric study

An international multicentric study of GIFT was initiated by Dr Ricardo Asch in 1985 to evaluate this new reproductive technique. To obtain sufficient data for this purpose, a large number of treatment cycles over a short period of time was required. Therefore, 12 centres were identified around the world. The centres and their participating investigators were:

(1) R.H. Asch, USA
(2) E. Cittadini, Italy
(3) De Cecco, Italy
(4) De Vroey, Belgium
(5) V. Gomel, Canada
(6) Hohl, Switzerland
(7) I. Johnston, Australia
(8) J. Leeton, Australia
(9) Noss, FRG
(10) Rodriguez-Escudero, Spain
(11) P.C. Wong, Singapore
(12) J. Yovich, Australia

A total of 2092 treatment cycles were pooled together. Of these, 601 women became pregnant (28.7 per cent) (Asch, 1987). The pregnancy rate by the different etiological groups is shown in Table 8-7. The overall incidence of miscarriage was 16.8 per cent, ectopic pregnancy 3.9 per cent, and multiple pregnancy 15.4 per cent.

Directions for the future

From our study, the pregnancy rates in the male factor category with oligoasthenospermia was 17.1 per cent, compared with 31.4 per cent in the unexplained, and 26.7 per cent in the endometriosis groups. Data from the multicentric study also supported this observation ie. male factor 15 per cent compared with 31 per cent, and 32 per cent in the unexplained and endometriotic groups respectively. This is due to low fertilisation rates from the use of inferior quality sperm from the male factor group. This observation also concurs with Matson (1987). To overcome this problem, the oocyte should be fertilised initially in vitro and then transferred to achieve higher pregnancy rates. Yovich et al (1988) therefore reported their technique of pronuclear stage tubal traansfer (PROST) in couples with oligospermia, asthenospermia and antispermatozoal antibodies. They obtained 30 pregnancies from 81 transfers (31.0 per cent). The pregnancy rates were 16.7 per cent, 43.5 per cent, 41.2 per cent, 47.4 per cent and 25.0 per cent when one, two, three, four and five embryos were transferred respectively. It appears therefore that PROST may be applicable to couples with male factor problems. Its value for other categories of infertility remains to be seen.

With the advent of ultrasound directed oocyte recovery procedures, in vitro fertilisation and embryo replacement (IVF-ER) techniques have become outpatient procedures, reducing patient inconvenience and cost. The GIFT procedure may follow suit. Oocyte recovery may be carried out by ultrasound guidance and the gametes transferred by hysteroscopy into the fallopian tubes. Recently, Jansen and Anderson (1987) have demonstrated catheterisation of the fallopian tubes retrograde from the vagina. They reported pregnancies after ultrasound guided fallopian insemination with cryostored semen (Jansen, 1988). This technique may enable GIFT to be performed without the need for laparoscopy, on an outpatient basis.

Acknowledgement

The authors would like to thank Drs E.L. Yong, F.K. Lim, A. Kurup and S. Davendra, the nursing and the technical staff for their assistance, and Ms Asma Bevi for typing the manuscript.

Table 8-1
GIFT pregnancies

	Number	Per cent
No. of treatment cycles	138	
No. of conceptions	41	(29.7)
Biochemical pregnancy	7	
Clinical pregnancy	34	(24.6)
Delivery	27	
Abortion	7	(29.2)

Table 8-2
Stimulation regimens

	N	*Mean No. oocytes*	*No. pregnancy*	*Per cent*
CC - hMG	9	3.8	1	11.1
FSH - hMG	109	6.9	27	24.8
GnRHa - hMG	2	7.5	1	50.0
hMG	18	5.3	5	27.8

Table 8-3
Pregnancy by etiology

Etiology	*N*	*Clinical pregnancy*	*Per cent*
Unexplained	51	16	31.4
Endometriosis	30	8	26.7
Oligospermia	35	6	17.1
Oligospermia + endometriosis	4	0	0
Others	18	4	22.2

Table 8-4
Multiple pregnancies

	Number	*Per cent*
No. of treatment cycles	138	
Clinical pregnancy	34	
Singleton	27	
Twins	6	} 20.6
Triplets	1	

Table 8-5
Pregnancy rates (including multiple pregnancies) by number of oocytes transferred

No. of oocytes transferred	No. of cycles	No. of pregnancies	Per cent	No. of multiple pregnancies	Per cent
0	4	0	0	0	0
1	2	0	0	0	0
2	12	1	8.3	0	0
3	20	5	25.0	1	20.0
4	100	28	28.0	6	21.4

Table 8-6
Correlation of IVF of excess oocytes with outcome of GIFT

IVF of excess oocytes	*Pregnant with GIFT*	*Not pregnant with GIFT*	*Total*
No fertilisation	5 (20.8%)	19 (79.2%)	24
Fertilisation	16 (41.0%)	23 (59.0%)	39

Table 8-7
Pregnancy rates by etiological groups

Etiology	*No. of cases*	*No. pregnant*	*Per cent*
Unexplained	796	247	31
Mole	397	61	15
Endometriosis	413	132	32
Failed AID	160	66	41
Tubal peritoneal	210	61	29
Cervical	68	19	28
Immunological	30	5	10
Premature ovarian failure	18	10	56
Total	2092	601	28.7

References

Asch, R.H., *GIFT: A multicentric international study.* VIth World Congress on Human Reproduction, Tokyo, 1987.

Asch, R.H., Ellsworth, L.R., Balmaceda, J.P. and Wong P.C. Pregnancy following translaparoscopic gamete intrafallopian transfer. *Lancet*, 1984; 2: 1034.

Asch, R.H., Ellworth, L.R., Balmaceda, J.P. and Wong P.C. Birth following gamete intrafallopian transfer. *Lancet*, 1985; 2: 163.

Borrero, C., Ord, T., Balmaceda, J.P., Rojas, F.J. and Asch, R.H. The GIFT experience: An evaluation of the outcome of 115 cases. *Human Reproduction*, 1988; 3: 227.

Confino, E., Friberg, J. and Gleicher, N. A new stirrable catheter for gamete intrafallopian tube transfer (GIFT) communications-in-brief. *Fertility and Sterility*, 1986; 46: 1147.

Corson, S.L., Batzer, F., Eisenberg, E et al. Early experience with the GIFT procedure. *Journal of Reproductive Medicine*, 1986; 31: 219.

Guastella, G., Comparetto, A.G. and Gullo, D. Gamete intrafallopian transfer (GIFT): A new technique for the treatment of unexplained infertility. *Acta Europaea Fertilitatis*, 1985; 16: 311.

Guastella, G., Comparetto, A.G., Palermo, R., Cefalu, E., Ciriminna, R. and Gittadini, E. Gamete intrafallopian transfer in the treatment of infertility: The first series at the University of Palermo. *Fertility and Sterility*, 1986; 46: 417.

Jansen, R.P.S., Anderson, J.C. Catheterisation of the fallopian tubes from the vagina. *Lancet*, 1987; 2: 309.

Jansen, R.P.S., Anderson, J.C., Radonic, I., Smit, J. and Sutherland, P.D. Pregnancies after ultrasound-guided fallopian insemination with cryostored donor semen. *Fertility and Sterility*, 1988; 49: 920.

Lim-Howe, D., Studd, J. and Dooley, M. Gamete intrafallopian transfer (GIFT). *British Journal of Hospital Medicine*, 1987; March: 241.

Madden, J.D., Bookout, D.M., Siverstein, E.H. et al. GIFT — Pregnancy by translaparoscopic gamete intrafallopian transfer. *Dallas Medical Journal*, 1986; 72: 15.

Matson, P.L., Blackledge, D.G., Richardson, P.A., Turner S.R., Yovich, J.M. and Yovich, J.L. The role of gamete intrafallopian transfer (GIFT) in the treatment of oligospermic infertility. *Fertility and Sterility*, 1987; 48: 608.

Molloy, D., Speirs, A., du Plessis, Y., McBain, J. and Johnston, I. A laparoscopic spproach to a program of gamete intrafallopian transfer. *Fertility and Sterility*, 1987; 47: 289.

Wong P.C., Ng S.C., Hamilton, M.P.R., Anandakumar, C., Wong Y.C. and Ratnam, S.S. Eighty consecutive cases of gamete intrafallopian transfer. *Human Reproduction*, 1988; 3: 231.

Yovich, J.L., Yovich, J.M. and Edirisinghe, W.R. The relative chance of pregnancy following tubal or uterine transfer procedures. *Fertility and Sterility*, 1988; 49: 858.

9

Laboratory IVF technology

A. Bongso, S.C. Ng and S.S. Ratnam

Introduction

> "On the 27th of April, 1890, two ova were collected from an Angora doe rabbit which had been fertilised by an Angora buck 32 hours previously; the ova were undergoing segmentation into 4 segments. These ova were immediately transferred into the upper end of the Fallopian tube of a Belgian doe rabbit which had been mated 3 hours before by a buck of the same breed as herself. . . . In due course the Belgian doe gave birth to 6 young: 4 of these resembled herself and her mate while 2 were undoubtedly Angoras" . . . . . (W. Heape, 1890).

This was the first report of a successful embryo transfer. The experiment was designed to determine (i) the effects, if any, of a foster mother on her foster children and (ii) whether the presence and development of foreign ova in the uterus would have any effect on the offspring of that mother.

From this experience, embryo transfer was extended to the animal farm industry by veterinarians to accelerate genetic progress in livestock by transferring embryos from genetically superior donors to inferior recipients. Basically, superior donor animals were superovulated, inseminated artificially using superior sperm and the embryos flushed out non-surgically via a transvaginal approach. The embryos were then non-surgically transferred to inferior recipients who take on the role of surrogate mothers. The offspring then formed a gene pool for future breeding.

As far back as 1949, Rowson and Dowling had already designed an apparatus for the non-surgical collection of cattle embryos. Later, in 1950, Rowson reported the first stimulation regime for cattle. In 1955, Averill and others described the use of the rabbit oviduct as an "incubator" for the aerial transport of sheep embryos. It is estimated today that in Europe, Australia and U.S.A. at least 50,000 to 100,000 embryos transfers are carried out annually. This technique has been extended to horses, sheep, goats, pigs, and zoo animals with variable success.

The first confirmed success of in vitro fertilisation (IVF) was in 1959 in the rabbit (Chang, 1959) by M.C. Chang. Just before this, the observation was made (Austin, 1951; Chang, 1951) that sperm required pretreatment in the female genital tract (capacitation) before fertilisation. Successful IVF was also reported by Yanagimachi and Chang in the hamster in 1964 followed by the mouse in 1968 by Whittingham. These discoveries set the stage for human IVF. In 1969, Edwards and others reported the successful fertilisation of human oocytes leading to the birth of the first test tube baby in February 1978 (Edwards et al, 1980). However, IVF in non-human primates lagged behind the work carried out in man. The first successful IVF in the non-human primate was the squirrel monkey in 1973 (Gould, 1973) followed by the baboon in 1979 (Gould, 1979) and the chimpanzee in 1983 (Gould, 1983).

Today, IVF has become routine for the treatment of infertility. It has also become commercial. Trounson (1986) very aptly stated that in the pursuit of increasing numbers of IVF pregnancies, there has been little rationalisation of progress, on occasions misrepresentations of results, a loss of fundamental scientific design in studies presented, and a failure to properly address the ethical implications of experimental embryology.

Laboratory design, equipment and procedures for IVF

The physical arrangement, laboratory setup, and culture procedures for an IVF laboratory are now standardised, and excellent reviews have been published. Table 9-1 summarises the various steps used in IVF, from collection of oocytes to the 4-cell stage of embryonic stage before replacement. Each laboratory may individualise its technique, depending upon its experience. The objective should be the simplification of the various laboratory procedure without compromising quality control, fertilisation rate and pregnancy success.

Innovations in laboratory IVF technology

New techniques in laboratory IVF are being developed in order to improve fertilisation and pregnancy rates. The areas of interest include the improvement of sperm quality, overcoming intrinsic egg problems, predicting embryonic viability, studying implantation phenomena, quality control, and exploring alternatives should IVF fail.

Improvement of sperm quality

The husband is usually requested to abstain from sex 48–72 hours before producing a sample for IVF. Semen is collected in a sterile container by masturbation either two hours before insemination or before the pick-up. Some laboratories prefer a split ejaculate collected in two containers, as the first emission has a higher percentage of motile sperm. If the husband has a problem in producing a sample, semen could be collected earlier and stored forzen. In most IVF laboratories semen is processed by the "swim-up" technique. Briefly, the seminal plasma is removed from the sample by washing with culture medium containing 7.5 to 10 per cent of the wife's serum, and centrifugation. The procedure is repeated again and the sperm pellet gently layered over with medium. The preparation is incubated for half to one hour at 37°C in five per cent of CO_2 to allow motile sperms to swim-up into the medium. Approximately 100,000 sperms from the layer is used for insemination per egg.

Sperm density and motility are two most important criteria for successful fertilisation. Approximately 500,000 sperms per egg has been recommended for asthenozoospermic samples. Recent studies using the 1987 WHO ratings (0–4) for forward progressive motility showed that a motility rating of two was the cutoff point for successful fertilisation. Sperm with motility ratings of ≥ 2 yielded over 70 per cent fertilisation rates per cohort of eggs compared with ≤ 10 per cent for ratings less than two. Further studies by Mahadevan and others (1987) on sperm binding to eggs also revealed that forward progressive motility was the single most important factor influencing successful fertilisation. The recommended minimum semen quality is 2,500,000 motile sperms in the entire ejaculate with a swim-up motility rating of two or greater.

Density gradients

If these criteria are not met, other semen preparation techniques may have to be employed. These include the Percoll gradient (Dravland et al, 1985), Ficoll entrapment (Cummins et al, 1984), glass bead column (Bongso et al, 1987) and glass woll filtration method (Neff et al, 1987). The Percoll gradient is the most popular. Briefly, the method involves the preparation of two gradients (45 per cent, 90 per cent) of Percoll (silica gel) layered one over the other in sterile tubes. The semen is layered on the surface of the upper 45 per cent gradient and the sample centrifuged. Centrifugation times vary with the quality of the semen sample. The motile sperms are recovered from the bottom (button), which is washed several times to rid the Percoll before use. Recovery of sperm seems to be better by this method for very poor samples. Some laboratories find the Percoll gradient technique unreliable.

Microfertilisation (Microinjection)

If the minimum semen parameters for IVF are not attained with these methods, the next recourse is the microinjection of sperms into eggs (microfertilisation) using the micromanipulator. Successful microfertilisation of human oocytes with oligoasthenozoospermic sperm has been achieved by our group at the National University Hospital. Microinjection has found implications in the treatment of severe male infertility. Motility is not a prerequisite, as long as sperms are viable. The fertilisation of a human egg mechanically denuded of its zona and incubated with capacitated sperm from a patient with immotile cilia syndrome was reported (Ng et al, 1987). Recently, fertilisation of the same patient's oocytes was accomplished by our group with immotile sperm from her husband who was suffering from immotile cilia syndrome. Three 3–6 stage embryos were replaced, with no resulting pregnancy.

Sperm motility enhancing agents

Agents that could potentially enhance sperm motility in asthenozoospermic males are being investigated. Caffeine, hyaluronic acid (pure) and theophylline are known to increase the motility of bovine sperm. We showed a significant activation of sperm exposed to caffeine or cyclic AMP, but forward progressive motility was not enhanced. Preliminary observations on fertilisation rates using caffeine treated sperm did not yield significantly better results although lateral displacement of the head of sperm was greatly increased. A comparative study of fertilisation rates was undertaken by Steen et al (1986) between the conventional "swim-up" procedure and sperm layered directly with pure high molecular weight hyaluronic acid without centrifugation. In the HAPP (Hyaluronic Acid Penetration, Pharmacia) group, 56 per cent eggs fertilised and cleaved compared with 53 per cent for the "swim-up" group. The authors concluded that it was possible to prepare sperms for IVF without the use of centrifugation and still achieve an acceptable fertilisation rate. It was speculated that centrifugation could damage sperm.

"Cell-soft"

Many established IVF laboratories are now using computer automated semen analysis ("Cell-soft"). Semen samples (fresh and after "swim-up") can be analysed both by manual microscopic methods and "Cell-soft". Linearity, velocity, amplitude of lateral head displacement (ALH) of sperm motion, percentage motile sperm and sperm counts can all be assessed through image analysis using a computerised microscope. The machine is easy to operate and results are rapid. Subjective motility ratings can be transformed into numerical values and a histogram of linearity and velocity of groups of sperms obtained. The "Cell-soft" system provides more detailed information on male factor patients and improves selection criteria for couples before being admitted for IVF programmes. The system can transform forward progressive motility ratings in microns/sec to the standard 1987 WHO scale of 0–4.

Sperm agglutination

Sperm agglutinating antibodies seem to interfere with fertilisation and subsequent cleavage. The problem is immunological and these antibodies are derived in the serum or seminal plasma. These antibodies coating the sperm has been reported as a cause of immunological infertility (Jones, 1986). Sperm antibodies belong to the IgA and IgG classes. The presence of these antibodies can now be tested using the mixed antiglobulin reaction (MAR) test or the immunobead method. The immunobead method is popular and simpler to use. Immunobeads are polyacrylamide spheres bound covalently with rabbit anti-human immunoglobulin. Motile sperm with surface antibodies adhere to the immunobeads. The proportion of sperm with surface antibodies and class of antibodies responsible are determined using the specific immunobead. If the patient's serum is positive, donor serum is used for preparing both insemination and growth media for IVF.

Sperm capacitation

Sperm capacitation is an essential prerequisite for mammalian fertilisation. Assessment of the degree of capacitation of a sperm sample can predict the outcome of fertilisation and the number of embryos available for replacement. Bioassays have been the traditional methods of assessment of capacitation. They include the penetration of zona free hamster eggs, the penetration of zona of non-living oocytes, or a combination of both approaches. These assays are laborious and do not reflect the actual physiological events of fertilisation. Alternatively, a qualitative estimate of the percentage acrosome reaction (AR) in a sperm population can performed. A triple stain method is used to differentiate between intact acrosome and AR sperm (Tablot et al, 1981). Some laboratories use a monoclonal antibody against the human acrosome (HS19 and HS21) (Wolf et al, 1985). The antibody binds to sperm with intact acrosomes and is detected by immunofluorescence. Recently, a clortetracycline (CTC) fluorescence assay was developed for capacitation and AR in human sperm (Lee et al, 1987). When capacitated sperm was treated with either ionophore A23187 or acid solubilised mouse zona pellucidae to induce AR, the CTC assay identified AR sperm by lack of fluorescence on the head.

Sperm binding

Sperm binding on the zone of human oocytes has been shown to provide information that is indicative of sperm function. A hemi-zona assay (HZA) was developed to assess IVF potential (Burkman et al, 1987). Hemi-zonas (HZ) were obtained from human eggs bisected by micromanipulative surgery to provide equal functional surfaces. HZ were incubated with fertile sperm and a matching HZ exposed to a subfertile sample. After three to four hours sperm that were firmly attached were counted following vigorous micropipetting of the HZ. The mean number of firmly attached sperm was found to be significantly greater for fertilised versus non-fertilised groups (8.7:1) Sperm motility and the number of motile sperm used to inseminate oocytes were correlated significantly with the number of sperm bound to the zonae whereas sperm morphology and sperm concentration did not. The authors concluded that sperm motility was the single most important factor influencing fertilisation of human oocytes in vitro.

Intrinsic egg problems

Chromosome analysis of oocytes

Three hundred and two unfertilised oocytes left over from successful IVF attempts in 143 women showed a 21 per cent chromosomal aneuploidy (Bongso et al, 1988a): 13 per cent hypohaploid (n=19 to 22), 8 per cent were hyperhaploid (n=24 to 26), 2 per cent were diploid and 0.4 per cent had structural rearrangements. Chromosomes were missing or extra in the A, B, C, D, E and G, groups of the human karyotype. The mean age of the patients showing aneuploid oocytes was 36.7 years, which was above the mean for the entire group. It was postulated that the aneuploidy was the result of errors in oogenesis (anaphase lagging or non-disjunction). Aneuploidy percentages of 21 to 57 per cent were also observed by other workers. (Plachot et al, 1986; Wramsby et al, 1987). These percentages were found in patient exposed to three conventional stimulation regimen. It is tempting to suggest that such abnormal chromosomal behaviour may be directly related to the stimulation regimen. The report offers one possible explanation for fertilisation failure in vitro and the overall low pregnancy rates in IVF programme. A 10 per cent incidence of premature chromosome condensation (PCC) has also been observed in human oocytes failing to fertilise in vitro (Bongso et al, 1987). This segregation distortion of chromosomes was suggested to be related to maturation problems in vitro, possibly caused by inadequate levels of a chromosome condensation factor (CCF) or maturation inhibition factor (MIF).

Oocyte maturation

All oocytes obtained at laparoscopy may not have completed maturation despite the appearance of cimulus, absence of germinal vesicle and nuclear chromatin changes. Studies on the maturation of sheep oocytes have conclusively shown that delay in insemination gave a dramatic improvement in the fertilisation of oocytes, their development to blastocycsts, and the birth of live young (Trounson, 1982). Human oocytes in IVF programmes are incubated in vitro at 37°C in culture media for five to six hours after collection, before insemination. This enhances fertilisation rates by maturing the oocyte and decreases the incidence of polyspermy because of maturation of the cortical granules. Delay in insemination of up to 12 hours or longer has been shown to cause delayed cleavage, increased fragmentation, and retarded embryo development (Trounson, 1982). The laborious task of examining eggs every four hours for maturation before insemination is no longer practised, since a single cohort of eggs will have matured in five to six hours in vitro.

Zona drilling and zona cutting

Zona drilling (Gordon et al, 1986) and zona cutting (Tsunoda et al, 1986) are two innovative techniques that have been successfully carried out in mice and may assist fertilisation in man. These techniques have potential for use in women with intrinsic egg problems (eg. zona hardening) when fertilisation fails even though the semen is of good quality. Zona drilling and zona cutting may be attempted before resorting to microinjection of sperm. Drilling of the zona of the mouse oocyte using the micromanipulator and acidified Tyrode's medium was shown to assist fertilisation at low sperm concentration without compromising embryonic development. Cutting of the zona of mouse oocytes with the micromanipulator also resulted in increased fertilisation rates. In another study, mouse zonae were cracked using two fine glass hooks fitted to a micromanipulator and exposed to mouse epididymal sperm (Odawara et al, 1987). This resulted in significantly higher fertilisation rates and a low incidence of polyspermy. Unlike micro-injection, these techniques allow natural in vitro fertilisation with poor quality sperm while retaining a degree of sperm self selectivity.

Embryo banks

Excess embryos obtined in an IVF or GIFT programme are usually frozen for later replacement in unstimulated cycles. A slow programmed freezing has been the method of choice using dimethylsuphoxide (DMSO), or 1, 2 propanediol (PROH) as cyroprotectants. The freezing equipment is expensive and the technique time consuming, as the temperature of the embryo has to be gradually brought down through several steps before plunging into liquid nitrogen at −196°C. Recently, Trounson and others (1987) reported a simple, inexpensive method (ultrarapid) of freezing using DMSO on mouse embryos without recourse to a freezing machine. The authors obtained an over 80 per cent embryo survival, and healthy offspring were produced through pseudopregnant foster mothers. The technique involved exposing the embryos to 3.5M DMSO for three minutes, loading in straws and plunging directly into liquid nitrogen without seeding.

Similar survival rates were also obtained by Bongso and others (1988b) when either DMSO or PROH were used as cryoprotectants. However, in this study, a 3.5 per cent incidence of chromosomal mitotic crossing over was observed in the DMSO ultrarapid group, which was not present in the PROH-ultrarapid group and the controls. This mitotic crossing over may result in the birth of offspring that are phenotypically normal but mosaics. The incidence of aneuploidy and polyploidy was the same as controls.

If the technique is to be used on human embryos with DMSO as a cryoprotectant, it may be necessary to identify the duration of the mitotic cycle of the blastomeres of the 2-cell embryo and freeze embryos at a particular stage in this cycle that will be least prone to chromosomal rearrangement. Alternatively, the PROH ultrarapid straw method may be a simplified freezing method for human embryos in the future. Although amniotic fluid has been used as a protein supplement for the growth of human and mouse embryos in vitro, it had no advantage with 1, 2 propanediol for the freezing of 2-cell mouse embryos (Ng et al, 1988).

Quality control

The development of the 2-cell mouse embryo to the expanded blastocyst or hatching stage has been the assay for water purity and suitability of reagents for human IVF. Over 75 to 90 per cent of embryos growing from 2-cell to blastocyst stage must be obtained before media and reagents can be used. Recent studies have shown that the 1-cell mouse zygote assay is more sensitive to culture conditions than the 2-cell assay and may be useful in evaluating media (Findley et al, 1987). Zygote blastulation rates were strongly correlated with the cleavage index (number of blastomeres X "grade" of embryo). Grade ranged from two (>50 per cent fragmentation) to five (distinct cell borders with no fragmentation). It was also shown recently that mouse embryos with intact zona were more resistant to suboptimal culture conditions than zona free embryos. The use of zona free embryos cultured to the morula and cavitation stages in small volumes of culture media may provide more stringent monitoring (Fleming et al, 1987).

Implantation and embryonic viability

Many embryos replaced in patients undergoing IVF fail to implant or to sustain implantation. Apart from technical problems in the replacement technique, there are two possible causes of implantation failure: (i) the condition of the endometrium and (ii) embryo quality or viability.

Endometrial cell lines

The molecular mechanisms of recognition, the adhesion of the blastocyst to the endometrial epithelum, and the embedding into the stroma are poorly understood. Direct microscopic in vivo studies on implantation mechanisms are not possible in man for ethical reasons. In vitro culture methods offer a useful tool for direct studies on the endometrium. Recently, epithelial and stroma cells of human endometrium from patients at different phases of the menstrual cycle were enzymatically separated and isolated by successive centrifugation and primary cultures established for in vivo studies (Bongso et al, 1988d). Gland and stromal monolayers were established in three to seven days and maintained alive as primary cultures for up to three to four weeks. Endometrial cells in culture showed remarkably similar structural features to those described for cells in situ. This allows comparative studies on blastocyst-endometrial interaction in stimulated and unstimulated cycles. A study on receptor site responsiveness in stimulated versus unstimulated endometrium is in progress at the National University Hospital.

Since a technique of maintaining endometrial cell lines is available, studies are in progress to evaluate endometrial and oviductal epithelial monolayers as support systems for human IVF and embryonic growth. Bovine endometrial fibroblast monolayers have proved to be excellent for short and long term cultures of halved bovine embryos, compared with Ham's F10 supplemented with 10 per cent foetal calf serum (Voelkel et al, 1984). It was also demonstrated that endometrial cell to embryo contact was required for enhanced in vitro development of pig embryos compared with endometrial cell cultural supernatants (Allen et al, 1984).

Priming of the embryo with implantation factors from secretary phase endometrial cells prior to replacement may yield better pregnancy rates. Studies have shown that pre-implantation mouse embryos took up or bound to at least eight proteins synthesised by endometrial cells when these embryos were co-cultured with endometrial cell monolayers (O'Fallon et al, 1984). The specific function of these proteins in in vitro development is still unknown.

Oviductal co-cultures

Newly fertilised eggs of farm animals cleave regularly only when transferred to the oviduct of a foster mother of the same or an appropriate species (Boland, 1984). These observations have led to the successful growth and development of sheep embryos co-cultured with sheep oviductal epithelial cells in vitro (Gandolfi et al, 1987). The authors concluded that during the first three days of fertilisation, cleavage progressed at a normal rate on different feeder layers but oviductal cells appeared to be required for the acquisition of full embryonic viability. It was hypothesised that potassium ions and specific glycoproteins secreted by the oviduct may play a role during fertilisation and cleavage (Brown et al, 1986).

Two interesting observations were made of the relationship between somatic cells and embryonic development when the co-culture period was extended from three to six days. Somatic cells differed in their ability to support embryonic development beyond the non-compacted morula stage: oviductal epithelial cells supported further development while fibroblasts did not. It was suggested that development of the sheep embryo from the morula to expanded blastocyst stage involved two critical phases, each with its own specific requirements (Gandolfi et al, 1987). The first occurred in the fourth cell cycle and was analogous to the 2-cell block in the mouse and gerbil and the 4-cell block in the pig.

These stages of restriction of development corresponds with the time at which the embryonic genome is activated and the first transcription occurs. Specific factors in the oviductal cells may facilitate passage through this restriction phase. Similar factors may be present in the human oviduct that may encourage viable 2-cell embryos to develop to the blastocyst stage without degeneration. Such factors need to be identified that many play an important role in developing viable embryos for replacement, thus increasing the IVF pregnancy rates.

Embryo viability

Embryo viability is a major factor affecting IVF pregnancy rates. It appears that the rate of cleavage of preimplantation embryos is an important variable for success. Significantly higher pregnancy rates were observed when one embryo at least had reached the 4-cell stage by 40–44 hours post-insemination (Claman et al, 1987). Oocytes not fertilised after a first attempt were considered unhealthy. One group reported higher pregnancy rates in patients receiving unfragmented embryos (Dor et al, 1985) while several others showed pregnancy rates to be unaffected when transferring fragmented embryos (Lopata, 1982; Mahr et al, 1987). The human embryo appears to be able to dispose of these enucleated cytoplasmic fragments. However, a very badly fragmented embryo may stand a poor chance of implantation compared to one with moderate fragments.

The need to develop culture media which will enable embryos to achieve their full developmental potential at rates comparable in vivo may increase their chances of viability. Currently, human embryos can develop in a wide range of media, with or without protein. The rate of development to blastocyst has varied. Caro and others (1987) suggested that preimplantation mouse embryos required a specific combination of hormones and growth factors to enable cleavage rates and development to match those occurring in vivo. An increased rate of embryonic development during culture in media containing insulin was obtained. Further, Chang's medium without any supplementation was shown to give significantly better fertilisation rates than Chang's medium with 10 per cent human serum of T6 and albumin (BSA) for mouse IVF (Bongso et al, 1988c).

Thus, 87.7 per cent of 2-cell mouse embryos developed to blastocyst stage in Chang's medium. After 72 to 96 hours in vitro, they hatched with their inner cell mass (ICM) and trophoectoderm (T) attached to the culture dish. Monolayers were formed among 30 per cent of embryos. However, the hatched ICM and T from blastocysts grown in T6 with or without BSA did not hatch and form monolayers (Bongso et al, 1988c). Chang's medium has as its formulation, dextrose, salts and other common components, eight per cent newborn calf serum, hormones, vitamins, amino acids, polypeptides and nucleosides which may play a vital role in embryo viability. It was recently shown that fertilised ova triggered platelet activation and caused a slight thrombocytopenia during the preimplantation phase of pregnancy. This provides a possible method for monitoring embryo viability (O'Neill et al, 1986). Assay for the presence of platelet activating factor (PAF) in the growth medium of embryos may be used as indicator of embryonic potential for pregnancy.

Acknowledgements

The authors thank Miss Harjeet Kaur for typing this manuscript.

Table 9-1
Laboratory steps for IVF

Culture medium:	
Type	— Earle's, Ham's F10, T_6, B2, Hoppe/Pitts, Tyrode's
Conditions	— pH, 7.3–7.5; 280–285 mOsmol Kg^{-1}
Sperm preparation:	
Time obtained	— before oocyte retrieval, 2 to 3 hrs before expected insemination
Wash technique	— "swim-up"
Oocyte maturation:	incubation 2 to 6 hrs
Culture conditions:	
Vessels	— tubes, paraffin oil in Nunc or Falcon wells
Gas Phase $CO_2/O_2/N_2$	— 5:5:90
CO_2/air	— 5:95
Sperm/ml	— $1–5 \times 10^5$
Cumulus, corona removal:	micropipetting, needling
Transfer to growth medium:	at 15 to 20 hrs
Growth medium (protein):	15% patient's or pooled serum
Expected cleavage:	4 cells at 48 hrs

References

Allen, R.L. and Wright Jr, R.W. In vitro development of porcine embryos in coculture with endometrial cell monolayers or culture supernatants. *Theriogenology*, 1984; 21: 219.

Austin, C.R. Observations on the penetration of the sperm into the mammalian egg. *Australian Journal of Scientific Research Serial B*, 1951; 4: 581.

Averill, R.L.W., Adams, C.E. and Rowson, L.E.A. Transfer of mammalian ova between species. *Nature*, 1955; 176: 167.

Boland, M.P. Use of a rabbit oviduct as a screening test for the viability of mammalian eggs. *Theriogenology*, 1984; 21: 126.

Bongso, T.A., Ng S.C., Wong P.C. and Ratnam, S.S. Premature chromosome condensation (PCC) in human occytes failing to fertilize in vitro. *Proceedings of XIth Asian Oceanic Congress of Obstetrics and Gynaecology*, December 1987, Hongkong.

Bongso, T.A., Ng S.C., Ratnam, S.S., Sathananthan, A.H. and Wong P.C. Chromosome anomalies in human occytes failing to fertilize after insemination in vitro. *Human Reproduction*, 1988a; 3: 645.

Bongso, T.A., Ng S.C., Sathananthan, A.H., Lim M.N., Mok H., Wong P.C. and Ratnam, S.S. Chromosome analysis of two-cell mouse embryos frozen by slow and ultrarapid methods using two different cryoprotectants. *Fertility and Sterility*, 1988b, 49: 167.

Bongso, T.A., Ng S.C., Mok H., Lim M.N., Wong P.C. and Ratnam, S.S. Evaluation of Chang's culture medium for mouse IVF and embryonic development. *Journal of In Vitro Fertilisation and Embryo Transfer*, 1988c; 5: 102.

Bongso, T.A., Gajra, B., Ng P.L., Wong P.C., Ng S.C. and Ratnam, S.S. Establishment of human endometrial cell cultures. *Human Reproduction*, 1988d; 3: 705.

Brown, C.R. and Cheng, W.K.T. Changes in composition of the porcine zona pellucida during development of the oocyte to the 2 to 4-cell embryo. *Journal of Embryology and Experimental Morphology*, 1986; 77: 411.

Burkman, L.J., Coddington, C.C., Kruger, T.F. and Hodgen, G.D. Hemi-zona assay: Is human sperm binding to the zona pellucida predictive of an IVF potential? *Proceedings of 43rd meeting of American Fertility Society*, 1987, 87.

Caro, C.M., Trounson, A.O. and Kirby, C. Effect of growth factors in culture medium on the rate of mouse embryo development and viability in vitro. *Journal of In Vitro Fertilisation and Embryo Transfer*, 1987; 4: 265.

Chang M.C. Fertilizing capacity of spermatozoa deposited into the fallopian tubes. *Nature*, 1951; 168: 697.

Chang M.C. Fertilization of rabbit ova in vitro. *Nature*, 1959; 184: 466.

Claman, P., Randall, Armant D., Seibel, M.M., Wang T., Oskowitz, S.P. and Taymor, M.L. The impact of embryo quality and quantity on implantation and the establishment of viable pregnancies. *Journal of In Vitro Fertilisation and Embryo Transfer*, 1987; 4: 218.

Cummins, J.M. and Breen, T.M. Separation of progressively motile spermatozoa from human semen by 'sperm-rise' through a density gradient. *Australian Journal of Medical Laboratory Science*, 1984: 5: 15.

Dor, J., Rudak, E., Mashiach, S., Nebel, L., Serr, D.M. and Goldman, B. Preovulatory 17B-estradiol changes and embryo morphologic features in conception and nonconceptional cycles after human IVF. *Fertility and Sterility*, 1985; 45: 63.

Dravland, J.E. and Mortimer D. A simple discontinuous Percoll gradient for washing human spermatozoa. *IRCS Medical Science*, 1985; 13: 16.

Edwards, R.G., Bavister, B.D. and Steptoe, P.C. Early stages of fertilization in vitro of human oocytes matures in vitro. *Nature*, 1969; 221: 632.

Edwards, R.G., Steptoe, P.C. and Purdy, J.M. Establishing full term human pregnancies using cleaving embryos grown in vitro. *British Journal of Obstetrics and Gynaecology*, 1980; 87: 737.

Findley, W.E., Pabon, J. and Besch, P.K. The efficacy of mouse zygote blastulation rates in evaluating media for embryo culture. *Proceedings of 43rd Annual Meeting of American Fertility Society*, 1987; 117.

Fleming, T.P., Pratt, H.P.M. and Braude, P.R. The use of mouse preimplantation embryos for quality control of culture reagents in human IVF programs: A cautionary note. *Fertility and Sterility*, 1987; 47: 858.

Gandolfi, F. and Moor, R.M. Stimulation of early embryonic development in the sheep by co-culture with oviduct epithelial cells. *Journal of Reproduction and Fertility*, 1987: 81: 23.

Gordon, J.W. and Talansky, B.E. Assisted fertilization by zona drilling: A mouse model for correction of oligospermy. *Journal of Experimental Zoology*, 1986; 239: 347.

Gould, K.E., Cline, E.M. and Williams, W.L. Observations on the induction of ovulation and fertilization in vitro in the squirrel monkey (*Saimiri sciurens*). *Fertility and Sterility*, 1973; 24: 260.

Gould, K.E. Ovum recovery and IVF in the chimpanzee. *Fertility and Sterility*, 1983; 40: 378.

Gould, K.G. Fertilization in vitro of non-human primate ova: Present status and rationale for further development of the technique. In *Report to the Ethics Advisory Board: HEW Support of Research Involving Hman IVF*, US Government Printing Office, Washington DC, 1979.

Heape, W. Preliminary note on the transplantation and growth of mammalian ova within a uterine foster mother. *Proceedings of the Royal Society London*, 1890; 48: 457.

Jones, W.R. Immunological factors in infertility. In Pepperell, R.J., Hudson, B. and Wood, C. (Eds), *The Infertile Couple*, Second edition, Chruchill Livingstone, London, 1986.

Lee, M.A., Trucco, G.S., Bechtol, B.K., Wummer, N., Kopf, G.S., Blasco, L. and Storey, B.T. Capacitation and acrosome reaction in human spermatozoa monitored by a chlortetracycline fluorescence assay. *Fertility and Sterility*, 1987; 48: 649.

Lopata, A. Factors influencing the growth of human preimplantation embryos in vitro. In Edwards, R.G. and Purdy, J.M. (Eds), *Human Conception In Vitro*, Academic Press, London, 1982, 207.

Mahadevan, M.M., Trounson, A.O., Wood, C. and Leeton, J.F. Effect of oocyte quality and sperm characteristics on the number of spermatozoa bound to the zona pellucida of human oocytes insemination in vitro. *Journal of In Vitro Fertilisation and Embryo Transfer*, 1987; 4: 223.

Mohr, L.R., Trounson, A.O., Leeton, J.F. and Wood, C. Evaluation of normal and abnormal human embryo development during procedures in vitro. In Beier, H.M. and Lindner, H.R. (Eds), *Fertilization of the Human Egg in Vitro*, Springer-Verlag, New York, 1983, 211.

Neff, M.R., Holmgren, W., Jeyendran, R.S. and Perez-Palaez, M. Glass wool filtration in the separation of a quality sperm aliquot. *Proceedings of 43rd Annual Meeting of American Fertility Society*, 1987; 243.

Ng S.C., Sathananthan, A.H., Edirisinghe, W.R., Kum Chue, J.H., Wong P.C., Ratnam, S.S. and Sarla, G. Fertilization of a human egg with sperm from a patient with immotile cilia syndrome: Case report. In Ratnam, S.S., Teoh, E.S. and Anandakumar, C. (Eds), *Advances in Fertility and Sterility*, Parthenon Publishing, 1987.

Ng S.C., Sathananthan, A.H., Bongso, T.A., Lee Mui-Nee, Helen Mok, Wong, P.C. and Ratnam, S.S. The use of amniotic fluid and serum with propanediol in freezing of murine 2-cell embryos. *Fertility and Sterility*, 1988; 50: 510.

Odawara, Y. and Lopata, A. Zona cracking: A new technique for assisted fertilization. *Proceedings of Australian Fertility Society*, Sydney, 1987, 73.

O'Fallon, J.V., Allen, R.L. and Wright Jr., R.W. Uptake of endometrial cell proteins by pre-implantation mouse embryos. *Theriogenology*, 1984; 21: 249.

O'Neill, C. and Saunders, D.M. Platelet activating factor — its assessment and interpretation. *Journal of In Vitro Fertilisation and Embryo Transfer*, 1986; 3: 188.

Plachot, M., Junca, A.M., Mandelbaum, J., Grouchy de, J., Salat-Barous, J. and Cohen, J. Chromosome investigations in early life 1. Human oocytes recovered in an IVF programme. *Human Reproduction,* 1986; 1: 547.

Rowson, L.E.A. Methods of inducing multiple ovulation in cattle. *Journal of Endocrinology,* 1950; 260.

Rowson, L.E.A. and Dowling, D.F. An apparatus for the extraction of fertilized eggs from the living cow. *Veterinary Record,* 1949; 61: 171.

Steen, Y., Wikland, M., Janson, P.O. and Wik, O. A new method for the treatment of sperm in an IVF programme. *Journal for In Vitro Fertilisation and Embryo Transfer,* 1986; 3: 173.

Tablot, P. and Chacon, R.S. A triple stain technique for evaluating normal acrosome reactions of human sperm. *Journal of Experimental Zoology,* 1981; 215: 201.

Trounson, A.O. The need for appropriate controls in studies on human IVF. *Journal for In Vitro Fertilisation and Embryo Transfer,* 1986; 3: 258.

Trounson, A.O. Factors influencing the success of fertilization and embryonic growth in vitro. In Edwards, R.G. and Purdy, J.M. (Eds), *Human Conception In Vitro,* Academic Press, London, 1982, 201.

Trounson, A.O., Peura, A. and Kirby, C. Ultrarapid freezing: A new low cost and effective method of embryo cryopreservation. *Fertility and Sterility,* 1987; 48: 843.

Tsunoda, Y., Yasui, T. and Nakamura, K. Effect of cutting the zona pellucida on the pronuclear transplantation in the mouse. *Journal of Experimental Zoology,* 1986; 240: 119.

Voelkel, S.A., Amborski, G.F., Hill, K.G. and Godke, R.A. Use of a uterine cell monolayer culture system for micromanipulated bovine embryos. *Theriogenology,* 1984; 21: 271.

Whittingham, D.G. Fertilization of mouse eggs in vitro. *Nature,* 1968; 220: 592.

Wolf, D.P., Boldt, J., Byrd, W. and Bechtol, K.B. Acrosomal status evaluation in human ejaculated sperm with monoclonal antibodies. *Biology of Reproduction,* 1985; 32: 1157.

Wramsby, H., Fredga, K. and Liedholm, P. Chromosome analysis of human oocytes recovered from preovulatory follicles in stimulated cycles. *New England Journal of Medicine,* 1987: 316: 121.

Yanagimachi, R. and Chang, M.C. In vitro fertilization of hamster ova. *Journal of Experimental Zoology,* 1964; 156: 361.

10
Cryopreservation in IVF

C. Chen

Introduction

Ideally one only requires a single embryo derived from a single egg to achieve a pregnancy. But in practice this is not so because the procedure of in vitro fertilisation (IVF) is not efficient enough to achieve such a result. With one embryo replaced, the pregnancy rate is only 9.5 per cent (Seppala, 1985). The rate is maximal with four embryos replaced, being 24 per cent. Replacing embryos in excess of four does not increase the pregnancy rate — in fact, there appeares to be a decline. On the other hand, the frequency of occurrence of multiple pregnancy increases significantly with the numbers of embryos transferred, resulting in twins and triplets (Kerin et al, 1983; Chen et al, 1982). Thus with multiple embryos transferred, the twinning rate is 12 per cent and with triplets two per cent (Saunders et al, 1988). Such a situation created is clearly unacceptable. In spite of all these efforts, the overall take-home baby rate is less than 10 per cent.

It becomes obvious that to achieve an acceptable pregnancy rate, a reasonable harvest of eggs during any single IVF treatment cycle is required for the creation of embryos. This can now be achieved using a variety of ovarian stimulation regimens (Seppala, 1985). However, it is not possible to predict or control precisely the number of eggs produced following ovarian hyperstimulation. Eggs well in excess of the numbers required may be obtained.

It is also not possible to select reliably which eggs will fertilise following exposure to sperm, since an average fertilisation rate of 60 to 70 per cent may be anticipated. Hence there is a tendency to inseminate all eggs obtained. This results in an excess of embryos created. As only three or four are required for replacement into the uterus, the remaining spare embryos will have to be discarded or stored.

As embryos are regarded by members of the community as human life in its early form, complex ethical, legal and moral issues inevitably arise (Warnock, 1984). The preservation of these embryos through deep freezing is one apparent solution to this dilemma. Even then, there will still be embryo wastage as a proportion of the embryos will not survive the freezing process.

An alternative approach to the problem of spare or excess embryos is to inseminate the required number of eggs, and to store the excess by cryopreservation for later use, as and when the need arises. With the current controversy surrounding embryo freezing, there is a need to explore the possiblity of cryopreservation of the human oocyte as an alternative to embryo freezing in IVF programmes. Like sperm banking, oocyte storage should be more acceptable to the community, since the procedure involves only the gamete, and is therefore free of the encumbrances associated with the storage of frozen human embryos. Of equal importance is the need for research into cryopreservation of the human oocyte. Little is known of the effects of deep freezing on the oocyte, its survival after thawing, and its subsequent performance and development following exposure to sperm in the IVF system. The potential significance and clinical application of this research can be far-reaching.

Cryobiological principles

Before proceeding further with the discussion on cryopreservation in IVF it may be pertinent to consider the principles of cryobiology in broad outline. The concept of cryopreservation is one of preservation and storage through deep freezing to temperatures as low as −196 °C, a state that is obtained with liquid nitrogen. At this temperature life comes to a standstill, biological time becomes arrested and a state of suspended animation prevails. Life can thus be preserved indefinitely.

Cryobiological concepts in freeze-thawing

Before undertaking work on cryopreservation, an understanding of cryobiological concepts in cell freezing is essential. Successful preservation is attributable to the application of theoretical considerations and empirical observations derived from studies in other species and cellular systems. There are two factors of importance in cryopreservation work; the presence of molar concentration of a protective solute or cryoprotectant, and appropriate rates of cooling and warming. Cryoprotective solutes which are of low molecular weight are thought to prevent the potentially deleterious exposure of cells to elevated concentrations of electrolytes by their colligative action in reducing the quantity of ice formed intracellularly at any sub-zero temperature. Also, precise control of the cooling rate and warming rate determines the ultimate fate of water present intracellularly during the cryopreservation process.

If during freezing the rate of cooling is sufficiently slow, cytoplasmic water will be permitted to flow out of the cell and freeze extracellularly, resulting in a gradual dehydration of the cell. However, damage to the cell at slow rates of cooling may be caused by solution effects, which in turn can be reduced by the use of cryoprotective media. On the other hand, if cooling is too rapid, the cytoplasm will not have sufficient time to dehydrate, it will supercool, and eventually freeze. The formation of intracellular ice is thought to lead to cell damage and death. For different cells there is an optimal cooling rate which varies according to the cell type.

The cell therefore suffers cryodamage due to three factors: (1) the formation of ice crystals inside the cell from water which is normally present in the cell; (2) the osmotic changes resulting from water draining out of the cell during the freezing process; (3) the release of latent heat of fusion, producing a shift in thermal equilibrium.

Cellular events during cryopreservation

When a cell suspended in a physiological medium is cooled down to a temperature slightly below 0 °C, ice forms first in the extracellular solution. The dissolved solutes become more concentrated as water is removed in the form of ice. As the temperature of the cell suspension is lowered further, more ice forms, resulting in a progressively more concentrated extracellular solution. The higher the concentration, the lower the chemical potential of water. The cell responds osmotically to equalize the chemical potentials of water across its membranes, hence during freezing, it loses water extracellularly. If the cell is cooled sufficiently slowly, it will progressively lose more water as the temperature is lowered so as to maintain an osmotic equilibrium with the extracellular solution. On the other hand, if a cell is cooled at high enough rates, there will be insufficient time for the cell to remain in osmotic equilibrium and, as the temperature falls, the cell contents will become increasingly supercooled, until suddenly the cell water freezes within the cell itself, thereby resulting in cell death. Seeding, or the induction of ice formation in the medium, overcomes this problem of supercooling and the deleterious effect of thermal changes following the release of the latent heat of fusion.

As cooling proceeds further, and the temperature reaches −40 °C, 74 per cent of the solution becomes crystallised and the solute concentration in the remaining liquid increases to 47 weight per cent (Rall et al, 1984). Many small ice crystals form and surround the cell, thereby obscuring it from view on cryomicroscopy. The next phase is a critical one where cell death can occur. As the temperature falls further, the intracellular contents freeze and the cell suddenly reappears. This is caused by diffraction of light by the ice crystals formed intracellularly — a phenomenon termed "blackening out" or "flashing". If the cell is now cooled rapidly by plunging it into liquid nitrogen at −196 °C, there is no additional crystallisation, that is, a "glass" forms and the residual liquid "vitrifies". Cooling to −196 °C results in an arrest of biological time for the cell, which can then be stored virtually indefinitely.

On thawing, the physical events depend on whether warming is slow or rapid. Slow warming is accompanied by a complex series of changes; a "flashing" of the cytoplasm at −90 °C, "first flash", the gradual growth of a dark crystalline material extracellularly between −90 °C to −70 °C, gradual disappearance of the dark material between −70 °C to −42 °C, and a "second flash" at −55 °C. With rapid warming, that is rates above 100 °C/minute, the extracellular ice merely melts when the temperature increases above −40 °C. There is insufficent time for the formation of ice nuclei or "devitrification" and the glossy solid therefore "liquefies". The final step is a critical one of diluting out the cryoprotectant and a return to physiological conditions.

These cryobiological concepts described are clearly of importance. The role of the cryoprotectant in protecting the cell during freezing, the avoidance of supercooling by seeding, careful control of the rate of cooling, the prevention of significant intracellular ice formation, the establishment of osmotic and thermal equilibrium during freezing, and the control of warming rates are of concern. Both an understanding of these concepts, and meticulous attention and control of these factors during freezing and thawing determine the successful outcome of the cryopreservation process.

Embryo cryopreservation

Wilmut (1972) and Whittingham et al (1972) independently initiated the cryopreservation of mammalian embryos. Their experiments demonstrated that the slow cooling of mouse embryos to low sub-zero temperatures in the presence of a cryoprotectant, and their slow thawing, resulted in embryo survival. Embryos of many other species have since been frozen successfully using minor variations of this technique. Thus human embryos have been successfully cryopreserved by Trounson and Mohr (1983) also using a modification of this freezing procedure. Human embryo cryopreservation has since been introduced into IVF programmes as a means of dealing with the problem of excess embryos.

Factors influencing successful embryo cryopreservation

Various factors affect the success of embryo preservation. They include: (1) the stage of embryonic development; (2) the degree of prefreeze fragmentation (ie. embryo quality); (3) the degree of blastomere postfreeze damage (ie. embryo survival); (4) the number of embryos frozen; (5) the freezing technique; and (6) the time of embryo transfer in relation to the embryonic age.

Embryonic stage at cryopreservation

Attempts have been made to cryopreserve embryos at different stages of their development, ranging from the pronucleate, two-cell, three-cell, four-cell, eight-cell, and even blastocyst stages. The results obtained have been variable. However, consistent and acceptable successes have been achieved with the two-, four-, eight-cell, and blastocyst stages. Embryos are best preserved at the interphase stages as in two-, four- and eight-cell stages with 67 per cent survival (Testart et al, 1986). Cryopreservation at other stages, as in three, five- and seven-, apparently result in a significant three-fold decrease in survival. The individual blastomeres seem more stable during the interphase stages.

Embryo quality

There is no doubt that embryo quality has a significant influence on survival with freeze-thawing. It is therefore necessary to grade embryo quality morphologically from the degree of fragmentation observed, 0 to one+, two+, and three+. This is illustrated by the results of freezing 225 embryos (Freeman et al, 1986). The pregnancy rate obtained after replacing frozen embryos is 15 per cent where their quality is excellent. The presence of minor fragments does not alter the chances of pregnancy. This chance is reduced to five per cent where fragmentation is moderate. But where fragmentation is extensive, pregnancy does not occur.

Number of embryos stored and replaced

As with regular IVF, the prospects of obtaining pregnancy are enhanced by the number of frozen embryos replaced (Freeman et al, 1986). The optimal opportunity is three or four, with rates of around 30 per cent. Replacing fewer or more appears to have an adverse effect, with the added disadvantage of increasing the chances of multiple pregnancy occurring. There is also a direct relationship between the chances of embryo replacement for any patient treatment cycle and the number of embryos stored frozen. This means that each patient will have a greater chance of getting frozen embryos back if she had two, three or four embryos frozen. This opportunity is influenced by the relatively high risk of embryo mortality from the freeze-thawing process itself.

Cryoprotectants

There are three cryoprotectants frequently used in embryo cryopreservation, namely dimethyl sulphoxide (DMSO), propanediol (PROH), and glycerol. Earlier cell stages are better protected against cryodamage when DMSO or PROH are used, whereas glycerol is best for the blastocyst stage. The addition and removal of cryoprotectant are crucial steps for cryoprotection of the cell. This is because cryoprotectants are cytotoxic and their careful removal is an important step in the cryopreservation process. There are two methods: step-wise, or as a single step.

Embryo cryopreservation techniques

There are four published techniques available for the cryopreservation of human embryos. Two of these use the slow-freeze approach and are widely used. The remaining two are not established; namely, the ultrarapid, and vitrification. Experience has shown that slow-freezing and halting the process at low sub-zero temperatures (eg. −80°C) prior to plunging into liquid nitrogen for storage, should be accompanied by slow-thawing. On the contrary, stopping at high sub-zero temperatures (eg. −40°C), should be accompanied by a fast-thaw. With ultrarapid and vitrification procedures, the cells should be thawed rapidly as well.

Ultrarapid freezing

Ultrarapid embryo freezing is experimental and has been applied to mouse embryos (Trounson, 1987). It involves exposure of the cell to 3.5M DMSO in 0.5M sucrose for three minutes and then plunging into liquid nitrogen. Thawing is rapid at 37°C. The results with eight cell mouse embryos look promising, with a 94 per cent survival and a 97 per cent blastocyst development rate.

Vitrification

Vitrification or freezing without ice formation is achieved by using very high concentrations of cryoprotectants such as a 40 per cent strength. Three cryoprotectants are used, DMSO, PROH, and acetamide. The potential dangers are toxicity and osmotic injury. However, eight-cell mouse embryos appear to give an 85 per cent survival (Rall, 1987).

Duration of embryo storage

From the practical point of view, once embryos are stored, most (ie. 64 per cent) can be expected to be used within six months (Freeman et al, 1986). However, 10 per cent are not used even after two years and therefore do present storage problems for busy IVF units. Besides, some patients may not return to the unit to claim their embryos, thereby raising difficult legal and moral problems on the question of their disposal.

DMSO technique

Three commonly used embryo freezing techniques will be discussed. The first is the Monash embryo freezing procedure, since it is the longer established and more widely used (Trounson & Mohr, 1983). The cells are suspended in phosphate buffered saline (PBS) containing 10 per cent foetal calf serum for 10 minutes, and then exposed to increasing concentrations of DMSO from 0.25M to 1.5M in 10 minute steps at room temperature. They are then cooled in glass ampoules, again in step-wise fashion, at 2 °C/minute to a temperature of −6 °C, seeded, and held for 30 minutes before slow cooling at 0.3 °C/minute to −32 °C, then 0.1 °C/minute to −35 °C, and 0.3 °C/minute to −80 °C. Thereafter cooling proceeds at 10 °C/minute until −110 °C before final storage in liquid nitrogen at −196 °C. Thawing is slow: the cell is taken out of storage and held at −80 °C for two minutes, before slow warming at 8 °C/minute to −4 °C, and then left at room temperature. Removal of DMSO is again step-wise from 1.5M to 0.25M, at decreasing holding intervals from 15 minutes to five minutes. Using this method, Freeman (1986) found the pregnancy rate obtained was 32 per cent for eight-cell embryos compared with 8 per cent among the four-cell stages. The overall survival rate of 402 embryos frozen was 58 per cent, with 70 per cent of patients who have had embryos frozen achieving embryo transfer, and only 11 per cent becoming pregnant. An analysis of 20 such pregnancies show a 25 per cent loss as biochemical pregnancies or spontaneous abortions. One pregnancy was terminated because of a missing limb, although the chromosomes were normal. The remaining 14 culminated in one twin birth, one stillbirth due to amnionitis, and the rest normal.

Glycerol technique

Cryopreservation of the blastocyst is the next option and is best performed at a stage when cavitation is complete and expansion has taken place (Ashwood-Smith & Simons, 1986). Stages earlier than this yield poor results. A serious limitation in using this approach for embryo cryopreservation is the fact that only about 30 per cent of embryos do eventually reach the blastocyst stage in in vitro culture. Glycerol is the cryoprotectant of choice and is added step-wise in increasing concentrations varying from one per cent to eight per cent at 10 minute intervals. The freezing procedure involves slow cooling at 1°C/minute to −7°C, then seeding is performed, with further cooling at 0.3°C/minute to −36°C before immersion and storage in liquid nitrogen. Thawing is achieved rapidly by immersion in a 30°C bath. Removal of glycerol is again done step-wise from eight per cent, decreasing at intervals varying from 10 to 20 minutes to a final concentration of one per cent.

Propanediol technique

More recently, propanediol has been employed in freezing embryonic stages of one to two day old embryos with promising results (Testart et al, 1986). Penetration of the cryoprotectant into the embryo is supposedly more efficient and hence better cryoprotection is obtained. The embryo is suspended in PBS containing 20 per cent human cord serum and a one-step exposure to 1.5M PROH and 0.1M sucrose performed. Sucrose is added because it appears to give additional cryoprotection. Cooling proceeds at 2°C/minute to −7°C, with seeding and a 10 minute hold at this temperature. Further cooling occurs at 0.3°C/minute to −30°C, then rapid cooling at 100°C/minute to −190°C before storage at −196°C in liquid nitrogen. Thawing is achieved by holding the sample at room temperature for 40 seconds, then rapid warming in a 30°C bath. Propanediol is removed step-wise by five minute holding intervals in IM PROH containing 0.2M sucrose, then 0.5M PROH in the same strength of sucrose, and finally in 0.2M sucrose alone before transfer into PBS containing 20 per cent human cord serum.

Timing of embryo transfer

The timing of embryo replacement is dependent on the technique of freezing used. With the Monash procedure, the embryos are replaced in a natural cycle at exact synchrony with the events of the previous treatment cycle. Ovulation is deemed to have occurred 40 hours from the onset of a blood LH surge, confirmed by blood progesterone assays. On the other hand, in the case of blastocysts, natural cycles are used and either an LH surge or hCG administered. Embryo replacement is performed on the fourth day after presumed ovulation. With PROH frozen embryos, natural cycles are also used for embryo transfer which varies between one and four days after presumed ovulation. Contrary to the Monash experience, using PROH, embryos are best transferred as day one or two embryos. Survivals of 83 per cent can be expected, compared with 58 per cent in the Monash series. The older the embryo, the poorer the survival.

Results of embryo cryopreservation

Comparing the pregnancy rates of the three methods of embryo cryopreservation revealed very promising results with blastocysts frozen in glycerol, and one to two day old embryos in which PROH was used (Astwood-Smith & Simons, 1986; Testart et al, 1986; Freeman et al, 1986). The pregnancy rates varied between 18 to 20 per cent. With DMSO and using the Monash technique, the pregnancy rate was half that obtained using the two other methods. Perhaps the method of choice should be PROH freezing since blastocysts are somewhat difficult to culture in vitro and there is a high embryo loss rate during culture. The abortion rate following embryo cryopreservation is around 30 per cent regardless of the stage of embryonic development.

Oocyte cryopreservation

From the point of view of oocyte freezing, an important feature is the size of the mammalian egg. The oocyte at the time of ovulation is generally the largest cell found in most mammals, being a sphere varying in diameter from about 70 to 80 μm in the mouse to about 130 μm in the human. During intra-uterine life, oocytes enter the prophase of the first meitoic division, and then become arrested in the diplotene stage. With the onset of reproductive life, the meiotic process is resumed and the first meiotic division is then completed. The second meiotic division occurs and the oocyte is ovulated at the metaphase II stage, with the first polar body extruded, and the chromosomes arranged on a spindle at the second meiotic metaphase. During this stage the oocyte may be regarded as relatively unstable. It is fairly characteristic of ovulated eggs that if fertilisation does not occur, the spindle subsequently breaks down, the chromosomes forming micronuclei. It is the view of cryobiologists that the oocyte should best be cryopreserved at the ovulated phase (Polge, 1977). Following fertilisation, resumption of meiotic maturation occurs, and the second polar body is extruded.

Feasibility of oocyte cryopreservation

Little is known about the feasibility and effects of deep freezing on the human oocyte, its survival after thawing, and its subsequent performance and development following exposure to sperm in the IVF system. There is, however, evidence in the literature in support of the feasibility of oocyte cryopreservation among a variety of mammalian species (Parkes, 1958; Leibo, 1977; Tsunoda et al, 1976; Quinn et al, 1982; De Mayo et al, 1985). The most important study was that of Whittingham (1977) who, using dimethyl sulphoxide (DMSO) as cryoprotectant, succeeded in freezing unfertilised ovulated mouse oocytes to a temperature of −196°C, and obtained 70 per cent survival after storage of these oocytes for periods varying between 24 hours to three months, clearly demonstrating the feasibility of oocyte cryopreservation. Fertilisation in vitro of the frozen-thawed oocytes was observed to be significantly lower than that of freshly collected control oocytes. However, live, healthy, normal young were obtained after transfer of the oocytes into the oviducts of recipient females mated with fertile males. While animal studies have clearly shown that the mammalian oocyte can be successfully frozen and stored, little evidence indicates that this can be feasible in man. Indeed, it was thought by some IVF researchers that cryopreservation of the human oocyte was extremely difficult, if not technically impossible, because of the potential instability of the oocyte chromosome spindle when subjected to freezing and thawing. In one study, Trounson (1984) obtained more than 80 oocytes from ovarian wedge samples and cultured them for 48 hours in vitro. Only four oocytes survived freezing and subsequent thawing. In another study, Bernard et al (1985) using glycerol as cryoprotectant, found that none of the oocytes were fertilisable after freeze-thawing. In the same study in which 1, 2-propanediol was used instead, both fertilisation and cleavage to the eight-cell stage occurred in one egg before the experiment was terminated.

Developing oocyte cryopreservation

In order to develop oocyte cryopreservation, the author initially used a murine model. Female mice belonging to an F1 hybrid strain were superovulated with pregnant mare's serum gonadotrophin and human chorionic gonadotrophin (hCG). Ovulated oocytes and fertilised oocytes were harvested after hCG administration and used for freezing. Dulbecco's PBS was the freezing medium. A programme of IVF established within the Department of Obstetrics and Gynaecology supported the study. Women were stimulated with clomiphene citrate given either alone or in combination with human menopausal gonadotrophin (hMG) to achieve ovarian follicular development. A typical regimen involved the use of 100 mg of clomiphene citrate given daily for five days from day four of the cycle together with 150 IU or more hMG also given daily from day six until a satisfactory serum estradiol response was obtained. The pattern of this response together with ultrasound evidence of follicular growth was used to time the administration of 5000 IU of hCG. Ooctye retrieval was performed by laparoscopy about 34 hours after the administration of hCG. When an endogenous surge of luteinising hormone (LH) occurred, as revealed in either serum or third-ourly urine samples, then retrieval was performed 26 hours from the time of the urinary LH surge.

The oocytes obtained were incubated at 37°C in a medium modified from Whittingham's formula and supplemented with sodium bicarbonate, penicillin, and streptomycin. The medium used for fertilisation and cleavage was supplemented with human serum, while the gas phase used during culture consisted of a mixture of five per cent carbon dioxide, five per cent oxygen, and 90 per cent nitrogen. Insemination of the oocyte was usually delayed over several hours in order to allow oocyte maturation in vitro. Fertilisation was usually assessed between 12 and 18 hours after insemination, at which time the medium was changed to one of higher serum concentration. Embryos were regularly transferred back to the patient at between the two- and six-cell stages, no more than four being replaced at any time. Oocytes in excess of those required to establish four embryos were then used for freezing.

Factors influencing successful freezing

A study was made of various factors seemingly influencing the successful outcome of human oocyte freezing. The factors included the volume for PBS for suspending the oocytes during freezing, the concentration of DMSO as cryoprotectant, the method of seeding, the temperature at which seeding was induced, the rate of freezing, the rate of thawing, and the final removal of DMSO before culture in vitro.

Oocyte selection

Not all oocytes were found suitable for freezing. Those that were preovulatory, appeared morphologically normal, with a well dispersed cumulus, and had good hormonal profiles during ovarian stimulation in the treatment cycle performed well.

Volume of medium for freezing

Oocytes were frozen in a 1.2ml cryule. A volume of 0.3ml was found most satisfactory, permitting seeding to be completed rapidly and efficiently. Volumes in excess of this failed to freeze quickly at the seeding temperature. Seeding induced at temperatures above −5°C were unsatisfactory, whereas at −7°C freezing of the buffer was both rapid and efficient.

Exposure to DMSO

Although the addition of cryoprotectant as a one-step procedure was found to give acceptable results, the rapid, step-wise addition of prechilled DMSO appeared more satisfactory. The final optimal concentration of DMSO in the suspending medium within the cryule was 1.5M. Following transfer of the oocyte into the cryule, the oocyte was then equilibrated at 0°C within an automatic cell freezer (model R204, Planner Products Ltd) for 20 minutes.

Seeding

The temperature was later rapidly decreased to −70°C at which point seeding of the sample was induced. Seeding occurred best at −7°C.

Rate of freezing

The oocyte was then slowly cooled at 0.5°C per minute to −40°C when it was then rapidly cooled to −196°C by imerssion in liquid nitrogren before storage. Cessation of slow cooling at temperatures below −40°C seemed to result in poor survival. Cooling rates that were too rapid resulted in cell death.

Rate of thawing

Thawing of the oocyte was achieved rapidly at rates exceeded 500°C per minute. Slower rates of warming were detrimental to the oocyte. Removal of the cryoprotectant from the oocyte was performed as a step-wise procedure by the addition of four times the sample volume of PBS, and the oocyte examined for morphologic evidence of survival.

Oocyte assessment and culture

Signs of oocyte damage included zonal fracture, discoloration of the ooplasm, oocyte disruption, and pyknosis. Further assessment of the oocyte required transfer into the regular culture medium, and at the appropriate time insemination was performed. Assessment of fertilisation and cleavage were made later.

Results of human oocyte cryopreservation

The results obtained in a study of human oocytes using the slow-freeze and rapid-thaw technique showed that at least 75 per cent of the oocytes survived freezing and became fertilised on exposure to sperm, with 60 per cent proceeding to cleavage division of six- to eight-cell stages (Chen, 1986). Both the time of appearance of the pronuclei and cleavage rates were nearly similar to those of unfrozen fertilised oocytes. Embryo transfers of between two and three embryos derived from frozen-thawed oocytes were performed in seven patients and two pregnancies resulted.

The first patient to conceive was 29 years old, with primary infertility due to severe pelvic inflammatory disease. She failed to conceive despite pelvic microsurgery. She then underwent an IVF treatment cycle which led to a laparoscopy on day 14, with the recovery of six oocytes that were cryopreserved five hours after culture in vitro. Three of the oocytes were subsequently thawed, and after a further four hours of culture, were inseminated. The three frozen-thawed oocytes became fertilised and were replaced in utero on day 16 at the three- to four-cell stage. A βhCG test gave a positive result by day 27 of her cycle and a healthy twin gestation was confirmed by ultrasound examination on day 49.

The pregnancy progressed completely uneventfully, and she was delivered of a healthy set of twins on the fourth of July 1986 by elective caesarean section at 38 week's gestation. The boy weighed 6 lbs 4 ozs, and the girl weighed 6 lbs 5 ozs. Chromosomal studies of their cord blood leukocyte cultures showed a normal male and female karyotype, respectively, with banding studies confirming the results.

A second woman, aged 37 years, conceived with the same technique. Her spare eggs, which were frozen for four months, were implanted during a natural cycle. Both her βhCG profile and ultrasound examination confirmed the presence of a developing singleton pregnancy. Subsequently amniocentesis revealed a normal female karyotype. The pregnancy progressed uneventfully to term, and she was delivered of a healthy female infant by caesarean section.

Comments

These results, although preliminary, demonstrate that the human preovulatory oocyte can be successfully frozen and stored. It retains its fertilising capacity after thawing, despite the potentially damaging effects of the freezing process. With oocyte freezing, animal studies have not substantiated any harmful effects on the offspring. The slow-freeze and slow-thaw technique described by Whittingham gave optimal rates of survival for both oocytes and embryos in the mouse. The method may not be applicable to the human oocyte, presumably because of species difference. It is recognised that there are structural differences between mouse and human chromosomes. Presently, the only practical means of assessing survival and subsequent performance of the fertilised frozen-thawed human oocyte is by its morphologic appearance on light microscopy.

The risk of foetal malformation resulting from freeze-thawing of the human egg is unknown. However, the findings of a normal karyotype among both frozen egg twins and the second singleton pregnancy are encouraging and reassuring. The studies of other species in which freeze-thawing has been successful have also shown no increased risk of foetal malformation. It is probable that only the more robust eggs survive and malformation may therefore be uncommon; certainly there is no evidence of an increased risk of malformation among mammalian or human embryos after freeze-thawing.

As this study is preliminary, the efficiency of this method of human oocyte cryopreservation must await further study. However, the establishment of human oocyte cryopreservation has important implications. It provides the means for storing surplus oocytes for use in subsequent unstimulated IVF cycles. The prospect is also favourable for the future establishment of oocyte banking. Thus women who suffer from diseases that endanger the life of the ovaries (such as cancer, endometriosis, recurrent cysts, and infection) should be able to store their oocytes for future use. Should the ovaries require removal to treat the disease, she could still become pregnant through IVF, using her stored oocytes. Oocyte freezing may find application in family planning. Women who defer childbearing because of the pursuit of a career, the unavailability of a marriage partner, or ill health at a young age may opt to have their oocytes stored for later use. The storage of oocytes at the time of sterilisation may also be an important method of conception for those women who later regret such a step, particularly if reversal is difficult or fails. Stored oocytes may also find use in oocyte donation programmes.

As regimens for stimulating the production of more than one oocyte improve, it is commonplace for three or more oocytes to be collected in a treatment cycle. If more than three oocytes are obtained, then the excess can be frozen and used to attempt conception at a later date. This has the advantages of a reduction in risk of multiple pregnancy, the number of anaesthetic procedures and egg pickups a woman needs to undergo to achieve a pregnancy, and a greater chance of success from embryo implants in a natural cycle, with a significant reduction in costs to the patient. Oocyte freezing is expected to increase the efficiency of IVF by increasing the number of pregnancies from several eggs obtained in any single IVF treatment cycle. It also improves the patient's pregnancy potential since several eggs obtained can be used in several future cycles. It may provide an alternative to embryo freezing, ultimately assisting in alleviating some of the serious objections and concerns related to human embryo storage. Oocyte freezing can therefore be expected to become more acceptable to the community.

References

Ashwood-Smith, M.J. and Simons, R. The freezing of early human embryos and blastocysts. In Feichtinger, W. and Kemeter, P. (Eds), *Future Aspects in Human Reproduction*, Springer-Verlag, Berlin, 1987, 97.

Bernard, A., Imoedemhe, D.A., Shaw, R.W. and Fuller, B. Effects of cryoprotectants on human oocyte. *Lancet*, 1985; 1: 632.

Chen, C., Jones, W.R. and Mudge, T.J. The development of an in vitro fertilisation programme within an infertility service. *Clinical Reproduction and Fertility*, 1982; 1: 327.

Chen, C. Pregnancy after human oocyte cryopreservation. *Lancet*, 1986; 1: 884.

De Mayo, F.J., Rawlins, R.G. and Dukelow, W.R. Xenogenous and in vitro fertilisation of frozen/thawed primate oocytes and blastomere separation of embryos. *Fertility and Sterility*, 1985; 43: 295.

Freeman, L., Trounson, A. and Kirby, C. Cryopreservation of human embryos: Progress on the clinical use of the technique in human in vitro fertilisation. *Journal of In Vitro Fertilisation and Embryo Transfer*, 1986; 3: 53.

Kerin, J.F., Quinn, P.J., Kirby C., et al. Incidence of multiple pregnancy after in vitro fertilisation and embryo transfer. *Lancet*, 1983; II: 537.

Leibo, S.P. Fundamental cryobiology of mouse ova and embryos. In Elliot, K. and Whelan, J. (Eds), *The Freezing of Mammalian Embryos*, Elsevier Excerpta Medica, Ciba Foundation 52 (new series), Amsterdam 1977; 69.

Parkes, A.S. Factors affecting the viability of frozen ovarian tissue. *Journal of Endocrinology*, 1958; 17: 337.

Polge, C. The freezing of mammalian embryos: Perspectives and possibilities. In Elliot, K. and Whelan, J. (Eds) *The Freezing of Mammalian Embryos*, Elsevier Excerpta Medica, Ciba Foundation 52 (new series), Amsterdam, 1977, 3.

Quinn, P., Barros, C. and Whittingham, D.C. Preservation of hamster oocytes to assay the fertilising capacity of human spermatozoa. *Journal of Reproduction and Fertility*, 1982; 66: 161.

Rall, W.F., Reid, D.S. and Polge, C. Analysis of slow-warming injury of mouse embryos by cryomicroscopical and physiochemical methods. *Cryobiology*, 1984; 21: 106.

Rall, W.F., Wood, M.J. Kirby, C. and Whittingham, D.G. Development of mouse embryos cryopreserved by vitrification. *Journal of Reproduction and Fertility*, 1987; 80: 499.

Saunders, D.M., Mathews, M. and Lancaster, P.A.L. The Australian register: Current research and future role. In Jones J.C., H.W. and Schrader, G. (Eds), *In Vitro Fertilisation and Other Assisted Reproduction*, Annuals of the New York Academy of Sciences, New York, 1988, 7.

Seppala, M. The World collaborative report on in vitro fertilisation and embryo replacement: Current state of the art in January 1984. *Annals of the New York Academy of Sciences*, 1985; 442: 558.

Testart, J., Lassalle, B., Belaisch-Allart, J., et al. High pregnancy rate after early embryo freezing. *Fertility and Sterility*, 1986; 46: 268.

Trounson, A. and Mohr, L. Human pregnancy following cryopreservation, thawing, and transfer of an eight-cell embryo. *Nature*, 1983; 305: 707.

Trounson, A. In vitro fertilisation and embryo preservation. In Trounson, A. and Wood, C. (Eds), *In Vitro Fertilisation and Embryo Transfer*, Churchill Livingstone, Edinburgh, 1984, 111.

Trounson, A., Peura, A. and Kirby, C. Ultrarapid freezing: A new low-cost and effective method of embryo cryopreservation. *Fertility and Sterility*, 1987; 48: 843.

Tsunoda, Y. Parkening, T.A. and Chang, M.C. In vitro fertilisation of mouse and hamster eggs after freezing and thawing. *Experentia*, 1976; 32: 223.

Warnock, M. *A Question of Life: The Warnock report of human fertilisation and embryology*, Basil Blackwell UK., 1985.

Whittingham, D.G., Leibo, S.P. and Mazur, P. Survival of mouse embryos frozen to −196°C and −269°C. *Science*, 1972; 178: 411.

Whittingham, D.G. Fertilisation in vitro and development to term of unfertilised mouse oocytes previously stored at −196°C. *Journal of Reproduction and Fertility*, 1977; 49: 89.

Wilmut, I. The effect of cooling rate, warming rate of cryoprotectant agent, and stage of development on survival of mouse embryo during freezing and thawing. *Life Sciences*, 1972; 11: 1071.

11
Microfertilisation of human eggs

S.C. Ng, A. Bongso, H. Sathananthan and S.S. Ratnam

Introduction

The expectations of in vitro fertilisation (IVF) and gamete intrafallopian transfer (GIFT) in the treatment of cases of oligozoospermia, and other male factor problems (particularly multiple ones), have been disappointing (de Kretser et al, 1985). Indeed high fertilisation rates are obtained only when the sperm is normal according to very strict criteria (Asch, 1987), and is fulfilled in <10 per cent of "normal" semen samples (Rosenwaks, 1987). This has prompted the development of a new approach called "microfertilisation", a procedure in which one or more sperms are injected through the zona pellucida of the oocyte to assist the union of the male with the female gamete. This is achieved with the aid of a micromanipulator.

History and terminology

Microfertilisation was initially developed as a technique to investigate the various components involved in the fertilisation process and may find possible application for the treatment of male subfertility. It has not yet been applied to the animal industry. The first sperm-egg injection experiments were described by Hiramoto (1962) in the sea urchin, and the first mammalian egg injection was described by Lin (1966) in the mouse. Uehara and Yanagimachi (1976) reported the microinjection of human and golden hamster sperm into hamster eggs. Good recent reviews of the subject are given by Markert (1983) and Kishimoto (1986), who also reviewed sperm micro-injection into starfish eggs.

The term "microfertilisation" was used by Trounson (1987) but the first human report came from Metka et al (1985) who "injected" single sperms into nine human oocytes. One pronuclear oocyte was obtained, which cleaved to the 4-cell stage.

Sperm can be introduced into the egg either singly or multiply. When injected into the perivitelline space, the term "sperm transfer" applies; direct injection into the egg cytoplasm is called sperm injection.

Indications

Microfertilisation may find application in the human with the following conditions:

Immotile sperm

Immotility of sperm may be environmental or congenital eg. immotile cilia syndrome. Environmental problems eg. drug therapy, usually result in decreased motility and may be improved by stopping the drug or using additives during sperm washing procedures (see Bongso, Ng and Ratnam in this volume). Congenital causes are more difficult to treat and there is the ethical question of whether propagation of such genes is desirable.

The immotile cilia syndrome is one such issue and it is an autosomal recessive (Palmblad and Mossberg, 1984). The condition is compatible with a normal life span if preventive therapy is given to avoid respiratory complications. We feel that microfertilisation is therefore justified. There is a report of a man with a dissociation between the ultrastructural and functional defects in his respiratory cilia and spermatozoa (Jonsson et al, 1982). The man had Kartagener's syndrome but motile spermatozoa and successfully fathered a son.

Severe oligozoospermia

When the sperm count is less that five million/ml, the prospects of fertilisation in IVF is much reduced (Yovich and Stanger, 1984). However, recently Yovich et al (1987) have described the technique of pronuclear stage transfer (PROST) for oligozoospermia, with improved pregnancy rates. However, fertilisation still requires the initial semen sample to contain more than five million/ml. Microfertilisation may find application here.

Failure of penetration of egg investments by sperm

There are instances where fertilisation fails to occur in spite of the presence of mature oocytes and spermatozoa of good motility (Chia et al, 1984). The zona penetration test may assist with the investigation of this problem (Overstreet, 1983). "Spontaneous" hardening of the zona pellucida may be one explanation and this has been observed in mouse oocytes cultured in vitro, with increasing resistence to solubilisation by chymotrypsin (De Felicia and Siracusa, 1982). These authors later suggested that follicular fluid may contain factors (especially glycosaminoglycans) that help prevent such hardening (De Felicia et al, 1985). Microfertilisation techniques may be employed if fertilisation fails to occur despite repeated attempts at IVF among all eggs obtained.

Multiple male factor problems

When three or more defects are demonstrated by semen analysis, successful fertilisation in vitro diminishes to less than eight per cent (Kretser et al, 1985). Where repeated failed fertilisation in vitro is encountered, there may be justification to employ microfertilisation techniques.

Sperm injection

Direct injection of sperm into the egg cytoplasm bypasses any form of sperm selection, "selection" having been done by the operator of the micromanipulator. The more active sperm are usually chosen but as yet there is no means of identifying sperm that are genetically normal. Only one sperm needs to be injected in a very small amount of egg suspension medium containing 10–20 per cent poly-vinyl-pyrrolidone (PVP). Oocyte mortality is high (Markert, 1983). Despite using very fine micropipettes (4–6 μm diameter) and even under ideal conditions, only about 30 per cent of injected eggs survive the procedure (Thadani, 1981).

For the injected sperm nucleus to continue its development, the oocyte must be activated during the injection procedure. With hamster oocytes, activation can be induced by suction of some cytoplasm before the sperm nucleus is injected (Perreault and Zirkin, 1982). The sperm head has to be separated from its tail in the first instance. This is done by ultrasonication, thereby reducing the size of the sperm. This also removes the outer acrosomal membrane, producing partial demembranation of the sperm head, a necessary prerequisite for sperm nuclear decondensation, although Thadani (1980) reported formation of the male pronucleus among 67 per cent following injection of "uncapacitated" mouse sperm into rat eggs. The sperm nucleus can also be treated with various detergents before microinjection, to study the effect of reduction of -S-S- bonds following sperm entry into the egg (Perreault et al, 1984).

Microinjection may be used to study heterospecies fertilisation, bypassing any species specific block. In 1976, Uehara and Yanagimachi reported the microinjection of human and golden hamster sperm into hamster eggs. The male nucleus decondensed in 11 of 16 hamster oocytes microinjected with hamster sperm nuclei, and in eight of 16 hamster oocytes with human sperm nuclei. Interspecies microfertilisation was also described by Thadani (1980) who injected mouse and deer mouse sperm into rat oocytes. "Capacitated" and "uncapacitated" mouse sperms were injected into unfertilised rat oocytes. Twelve of 14 and 17 of 20 eggs that survived the injection of capacitated and uncapacitated sperms, respectively, developed normal pronuclei. Similarly 17 of 20 eggs that survived the injection with "incubated" deer mouse sperm had normal pronuclei. The first cleavage division was similar to that of zona free rat oocytes fertilised with mouse sperm in vitro.

Naish et al (1987) injected hamster, mouse, rabbit and fish sperm nuclei, hamster hepatocyte nuclei into hamster eggs to investigate the ability of the egg to initiate DNA synthesis in nuclei differing in basic protein content. They reported that within six hours of the injection, nuclei of each type underwent transformation into pronuclei and DNA synthesis, with the male pronucleus being formed from 87 per cent of hepatocyte nuclei, 78 per cent of fish nuclei, 79 per cent of rabbit nuclei, 96 per cent of mouse nuclei, and 95 per cent of hamster nuclei. The authors concluded that non-specific mechanisms were involved within the hamster oocyte to convert sperm nuclei into pronuclei and to effect DNA synthesis, though the mechanisms, especially DNA synthesis, were more efficient with the hamster sperm nucleus rather heterologous sperm nuclei. Direct sperm injection of human oocytes appears to be proceeding in Norfolk, USA (Malloney M, 1987 — personal communication).

Sperm transfer

Sperm transfer is technically easier to perform and has much higher egg survival. To avoid polyspermy, single sperms are introduced into the perivitelline space (PVS). The PVS can be widened to improve the sperm transfer (Yang et al, 1988). Fusion of the sperm with the oocyte requires the sperm to be acrosomally reacted in the first instance (Yanagimachi and Noda, 1970; Yanagimachi, 1988). Therefore, for single sperm transfers to be performed efficiently, the proportion of acrosomally reacted sperm needs to be high. With rodents, the acrosome reaction is more uniform: eight per cent of mouse sperms collected from the epididymis and incubated in capacitating medium are already acrosomally reacted after half an hour, with the percentage increasing to 25–40 per cent by two hours (Fraser, 1983; Ward and Storey, 1984). Human sperm shows a much lower percentage of acrosome reaction, with only 10–30 per cent acrosomally reacted six hours after incubation in capacitating medium (Lee et al, 1987; Byrd and Wolf, 1986). Techniques to improve or synchronise acrosome reaction are therefore required in single sperm transfers in the human. This was reported by Laws-King et al (1987), where a calcium depleted strontium based medium was employed for overnight sperm incubation. A similar approach was used in the TEST-yolk buffer at 4°C (Johnston et al, 1984; Chan et al, 1987). Laws-King et al (1987) reported seven human eggs which had single sperm transfers six to nine hours after collection. Five became fertilised; three were cultured further in vitro before subjecting to transmission electron microscopy or karyotyping, and the remaining two showed normal cleavage. A further 12 human oocytes were cultured for 23 to 28 hours to enable the oocytes to reach metaphase II before single sperm transfers. Three fertilised but a further three showed parthenogenetic activation.

Single sperm transfer in the mouse has been used as a model for human sperm transfer (Mann, 1988). He observed two pronuclei and a second polar body eight hours after sperm transfer among 22 per cent (33/151) of his mouse eggs where a single sperm was introduced into the PVS. After transfer into pseudopregnant recipients, 54 per cent (26/48) of those that become fertilised developed into live fetuses.

There is possible advantage in the transfer of multiple sperm so that selection may occur at the level of the oolemma membrane containing sperm receptors and where a membrane block seems to occur (Wolf, 1978). When sperm transfer is performed because of poor sperm counts or decreased sperm motility, there is the potential risk of picking up chromosomally abnormal sperm. However, there is no unequivocal evidence that a correlation between genetic abnormality and decreased sperm motility exists. There is also no evidence suggesting the existence of oolemma membrane "selection", although Lazendorf et al (1987) reported 97 per cent of human sperm nuclei from donors who had poor penetration of zona free hamster eggs (ie. <10 per cent eggs penetrated) underwent decondensation after direct cytoplasmic injection into hamster oocytes.

Multiple sperm transfer of human sperms into human and golden hamster eggs were reported by Lassalle et al (1987). They injected sperm from three normal donors who gave a >20 per cent oocyte penetration rate in the sperm penetration assay using zona free hamster eggs. With one to four sperms transferred, up to nine per cent of hamster eggs were penetrated. With five to 12 sperms, the penetration was 36–37 per cent. With 12 or or more sperms transferred, penetration decreased to between zero and 6.6 per cent. No polyspermy was observed when one to four sperms were transferred, but polyspermy occurred in 55 per cent (10/18) when five to 12 sperms were transferred, and 100 per cent (2/2) when >12 sperms were transferred. Unfortunately, there was no description of the degree of polyspermy. Lassalle et al (1987) also reported multiple sperm transfer in human oocytes: three to five sperms were transferred into seven oocytes resulting in three monospermic fertilisations. When the sperms transferred were increased to 10–12 sperms per egg, polyspermy occurred in two of three eggs fertilised.

Whole immotile sperms have been transferred into human eggs, especially in the immotile cilia syndrome. Ng et al (1987) reported fertilisation of a donated egg by sperms from a patient with immotile cilia syndrome, after tearing the zona pellucida in the presence of the immotile sperms without the micromanipulator. Two pronuclei and an abnormal sperm tail next to one of the pronuclei were observed on transmission electron microscopy. The wife's eggs were later subjected to multiple sperm transfer. Of five eggs treated, only three became fertilised and were transferred but no pregnancy resulted (Bongso et al, 1989). The introduction of immotile sperms into the PVS can therefore result in fertilisation. Similar work in the mouse by Barg et al (1986) does not support this observation.

Sperm receptors on the oolemma membrane

There is increasing evidence to suggest the existence of some sort of sperm receptor on the oolemma membrane. Earlier studies on zona free eggs suggested some form of block to excessive polyspermy (Pavlok and McLaren, 1972; Toyoda and Chang, 1968; Niwa and Chang, 1975). In a study of murine gametes, Ng and Solter transferred between three and five motile sperms into eggs before and after ethanol activation of the eggs (see Cuthbertson, 1983). Of 101 eggs in which there was no ethanol activation, 32 (31.7 per cent) developed two pronuclei and a second polar body at eight hours. There was a very low polyspermy rate: only two eggs with three pronuclei, and none with more than three pronuclei by eight hours (Table 11-1). The fertilisation rates (monospermic and polyspermic) were not significantly different from eggs that were exposed to ethanol one to two hours after the multiple sperm transfer. However, when the eggs were exposed to ethanol half to one hour before the sperm transfer, only eight of 60 eggs were fertilised.

These observations support the hypothesis that sperm receptors are present on the oolemma membrane of zona intact eggs because the polyspermy rates were low despite transfer of three to five sperms; moreover, ethanol activation prior to sperm transfer probably caused removal or inactivation of sperm receptors thus resulting in low fertilisation rates. The presence of sperm receptors on the oolemma membrane may explain the low fertilisation rates of inter-species fertilisation in zona free eggs, with the exception of rat and golden hamster eggs (Yanagimachi, 1984). In both these species, it is possible that the sperm receptors are not specific.

When large numbers of sperm are transferred into the PVS, there is a greater chance of polyspermy (Lassalle et al, 1987). This occurrs despite the presence of sperm receptors on the oolemma membrane. With high sperm concentration, it is conceivable that more than one sperm could be attached to the receptors on the oolemma membrane before these receptors become inactivated, possibly by cortical granule release.

The risk of chromosomal abnormality

Male subfertility may be associated with a higher percentage of chromosomally or genetically abnormal sperm. In a survey of male patients attending a subfertility clinic. Chandley et al (1975) reported a frequency of two per cent chromosomal abnormality, a frequency that rose to six per cent when the mean sperm count was less than 20 million per ml, and 15 per cent in the azoospermic men. Earlier studies by Kjessler (1972) also revealed that the majority of chromosomally abnormal infertile men were oligospermic or azoospermic. In a study on 1000 human sperm pronuclear chromosome complements from 33 normal donors, Martin (1983) reported an abnormality rate of 8.5 per cent with 5.2 per cent aneuploidy and 3.3 per cent structural abnormalities. There is also an increased incidence of spina bifida and transposition of great vessels from babies born after IVF and GIFT in Australia and New Zealand (Lancaster, 1987). This may be related to the high incidence of chromosomal abnormality seen in human eggs collected after ovarian stimulation (Wramsby et al, 1987).

Fusion of the male germ cell with the metaphase II oocyte

Besides the introduction of the mature sperm into the metaphase II oocyte, it may be possible to use the male genome during its earlier stages of development. Fusion of the murine pachytene spermatocyte, Golgi phase spermatid, and male pronucleus with the metaphase II oocyte were recently performed by Ng and Solter. Besides chromosomal asynchrony, there may be important cytoplasmic effects on the nucleus. This may occur following spermatocyte and spermatid transfer. However, the technique of pronuclear transfer, originally described by McGrath and Solter (1983), allows only minimal transfer of cytoplasm in the creation of the karyoplast.

In the experiments of Ng and Solter, the pachytene spermatocyte had not undergone its first meiotic division, and the chromosomes were in tetramers. Eight hours after fusion, 22 zygotes from 30 oocytes developed one to three pronuclei. Whole mount spreads revealed that meiotic division of the male chromosomes occurred within the activated oocyte, and about 10 per cent of the resulting embryos were diploid. This observation led the authors to believe the existence of factors/proteins within the oocytes that acted on the male chromosomes whilst completing the meiosis of the female chromosomes. This also suggested that the factors/proteins involved were not specific to the second meiotic division the oocyte. Interestingly, none of the embryos developed beyond the morula stage.

Golgi phase spermatids are haploid, but have not undergone spermiogenesis. Of 21 oocytes fused, none were diploid; chromosomal preparations showed that the chromosomes from the male remained as separate chromatin masses. The maximal development of these spermatid nuclei was that of a Stage I pronucleus.

Male pronuclear fusion resulted in multiple "pronuclei" at eight hours in one of 22 early male pronuclear transfers and four of 17 late male pronuclear transfers. On whole mount spreads, the male pronucleus could be seen to "break down" into multilobed nuclei, which were probably micronuclei. The authors believe there was spindle "fragility", perhaps due to spindle formation that was out of phase with kinetochore formation.

The results of the study showed that meiotic "asynchrony" is incompatible with normal embryonic development. It is unlikely that the treatment of male subfertility by fusion of the early male germ cell obtained perhaps from testicular biopsy with the mature oocyte is feasible.

Conclusion

While microfertilisation (especially sperm transfer) offers some hope for the treatment of male subfertility, there are severe limitations to its use. It requires special equipment and training besides being a time consuming procedure. Presently, the fertilisation rates are low. There is a need for more basic research and a deeper understanding of the process of fertilisation. As yet there has not been any report of a human pregnancy obtained with this procedure. Should pregnancy occurr then karyotyping of the fetus should be recommended to exclude chromosomal abnormality.

Acknowledgements

The senior author is grateful to Drs Davor Solter and John Aaronson of the Wistar Institute, Philadelphia, for their guidance in micromanipulation,, and to Dr Ryuzo Yanagimachi and Dr Cheng-Hsiung Yang of the University of Hawaii for their help in sperm injection of hamster oocytes.

Table 11-1
Fertilisation of mouse eggs after transfer of three to five sperms into the perivitelline space

Ethanol activation	n	2PN and 2nd PB	3PN and 2nd PB	>3PN and 2nd PB
Nil	101	32	2	0
After sperm transfer	137	43	1	0
Before sperm transfer	60	8	0	0

References

Asch, R. Results of the multicentric international cooperative study of GIFT. Plenary lecture 70, *5th World Congress of In Vitro Fertilisation*, Virginia, 1987.

Barg, P.E. Wahrman, M.Z., Talansky, B.E. and Gordon, J.W. Capacitated, acrosome reacted but immotile sperm, when microinjected under the mouse zona pellucida, will not fertilize the oocyte. *Journal of Experimental Zoology*, 1986; 237: 365.

Bongso, T.A., Sathananthan, A.H., Wong P.C., Ratnam, S.S., Ng S.C., Andandakumar, C. and Ganatra, S. Human fertilization by microinjection of immotile sperm. *Human Reproduction*, 1989, in press.

Byrd, W. and Wolf, D.P. Acrosomal status in fresh and capacitated human ejaculated sperm. *Biology of Reproduction*, 1986; 34: 859.

Chan, S.Y.W., Li S.Q. and Wang, C. TEST-yolk buffer storage increases the capacity of human sperm to penetrate hamster eggs in vitro. *International Journal of Andrology*, 1987; 10: 517.

Chandley, A.C., Edmond, P., Christie, S., Gowans, L., Fletcher, J., Frackiewicz, A. and Newton, M. Cytogenetics and infertility in man, Part 1: Karyotype and seminar analysis. *Annals of Human Genetics*, 1975; 39: 31.

Chia, C.M., Sathananthan, H., Ng S.C., Law H.Y. and Edirisinghe, W.R. Ultrastructural investigation of failed in vitro fertilisation in idiopathic subfertility. Abstract, *18th Singapore Malaysia Congress of Medicine*, 1984.

Cuthbertson, K.S.R. Parthenogenetic activation of mouse oocytes in vitro with ethanol and benzyl alcohol. *Journal of Experimental Zoology*, 1983; 226: 311.

De Felici, M. and Siracusa, G. "Spontaneous" hardening of the zona pellucida of mouse oocytes during in vitro culture. *Gamete Research*, 1982; 6: 107.

De Felici, M., Salustri, A. and Siracusa, G. "Spontaneous" hardening of the zona pellucida of mouse oocytes during in vitro culture II. The effect of follicular fluid and glycosaminoglycans. *Gamete Research*, 1985; 12: 227.

de Kretser, D.M., Yates, C.A., McDonald, J., Leeton, J.F., Southwick, G., Temple-Smith, P.D., Trounson, A.O. and Wood, E.C. The use of in vitro fertilization in the management of male infertility. In Rolland, R., Heineman, M.J., Hillier, S.G. and Vemer H. (Eds), *Gamete Quality and Fertility Regulation*, Excerpta Medica, Amsterdam, 1985.

Fraser, L. Potassium ions modulate expression of mouse sperm fertilizing ability, acrosome reaction and hyperactivated motility in vitro. *Journal of Reproduction and Fertility*, 1983; 69: 539.

Hiramoto, Y. Microinjection of the live spermatozoon into sea urchin eggs. *Experimental Cell Research*, 1962; 27: 416.

Johnson, A.R., Syms, A.J., Lipschultz, L.I. and Smith, R.G. Conditions influencing human sperm capacitation and penetration of zona free hamster ova. *Fertility and Sterility*, 1984; 41: 603.

Jonsson, M.S., McCormick, J.R., Gillies, C.J. and Gondos, B. Kartagener's syndrome with motile sperm. *New England Journal of Medicine*, 1982; 307: 1131.

Kishimoto, T. Microinjection and cytoplasmic transfer in starfish oocytes. *Methods in Cell Biology*, 1986; 27: 379.

Kjessler, B. Facteurs genetiques dans la subfertile male humaine. In *Fecondite et Sterilite du Male*, Acquisitions recentes, Paris, Masson, 1972.

Lancaster, P.A.L. Congenital abnormalities after in vitro fertilization. *Lancet*, 1987; 2: 1392.

Lassalle, B., Courtot, A.M. and Testart, J. In vitro fertilization of hamster and human oocytes by microinjection of human sperm. *Gamete Research*, 1987; 16: 69.

Laws-King, A., Trounson, A., Sathananthan, H. and Kola, I. Fertilization of human oocytes by microinjection of a single spermatozoon under the zona pellucida. *Fertility and Sterility*, 1987; 48: 637.

Lazendorf, S.E., Mayer, J.F., Swanson, J., Acosta, A., Hamilton, M. and Hodgen, G.D. The fertilizing potential of human spermatozoa following microsurgical injection into oocytes. Abstract, *5th World Congress of IVF & ET*, Virginia, 1987.

Lee, M.A., Trucco, G.S., Bechtol, K.B., Wummer, N., Kopf, G.S., Glasco, L. and Storey, B.T. Capacitation and acrosome reactions in human spermatozoa monitored by a chlortetracylcine flourescence assay. *Fertility and Sterility*, 1987; 48: 649.

Lin, T.P. Microinjection of mouse eggs. *Science*, 1966; 151: 333.

Mann, J.R. Full term development of mouse eggs fertilized by a spermatozoon microinjected under the zona pellucida. *Biology of Reproduction*, 1988, in press.

Markert, C.L. Fertilization of mammalian eggs by sperm injection. *Journal of Experimental Zoology*, 1983; 228: 195.

Martin, R.H. The chromosome constitution of 1000 human spermatozoa. *Human Genetics*, 1983: 63: 305.

McGrath, J. and Solter, D. Nuclear transplantation in the mouse embryo by microsurgery and cell fusion. *Science*, 1983: 220: 1300.

Metka, M., Haromy, T., Huber, J. and Schurz, B. Artificial insemination using a micromanipulator. *Fertilitat*, 1985; 1: 41.

Naish, S.J., Perreault, S.D. and Zirkin, B.R. DNA synthesis following microinjection of heterologous sperm and somatic cell nuclei into hamster oocytes. *Gamete Research*, 1987; 18: 109.

Ng S.C., Sathananthan, A.H., Edirisinghe, W.R., Ho K.C.J., Wong P.C., Ratnam, S.S. and Ganatra, S. Fertilization of an human egg with sperm from a patient with immotile cilia syndrome: Case report. In Ratnam, S.S., Teoh, E.S. and Anadakumar, C. (Eds), *Infertility*, Advances in Fertility and Sterility series Vol. 4, Parthenon Publishing Group, Lancaster, 1987, 71.

Ng S.C. and Solter, D. Fusion of male germ cells (from male pronucleus to pachytene spermatocyte) with the metaphase II oocyte in the mouse. In preparation.

Niwa, K. and Chang, M.C. Requirement of capacitation for sperm penetration of zona free rat eggs. *Journal of Reproduction and Fertility*, 1975; 44: 305.

Overstreet, J.W. The use of the human zona pellucida in diagnostic tests of sperm fertilizing capability. In Crosignani, P.G. and Rubin, B.L. (Eds), *In Vitro Fertilization and Embryo Transfer. Proceedings Serono Clinical Colloquia on Reproduction No. 4*, Academic Press, London, 1983, 145.

Palmblad, J. and Mossberg, B. Ultrastructural, cellular and clinical features of the immotile cilia syndrome. *Annual Review of Medicine*, 1984; 35: 481.

Pavlok, A. and McLauren, A. The role of cumulus cells and the zona pellucida in fertilization of mouse eggs in vitro. *Journal of Reproduction and Fertility*, 1972; 29: 91.

Perreault, S.D. and Zirkin, B.R. Sperm nuclear decondensation in mammals: Role of sperm associated proteinase in vivo. *Journal of Experimental Zoology*, 1982; 224: 253.

Perreault, S.D., Wolf, R.A. and Zirkin, B.R. The role of disulfide bond reduction during mammalian sperm nuclear decondensation in vivo. *Developmental Biology*, 1984; 101: 160.

Rosenwaks, Z. State of the art lecture: In vitro fertilization. *43rd meeting of American Fertility Society*, 1987.

Thadani, V.M. A study of hetero-specific sperm-egg interactions in the rat, mouse and deer mouse using in vitro fertilization and sperm injection. *Journal of Experimental Zoology*, 1980; 212: 435.

Thadani, V.M. *Study of Oocyte Interactions Using In Vitro Fertilization and Sperm Microinjection*, PhD Thesis, Yale University, 1981.

Toyoda, Y. and Chang M.C. Sperm penetration of rat eggs in vitro after dissolution of zona pellucida by chymotrypsin. *Nature*, 1968; 220: 589.

Trounson, A. Microfertilization. Plenary lecture 56. *5th World Congress of In Vitro Fertilization*, Virginia, 1987.

Uehara, T. and Yanagimachi, R. Microsurgical injection of spermatozoa into hamster eggs with subsequent transformation of sperm nuclei into male pronuclei. *Biology of Reproduction*, 1976; 15: 476.

Ward, C.R. and Storey, B.T. Determination of the time course of capacitation in mouse spermatozoa using a chlortetracycline flourescence assay. *Developmental Biology*, 1984; 104: 287.

Wolf, D.P. The block to sperm penetration in zona free mouse eggs. *Developmental Biology*, 1978; 64: 1.

Wramsby, H., Fredga, K. and Liedholm, P. Chromosome analysis of human oocytes recovered from preovulatory follicles in stimulated cycles. *New England Journal of Medicine*, 1987; 316: 121.

Yanagimachi, R. and Noda, Y.D. Physiological changes in the post nuclear cap region of mammalian spermatozoa: A necessary preliminary to the membrane fusion between sperm and egg cells. *Journal of Ultrastructural Research*, 1970; 31: 486.

Yanagimachi, R. Zona free hamster eggs: Their use in assessing fertilizing capacity and examining chromosomes of human spermatozoa. *Gamete Research*, 1984; 10: 187.

Yanagimachi, R. Mammalian fertilization. In Knobil, E. and Neill, J. (Eds), *The Physiology of Reproduction*, Raven Press, New York, 1988, 135.

Yang, X., Chen, J., Chen, Y. and Foote, R.H. Survival of rabbit eggs shrunken to aid in sperm microinjection. *Theriogenology*, 1988; 29: 336.

Yovich, J.L. and Stanger, J.D. The limitations of in vitro fertilization from males with severe oligospermia and abnormal sperm morphology. *Journal of In Vitro Fertilisation and Embryo Transfer*, 1984: 1: 172.

Yovich, J.L., Blackledge, D.G., Richardson, P.A., Matson, P.L., Turner, S.R. and Draper, R. Pregnancies following pronuclear stage tubal transfer. *Fertility and Sterility*, 1987; 48: 851.

12
Infertility due to sperm dysfunction

P.G. Wardle, W.C.L. Ford and M.G.R. Hull

Introduction

Sperm dysfunction represents one of the biggest and most elusive problems in infertility practice. Not only is it a major cause of infertility but diagnosis and treatment are largely ineffective. The only recent real advance has been the recognition of the dysfunction. With the exception of antisperm antibodies, and to a lesser extent infections, there is no diagnostic means of recognising the underlying cause. There is also virtually no treatment of proven effectiveness, and no advance is likely to be made until there is understanding of the fundamentals of sperm physiology and its disorder. Empirical treatment aimed simply at bringing sperm into close contact with the oocyte — by intrauterine insemination (IUI), GIFT and IVF — has not been entirely effective.

Donor insemination (DI) will remain the most effective treatment for some years to come, and although not a cure for the problem, but merely bypassing it, it also brings with it ethical difficulties. DI will at least become better accepted as society learns to distinguish between fertility and virility in men, and as sperm dysfunction becomes reliably definable in men with normal or only mildly reduced sperm "counts" as found by standard seminal analysis.

This chapter will therefore focus on the recognition of sperm dysfunction, starting with critical questioning of the accuracy of the standard seminal analysis and emphasising the need instead of testing for *function*. Basic aspects of sperm function and their laboratory investigation, to improve understanding of the fundamental problems affecting clinical practice will also be discussed. Treatment will be considered in a limited way as so much of it is undertaken hopefully and without proven benefit.

It has been estimated that in 25 to 50 per cent of infertile couples the cause lies wholly or partly with the male partner (Gottesman and Bain, 1980; Hull et al, 1985; Spira, 1986). In a population based study employing strict criteria for sperm dysfunction (Hull et al, 1985) the frequency of male infertility was 26 per cent. Only two per cent was due to azoospermia, whether caused by obstruction, spermatogenic failure, or gonadotrophin deficiency. The vast majority — 24 per cent of all infertile couples — was due to sperm dysfunction, often associated with normal sperm "counts" on standard seminal analysis.

Most male infertility is not absolute, there being some degree of subfertility. This can lead to difficulty in distinguishing between male and female underlying factors with dual abnormalities occurring fairly commonly. Complicated statistical calculations have been undertaken to take account indirectly of the past uncertainties in recognising both male and female subfertility (Aafjes et al, 1978; Comhaire, 1987), and in cases of apparent male infertility the need to attend to possible female factors has been emphasised (Steinberger and Rodriguez-Rigau, 1983). We agree strongly with the need to investigate both partners fully and to treat them both where appropriate. On the other hand we no longer agree with speculative treatment of the woman because of uncertainty of the male condition. Definition of sperm dysfunction causing severe male subfertility can now be made confidently. All of our studies (see below) on male fertility have been undertaken after rigorous exclusion of female infertility factors.

Standard seminal analysis

Microscopic assessment of semen has been a central element for the objective measurement of a man's fertility since a standardised technique was first described by Macomber and Sanders (1929). Their method was similar to that used for a blood cell count and, as preparations were fixed in formalin, only took account of sperm density. Refinement of the technique followed with the introduction of assessments of sperm motility and morphology, and several large studies have examined differences in reputedly fertile and infertile men (Page and Houlding, 1951; MacLeod and Gold, 1951 and 1953; Rehan et al, 1975; Zuckerman et al, 1977). In an attempt to standardise the techniques of semen analysis, the World Health Organisation (1980) recommended methods for measurement of seminal volume, sperm density, quantitative and qualitative assessment of motility, sperm viability, morphology, and agglutination. In addition, "normal" ranges and threshold values were suggested. However, despite the WHO recommendations, there is still considerable controversy about acceptable criteria for a "normal" semen analysis.

There is considerable variation in semen quality for any individual when successive samples are analysed (Hotchkiss, 1941; Freund, 1962; Poland et al, 1985). Whether studies have been undertaken on supposed fertile or infertile men, the duration of prior sexual continence has been shown to have a marked effect on sperm density (Schwartz et al, 1979; Baker et al, 1981; Levin et al, 1986), motility (Freund, 1962; Heuchel et al, 1981; Poland et al, 1985) and morphology (Baker et al, 1981; Schwartz et al, 1986). Some of these variables also appear to be subject to seasonal variation (Baker et al, 1981). Some authors advise analysis of several semen samples to take account of the degree of natural variation (Pryor, 1981; Poland et al, 1985). Although this may improve the prognostic value of seminal analysis for male fertility, there will still inevitably be some inaccuracy regarding the consistency of quality of subsequent ejaculates. The two most important criticisms of reported studies are a lack of control of female factors and a retrospective approach. The need for prospective study will be explained shortly.

Let us take a fresh approach to evaluating seminal analysis. Aitken et al (1982a) found that in couples with prolonged and apparently unexplained infertility, in whom the woman was normal and the man had a normal seminal analysis, the sperms lacked fertilising ability in one third of cases as demonstrated by the hamster egg penetration test. Thus, if it is accepted that some men with normal sperm counts are severely subfertile, it is less surprising that some men with low counts are in fact normally fertile. Therefore let us set aside present notions about what are critical sperm "counts" for normality and study the matter prospectively with an open mind.

Prospective study is essential. The usual retrospective studies of men whose wives have become pregnant, demonstrate what sperm "counts" are *possible* with which to achieve pregnancy, but not what is *probable.* This point is demonstrated in Figure 12-1 and explained in the legend. The typical sigmoid curve relating fertility to sperm "counts" is best demonstrated (see below) by studies of fertilisation rates in vitro. The relationship to natural pregnancy rates is less clearly demonstrated, being more remote due to the time span involved.

Wardle (1987) studied fertilisation rates in vitro in infertile couples in whom the woman had normal ovarian function, and ovarian stimulation for IVF treatment was standardised. Every seminal variable was studied after dividing the range of values into bands, as exemplified by the results for sperm density shown in Figure 12-2. Similar relationships were found for the other variables, principally the proportions with progressive motility and with normal morphology. The normal criteria derived from these results were: sperm density 40×10^6/ml (see Figure 12-2); progressive motility 40 per cent; normal morphology 40 per cent.

The relationship of fertilisation rates to combinations of abnormalities of one or more of these variables (or none, implying complete normality) is shown in Figure 12-3. This demonstrates a significant but only small reduction in fertility when only one or two variables are abnormally low, but a very large reduction when all three variables are abnormal. These findings are similar to those reported by De Kretser et al (1985).

Another way of taking account of all the variables in an individual is to calculate their product, ie. density × proportion progressive motility × proportion normal morphology, or the motile normal sperm density (MNSD). Although this derivation assumes equal distribution of morphology between the motile and non-motile fractions, which is unlikely to be true, it was found to be the most useful index of natural fertility by Glazener et al (1987a) as discussed below. Fertilisation rates in vitro related to the MNSD are shown in Figure 12-4.

Glazener et al (1987a) undertook prospective studies of natural fertility (in previously infertile couples) relating cumulative conception rates during 18 months to each seminal variable divided into banded values. Female infertility factors were carefully excluded. For every variable there was marked overlap in the results between the banded values and it was only possible eventually to distinguish significant differences between two main subgroups of values. This is exemplified in Figure 12-5 which shows the results for MNSD, which was found to be the most useful seminal predictor of pregnancy, the critical value being 4×10^6/ml. Nevertheless, although significant, the power of prediction is clearly weak both for conception and failure to conceive; only about 60 per cent of couples with a normal MNSD achieved pregnancy within 18 months, yet 30 per cent with a low MNSD achieved a pregnancy. This is only half the predictive power of the simplest test of sperm function — postcoital mucus penetration and survival — which Glazener et al (1987a) compared in the same study, as will be described later.

These findings confirm the conclusions of others (Smith et al, 1977; Glass and Ericsson, 1979; Aitken et al, 1984) that seminal analysis is of limited value in assessing a man's fertility. Perhaps that should not be surprising. Most sperm in a semen sample are redundant and examining sperm in semen can give no direct indication of the sperm's functional ability, which ranges from penetration of cervical mucus to fertilisation of the egg. Indeed, it is worth appreciating that seminal plasma is a relatively hostile environment for sperm and it is perhaps wrong to undertake seminal analysis some hours after ejaculation. The several constituents of seminal plasma are mixed with the sperm only at ejaculation and the fertilising ability of sperm diminishes substantially with time spent in semen (Kanwar et al, 1979), the reduction evident sometimes within 30 minutes (Rogers, 1985). Thus, it seems that seminal plasma acts essentially as a very brief transport medium and is an unfavourable medium in which to examine sperm.

It is now clear, as will be discussed, that it is the functional ability of sperm that must be assessed, limited to the best subpopulation of sperm, and carried out in supportive physiological media, whether natural cervical mucus or artificial media. Therefore, before discussing tests of function we would like to describe our clinical philosophical approach to such testing and to describe basic sperm phsyiology in some detail.

The philosophy of sperm function tests

At present the principal objective of semen analysis is to provide an accurate estimate of a man's fertility. Infertility or subfertility can only be ascribed to a defined defect in sperm function in very few patients and the responsible lesion in the male reproductive tract can be identified in fewer still. The introduction of sperm function tests based on our growing knowledge of sperm physiology is one approach which will contribute to assigning infertility to specific causes. Once this is achieved, the rational development of therapy will be possible and in some cases the occurrence of infertility may be prevented. A further advantage will be to replace subjective assessments by quantitative objective methods which are easier to standardise and should be more reproducible between different laboratories.

Sperm function tests range between those, such as the hamster egg test, which demand that the spermatozoa utilise a large proportion of the physiological systems required for fertilisation and others, eg. the measurement of free oxygen radical production, which focus on a single biochemical pathway. We hope that a rational system of seminology can be developed which will allow fertility to be estimated by a wide ranging test and the responsible lesion diagnosed by a series of more specific assays. However, many sperm function tests are relatively complex, time consuming, and expensive, and their adoption beyond the research laboratory will depend on whether the additional information they provide can justify costs involved.

The physiology of spermatozoa in the female reproductive tract

Transport of spermatozoa

Between 5 and 200 million spermatozoa are deposited in the vagina after coitus but only a few hundred of these will reach the oviduct where fertilisation occurs. In the rabbit, a population of spermatozoa reaches the oviduct one minute after coitus but most are damaged and are rapidly cleared off the peritoneal cavity and play no role in fertilisation (Overstreet and Cooper, 1978a). It is doubtful if rapid sperm transport occurs in the human (see Mortimer, 1983). The fertilising population of spermatozoa move up the female reproductive tract during a second sustained phase of transport. In the rabbit, the main barriers are the cervix and the utero-tubal junctions, and marked decreases in the number of spermatozoa occur as these are crossed (Figure 12-6). In the rabbit, no sperms (from this cohort) enter the tubal isthmus until six hours post-coitum and only about 150 are present in the ampulla at the time of ovulation. (Overstreet and Cooper, 1978b). A similar degree of attenuation occurs in the human (Ahlgren, 1975; see Mortimer, 1983). Evidence from large domestic animals suggests that the isthmus of the oviduct retains a population of viable sperms in a quiescent state which can be reactivated and released into the ampulla when the egg is ready to be fertilised.

Initiation of motility

Sperms are immotile in the human epididymis and in the epididymides of most species except the rabbit. They become motile after they come into contact with seminal plasma and are deposited in the female reproductive tract. In rats and hamsters, motility of spermatozoa in the cauda epididymis is restrained by the enormous viscosity of the cauda epididymal plasma (Usselman and Cone, 1983). In the bull, cauda epididymal sperms are immotile because their internal pH (pHi) is decreased by the low pH of cauda epididymal plasma and an unidentified factor, probably a weak acid (Acott and Carr, 1984; Carr and Acott, 1984). Human cauda epididymal plasma is similar to that of the bull but motility of the human sperm is less markedly decreased by low pHi than bull sperm (Carr et al, 1985; Turner and Reich, 1985). It is doubtful if low pHi alone would be sufficient to suppress its motility in the epididymis. The mechanism for the initiation of human sperm motility is unknown. The problem is further complicated by the coagulation of human semen, which itself restrains sperm movement. Failure of semen to liquefy may contribute to infertility (see Mann and Lutwak Mann, 1981).

Invasion and penetration of cervical mucus

The cervix is a site of entry of sperm into the female genital tract. Glands within the cervical canal produce mucus which undergoes cyclical changes both in its physical properties (Odelblad, 1978) and structure (Daunter et al, 1976; Gaddam-Rosse et al, 1980). Odelblad described two main types of mucus: "G" mucus, produced under progesterone influence, and is usually scanty, tacky, cellular, and relatively resistant to sperm penetration; "E" mucus, produced under the influence of oestrogens in the preovulatory phase, and is copious, clear, ductile, and favours sperm penetration and migration.

Cervical mucus contains both a liquid and a gel phase. At mid-cycle it is in the aqueous phase and contains about 98 per cent water, inorganic ions, enzymes, other proteins, sugars and amino acids. The gel phase of "E" mucus consists of micelles which form strings between which the sperm must migrate (see Fordney-Settlage, 1981; Chantler and Elstein, 1986). The structure of the micelles serve to direct sperm into the cervical crypts or to pass along the canal according to the velocity with which the sperm swims (see Odelblad 1986). Normal interaction between sperm and pre-ovulatory cervical mucus includes the penetration of the sperm into the mucus, its passage through the mucus and the maintenance of sperm motility (Kremer and Jager 1988).

Sperm penetration of mucus at the semen-mucus interface occurs in a characteristic pattern. As shown later in the section depicting the normal in Figure 12-9, mucus appears to form billowing projections into semen between which are formed clefts. The clefts of semen become densely colonised by motile progressive spermatozoa, which penetrate the mucus primarily at the apex of each cleft, forming a narrow phalanx from which they gradually fan out at random, further invading the mucus. Spermatozoa also penetrate the mucus at the interface between clefts, but to a relatively slight degree. Abnormalities of these various features at the sperm-mucus interface are associated with specific abnormalities of semen and mucus, which will be described later in the section on sperm function tests.

Sperm quality rather than mucus quality was the factor responsible for the failure of sperm to penetrate mucus. The success of sperm-mucus penetration can be predicted from quantitative measurements of sperm motility. In experiments with sperm from different semen samples, velocity (or the concentration of sperm with a velocity $>25\mu m/sec$ at 37°C) was the most important determinant. Velocity affects both the number of collisions between sperm and mucus and the chance that a collision will lead to penetration of the mucus. However, the possibility that a collision once it occurs will result in successful penetration is also strongly influenced by the lateral head displacement of the sperm, a displacement of <4.5 μm being a significant disadvantage (Aitken et al, 1985; Aitken et al, 1986). A possible criticism of these studies is that poor motility could be associated with some other deleterious property of the sperm, but we have confirmed the importance of sperm velocity by measuring the ability of sperm from the same ejaculate to penetrate cervical mucus at different temperatures. Over the range 18–37°C, sperm velocity increases up to twofold but there is comparatively little change in lateral head displacement (Alison Ponsford and WCL Ford, unpublished data). All these studies were done with washed spermatozoa in vitro and ignored both any influence of the seminal plasma on the mucus (eg. it may serve to increase the often acidic pH of endocervical mucus) and differences between mucus structure in vivo and in vitro.

The ability of spermatozoa to progress through the mucus may be predicted from their motility in semen or in artificial media. However, a complete correlation should not be taken for granted because the movement characteristics of spermatozoa can be modified in cervical mucus, eg. (i) flagellar beat frequency is greater in cervical mucus than in semen or Tyrode's solution, whereas the beat amplitude is decreased and velocity is little changed (Katz et al, 1978); (ii) vanguard spermatozoa are able to modify the structure of the mucus so that they can move more rapidly than "followers" (Katz et al, 1982); (iii) the percentage motility and the percentage of morphologically normal spermatozoa in cervical mucus are of course greater than in seminal plasma due to selective penetration of the mucus (Hanson and Overstreet, 1981). It is generally presumed that spermatozoa which enter the cervical crypts survive there for a considerable time and gradually escape to find their way to the oviduct to ensure that a small but changing population of spermatozoa is present there to fertilise the egg when it passes through the ampulla (eg. see Kremer and Jager 1988). Human spermatozoa deposited in the cervix for 80 hours or longer can remain motile and the penetrate denuded hamster eggs (Gould et al, 1984). The importance of various factors which determine sperm survival is unknown. The properties of the sperm plasma membrane are very important, both with respect to its physiological integrity and the presence of antigens which can determine the interaction between the sperm and the immunological defences of the female tract. The sperm must also be metabolically competent.

Transport of sperm through the uterus and fallopian tubes.

Spermatozoa entering the internal cervical os are probably evenly distributed within the uterus by contractions of the myometrium (see Mortimer 1983). The utero-tubal junction is a barrier to sperm transport but the physiological mechanisms controlling it are unknown.

There is good evidence in cows and sheep that the population of spermatozoa capable of fertilisation is established in the isthmus of the oviduct six to eight hours after coitus. They are sequestered there for 17 to 18 hours until the moment of ovulation, when they are then displaced into the ampulla. In the pig, spermatozoa can be sequestered in the isthmus for as long as 40 hours. In the hamster, nearly all the spermatozoa that enter the oviduct are retained in the caudal isthmus and are released into the ampulla at ovulation. Transport of sperm to the cauda isthmus is accelerated when mating takes place shortly before ovulation (Smith et al, 1987). In the mouse, spermatozoa can be observed through the transparent walls of the oviduct: no spermatozoa are seen in the ampulla until around the time of ovulation, when they have hyperactivated motility. By contrast, a population of sperm is established in the lower isthmus one to two hours post-coitum, and these sperms are immotile or sluggishly motile, with some adhered to the epithelium. The immotile sperms regain their motility when dispersed in artificial media (Suarez, 1987).

These data suggest that at least in some animals the isthumus of the oviduct is responsible for controlling the access of sperm to the egg. This is probably true in humans but there is only a little evidence in support (Mortimer 1983).

Capacitation

Freshly ejaculated spermatozoa cannot immediately fertilise an egg but must first undergo a series of changes referred to collectively as capacitation. Capacitation takes several hours but the exact time required varies between species (see Hunter, 1987) and in man may vary between individuals (see Rogers et al, 1983). The consequences of capacitation are: (i) the spermatozoa begin to move with "whiplash" or "hyperactivated" motility, ie. the amplitude of flagella bending greatly increases and the cells move along erratic trajectories rather than progressing smoothly in straight lines; (ii) the spermatozoa become capable of undergoing the acrosome reaction (see Fraser, 1984); (iii) the spermatozoa develop an enhanced ability to bind to the zona pellucida (Lambert and Le, 1984). In vivo capacitation is timed to coincide with ovulation and is probably achieved by a suppressive effect of the tubal isthmus. In the mouse, hyperactivated spermatozoa can be seen in the uterus but their capacitation is reversed once they enter the isthmus of the oviduct (Suarez and Osman, 1987; Hunter 1987). Human sperm can capacitate in cervical mucus (Lambert et al, 1985) but the physiological significance of this is unknown.

Penetration of the egg investments and the acrosome reaction

Once the sperm encounters the egg, it must penetrate the egg's investments. The first barrier is the cumulus oophorus, including the corona radiata. During in vitro fertilisation, the cumulus is dispersed by the acrosomal enzymes. When physiological numbers of spermatozoa are present, this does not occur. When very small numbers of capacitated acrosome intact sperm are incubated with fresh eggs, they penetrate the cumulus without dispersing them, as shown in hamster studies (Corselli and Talbot, 1986).

Once the sperm has traversed the cumulus oophorus, the next obstacle is the zona pellucida. The sperm first attaches to the zona in a loose non-specific way and then binds tightly in a species specific way. Binding is mediated by sperm receptors in the zona and by corresponding egg binding proteins present in the sperm plasma membrane. In the mouse, only acrosome intact sperm can attach to the zona and go on to fertilise the egg. The zona sperm receptor is a 83,000Mr glycoprotein, ZP3, which contains both "N" and "O" linked oligosacharides on a 44,000Mr polypeptide core. The specificity of binding is determined by some of the O-linked carbohydrate moieties attached to ZP3 (see Wassarman, 1987) but binding is a two step process and may involve a trypsin like active site (Benau and Storey, 1987). The sperm-egg binding protein has not been identified, but likely candidates are galactosyl transferase or a trypsin like protease (see Wassarman, 1987). In the boar, a polypeptide of 53,000Mr can be extracted with detergents from sperm and binds zona glycoproteins (Brown and Jones, 1987).

Once bound, the sperm undergoes the acrosome reaction. This is a regulatory event separate from binding (Endo et al, 1987) and requires the polypeptide component of ZP3 to initiate it (see Wassarman, 1987). The acrosome reaction involves the fusion of the outer acrosomal membrane with the sperm plasma membrane over a number of sites. This results in the breakdown of the membranes covering the acrosome and ultimately to the shedding of the acrosomal cap and most of its contents. The acrosome reaction is calcium dependent and can be induced with the calcium ionophore A23187 but changes in internal pH, cAMP concentration, prostaglandins and phospholipase activity have also been implicated (see Fraser, 1984; Working and Meizel, 1983; Hyne, 1984; Mrsny and Meizel, 1980; Meizel and Turner 1984; Joyce et al, 1987; Bent et al, 1987). The human sperm acrosome reaction occurs slowly in sperm suspended in suitable media and is broadly similar to that in the animal sperm (Nagae et al, 1986; Stock and Fraser, 1987). It is likely that the physiological acrosome reaction occurs once the sperm is bound to the zona in both humans and mice (Singer et al, 1985). Solubilised human zona proteins are capable of inducing the acrosome reaction in human sperm (Cross et al, 1987) as are intact oocytes (De Jonge et al, 1988). On the other hand, the percentage of acrosome reacted sperm on the zona and in free suspension is the same one minute after co-incubation between capacitated human sperm and non-viable human oocytes, suggesting that both acrosome intact and acrosome reacted sperm can bind to the zona (Morales et al, 1988).

At this stage, the sperm must penetrate the zona pellucida. Penetration is not accompanied by a general dissolution of the zona. The penetrating sperm forms a channel through the zona hardly greater than its own head diameter. There is dispute as to whether this can be achieved by a mechanical force alone or by partial activity of the residual acrosin bound to the sperm head after the acrosome reaction (see Bedford, 1982; Katz and Demestre, 1985; Green, 1987).

Fertilisation

The sperm, after penetration, lies on the surface of the oolemma, which is evenly covered with microvilli. Fusion between the membranes of the sperm and egg begins in the post-acrosomal region. Fusion triggers cortical granule release in the egg and the zonal reaction, preventing polyspermy (see Bedford, 1982; Wassarman, 1987). Following fusion, the sperm head becomes drawn into the cytoplasm of the egg and swells or decondenses (see Fraser, 1984).

Conclusions

In order to achieve fertilisation in vivo, spermatozoa must be motile and capable of surviving within the female reproductive tract until ovulation occurs. They must be capable of responding to signals from the female reproductive tract eg. to remain quiescent when stored in the isthmus of the oviduct or to initiate capacitation at the appropriate time. They must be capable of recognising the egg, binding to it, and penetrating the zona pellucida. Finally, they must be able to fuse with the oolemma and be drawn into the egg where the sperm nucleus decondenses and ultimately fuses with the egg nucleus.

Sperm function tests

Post-coital test

After normal intercourse, sperms swim actively into the cervical mucus and colonise the cervical crypts. Insemination studies have shown this to occur within two hours and that the number of sperms present remains unchanged for 24 hours (Insler et al, 1980). Their fertile life may last as long as 80 hours. The cervix acts as a reservoir from which sperms are released steadily into the uterine cavity, largely compensating for inadequate timing of coitus with respect to ovulation. The post-coital test (PCT) involves microscopic examination of cervical mucus after intercourse to identify and quantify the sperms present, principally those moving with straightforward progression.

The first PCT was reported by Sims in 1866. Huhner developed the method further and first incorporated the PCT as a clinical investigation of infertility (Huhner, 1913). However, much of the work relating PCT results to fertility has been retrospective, with inadequate criteria (eg. Kovacs et al, 1978), or failure to compare results with those of normal fertile couples (eg. Harrison, 1977). Prospective studies have generally shown significant correlation between the PCT result and subsequent pregnancy (Scott et al, 1977; Harrison, 1981; Kremer, 1981), especially when time specific conception rates have been used for proper statistical comparison (Hull et al, 1982; Glazener et al, 1987b).

Although widely used as a clinical test of sperm function, the methodology and interpretation of the PCT vary widely in reported studies despite the WHO recommendations over these aspects (WHO, 1980). Thus post-coital testing with suboptimal mucus, instead of fully developed preovulatory mucus, does not reflect sperm function. This is particularly relevant when interpreting a poor or negative test. A delay of 12 to 18 hours after intercourse, the quantitative recording of only those sperm showing forward progression in at least five representative high-power (×400) microscope fields, and strict criteria of cervical mucus quality are all necessary for consideration of a valid result. Cervical mucus should appear clear to the naked eye, copious in amount (with a volume of at least 0.3 ml), ductile (to 10 cm) (Hull et al, 1982), and with a pH greater than 6.0 as sperms are immobilised in more acidic mucus (McBain and Clarke, 1986; Peek and

Mathews, 1986). If timing of the PCT is inaccurate, most apparently negative or poor PCT will be found to give a normal result when performed in a different cycle (Matthews et al, 1980). A negative or poor result should not be accepted as valid unless the mucus is fully developed, or timing of ovulation confirmed in cases of specific mucus defects unrelated to ovulatory disorder. It may be necessary to monitor ovulation by ultrasonography (Hamilton et al, 1986) or by the detection of the LH surge, although this may not be practicable as a routine. Even when a valid negative or poor PCT result is obtained, it is advisable to have it repeated and confirmed in a separate cycle before the result is accepted as a failure of postcoital sperm-mucus penetration and survival.

Inadequate standardisation of the PCT seems to account for much of the confusion regarding the prognostic value of the PCT for fertility. However, where strict criteria for interpretation have been applied, there is a clear correlation between the PCT and subsequent fertility (Harrison, 1980; Hull et al, 1982; Portuondo et al, 1982; Glazener et al, 1987a), with the zona free hamster egg penetration test (Soules et al, 1982; Schats et al, 1984; Aitken et al, 1985), and with human in vitro fertilisation (Hull, et al, 1984; Wardle et al, 1985; Hull et al, 1987).

Glazener et al (1987a) have studied the prognostic value of the PCT in direct comparison with standard seminal analysis. Time-specific cumulative conception rates related to the best seminal criterion (an MNSD of 4×10^6/ml) are shown in Figure 12-5. In the same untreated couples, in whom the female partner's investigations of fertility were all normal, including apparently normal preovulatory cervical mucus production, the conception rates related to the PCT results six to 18 hours after intercourse are shown in Figure 12-7. The PCT results were originally divided into several bands according to the number and motility of spermatozoa found but they could be reduced to only three significantly distinct groups as shown. Compared with the results related to seminal analysis shown in Figure 12-5, the distinction of the PCT results into three groups suggests the PCT may be a more sensitive prognostic index. Furthermore, the predictive power between positive and negative PCTs can be seen to be twice that of seminal analysis, particularly because of the predictive power for severe subfertility; negative PCTs were associated with only about a 15 per cent pregnancy rate after 18 months.

Direct comparison of the seminal and PCT results (excluding for simplicity the minority poor-positive PCT group) is shown in Figure 12-8. It is evident that when the PCT is favourable, the seminal sperm "counts" are irrelevant, suggesting good sperm function irrespective of numbers. By contrast, negative

PCTs indicate fairly severe subfertility even when seminal sperm "counts" are normal. When both PCT and seminal sperm "counts" are abnormal, there is severe subfertility. In other words, seminal analysis provides independent useful information only after finding unfavourable PCTs.

Although the PCT results generally correlate with fertilising ability of the sperm (see above), indicating that impairment of the PCT result is usually due to sperm dysfunction rather than mucus "hostility" (as was usually assumed), other causes are possible in a minority of cases and further diagnostic evaluation is required. Impairment of the PCT may also be due to primary defects or dysfunction of cervical mucus, secondary effects in mucus due to an unfavourable vaginal environment, or unadmitted coital failure. Therefore the next logical step is to test sperm-mucus penetration and invasion in vitro, ideally undertaking a "crossed invasion test" employing normal donor mucus and semen samples as controls.

In vitro sperm mucus penetration

In vitro testing of sperm invasion of cervical mucus provides alternative methods of assessing sperm function. The simplest technique involves semen and mucus drops placed apart on a microscope slide and brought into apposition by spreading under a cover slip so as to achieve a vertical interface. This test was first described by Miller and Kurzrok (1932) (the "K–M test"). As described by those authors, the test is essentially quantitative, the density of sperms being assessed at a certain distance (a low power field diameter) from the sperm-mucus interface. Glazener and Hull (1987), however, demonstrated the diagnostic value of the distinct qualitative changes evident at the interface.

As shown in Figure 12-9, normal sperm invasion of the mucus follows a characteristic pattern of cleft formation, dense colonisation of the clefts by spermatozoa, initial penetration of the mucus by phalanges of spermatozoa, followed by distinct deep invasion of mucus, and subsequent survival with progressive motility within it. Glazener and Hull (1987) studied these features in relation to distinct sperm defects, antisperm antibodies, and mucus defects. As implied in Figure 12-9, they found (i) close correlation of sperm defects with failure to form semen clefts and of spermatozoa to colonise clefts, with a diagnostic accuracy (positive and negative) of 90 per cent — most of the discrepancies, in which sperm dense clefts developed despite low sperm counts, were due to antisperm antibodies in semen; (ii) when sperm dense colonisation of clefts occurred normally, usually with phalanx formation, but with failure to invade mucus, close correlation was found with the demonstration by the MAR or TAT of antisperm antibodies in semen with a diagnostic accuracy of 81 per cent; (iii) there was insufficient evidence to relate failure of sperm survival in mucus after normal invasion and antisperm antibodies in mucus or specific disorder of mucus, partly because such problems seem to occur very uncommonly when properly investigated. In a population study Hull et al (1985) found mucus defects or dysfunction accounted for only three per cent of cases of infertility.

These findings are supported by earlier less specific studies. Reduced or absent penetration of cervical mucus has been associated with high titers of antisperm antibodies in semen (Kremer and Jager, 1976; Morgan et al, 1977) and with poor semen quality (Joyce and Vassilopoulos, 1981). Furthermore, failure of sperm-mucus penetration has been found to be associated with a reduced fertilising ability of the spermatozoa (Hull et al, 1984; Schats et al, 1984). It appears that the quality of motility of the sperm to penetrate cervical mucus and its vitality to survive for long periods in the mucus seem closely related to the functional characteristics required to penetrate the egg-zona-cumulus complex.

Thus the qualitative test of sperm penetration and invasion of cervical mucus at the interface offers considerable diagnostic value because of its simplicity and accuracy compared with the relative complexity of other tests. It also offers more specific information than the purely quantitative tests aimed at measuring depth of penetration (invasion) of mucus. The "K–M" test is the simplest of those tests, as mentioned earlier.

A more complicated test using a capillary tube filled with cervical mucus with one end immersed in semen was first described by Kremer in 1965. An improvement of the technique, using a flat capillary tube to make visualisation of the sperm easier, was introduced by Katz et al (1980). Although commonly used, we see little value for such tests in clinical practice although they may be useful in quantitative research.

One possible important distinction between tests of sperm-mucus penetration in vivo (the PCT) and in vitro is that the latter fails to test prolonged sperm survival, unlike the PCT, which should be done about 12 hours after intercourse (the studies by Glazener et al (1987a) depicted in Figures 12-7 and 12-8 were based on a delay of six to 18 hours). Our studies of in vitro fertilisation show a discrepancy between the PCT and the in vitro sperm-mucus invasion test in a small proportion of cases (Glazener and Hull, 1987). There was generally good correlation between sperm-mucus penetration and fertilisation. In about 12 per cent of cases although the PCT was negative, the in vitro sperm-mucus invasion test was normal and there was a severe reduction in the fertilisation rates (from 71 per cent to 10 per cent)

(Hull et al, 1987). This implies that a normal in vitro sperm-mucus invasion test can sometimes be misleading.

The PCT seems preferable as the primary screening test of sperm and mucus function, using the in vitro sperm-mucus invasion test should the PCT show repeatedly negative or poor results. The in vitro test can be further enhanced by the inclusion of control semen and mucus samples in a "crossed invasion test".

Crossed in vitro sperm mucus invasion test

In couples with poor or negative PCTs or in vitro invasion tests, interpretation of the result may be improved by the use of normal donor cervical mucus and semen together with the samples of mucus and semen from the infertile couple using in four-way in vitro crossed invasion test. A slide or capillary tube method may be employed (Kremer, 1968; Moghissi, 1967). Strict criteria on cervical mucus quality from both patient and donor need to be adhered to if reliable results are to be achieved. Crossed invasion studies in couples with abnormal PCT results confirm that these are far more frequently related to sperm rather than cervical mucus dysfunction (Jonsson et al, 1986). True cervical mucus dysfunction seems uncommon (Hull et al, 1985). Despite its presence, sperm can still be recovered from the pouch of Douglas (Stone, 1983).

Antisperm antibody testing

The presence of antisperm antibodies may be suspected by the presence of agglutinated sperm during seminal analysis, or by the characteristic pattern of sperm-mucus interaction in the qualitative in vitro sperm mucus invasion test. Specific assays for antisperm antibodies should be undertaken to establish its causal relationship with infertility.

A possible role of antisperm antibodies in infertility was first suggested by Rumke and Hellinger (1959) and they occur in three to 13 per cent of infertile men (Aafjes and Van der Vijver, 1976; Hargreave et al, 1980). The mechanisms by which they cause infertility remain to be defined but they appear to interfere with sperm motility, capacitation and the acrosome reaction (Bronson et al, 1983).

The mixed agglutination reaction (MAR) and the tray agglutination test (TAT) are widely used as screening tests for antisperm antibodies. The MAR test has limitations in determining the site of antibody binding on the sperm surface, and the TAT has a relatively high incidence of false positive reactions of uncertain clinical significance.

Present evidence suggests that antibodies which bind to the sperm head have a greater inhibitory effect on sperm mucus interaction (Bronson et al, 1982) and sperm fertilising capacity in vitro (Mandelbaum et al, 1987). Identification of the site of antibody binding to the sperm is therefore important and is possible using immunoglobulin coated polyacrylamide beads (Bronson et al, 1981) or latex particles (Comhaire et al, 1987). These are currently the most useful tests for detecting antisperm antibodies which may be of clinical importance in an infertile couple.

Although immunosuppression with corticosteroids may reduce the titer of antisperm antibodies in some cases, this has given inconsistent pregnancy successes (Hendry et al, 1981; Hargreave and Elton, 1982; Baker et al, 1983). A controlled trial by Coulson et al (1986) failed to show any significant improvement in conception rates. The incidence of serious side effects with corticosteroid treatment for antisperm antibodies varies between two and six per cent (Hendry et al, 1981; Schulman and Schulman, 1982).

Quantitative sperm motility measurements

Sperm motility has long been considered to be the best single parameter of the standard semen analysis to assess fertility (see Mann and Lutwak-Mann, 1981; Blasco, 1984; Overstreet and Katz 1987). Attention is now focussed on objective methods which allow the quantitative measurement of velocity and other movement characteristics of sperm in artificial culture media. These methods look at the best subpopulation of spermatozoa from a selective process of sperm penetration of the culture medium from which they are recovered.

Although many parameters can be deduced from laser light scattering by sperm in free suspension (eg. Jouannet et al, 1977; Frost and Cummins, 1981) most methods depend on recording the movement of spermatozoa on a microscope slide. Movement of sperm can be recorded with a still camera and dark field illumination either by leaving the shutter completely open for a suitable period of time, usually one second, when motile sperm appear as continuous tracks ("time-lapse photography") (Overstreet et al, 1979) or by using stroboscopic illumination (Makler, 1980). Alternatively the sperm's position can be plotted from frame-by-frame analysis of cinefilm or videotape (Katz and Overstreet, 1981). The latter analysis can be carried out by computer (Holt et al, 1985; see Overstreet and Katz, 1987). Whatever method is used, the most important parameters are the sperm velocity and the amplitude of lateral head displacement, that is, the sideways displacement of the head about the sperm's mean path (see Aitken, 1988). It is important to realise that the results obtained are not uniform for all methods used, eg. stroboscopic or frame-by-frame methods give lesser values for lateral head displacement than the time-lapse method. This is partly because measurements are made from the centre of the head in the former and the tip of the head in the latter. It is also important to note the temperature at which the measurements are made, the medium used to suspend the sperm, and the precautions taken to prevent spermatozoa from sticking to the glass of the slide or coverslip.

The average velocity of fertile human sperm lies between 25 and 50μm/sec and the average lateral head displacement between four and 6μm. The average velocity is decreased in sperm from infertile or subfertile men and in sperm exposed to inhibitors (Table 12-1). Mean sperm velocity and amplitude of lateral head displacement show a high positive correlation with fertilising potential (Milligan et al, 1980; Aitken et al, 1984; Feneux et al, 1985; Holt et al, 1985; Jeulin et al, 1986; Irvine and Aitken, 1986). However, both are continuous variables and the faster sperm in most infertile cases move as fast as the average sperm in fertile cases. So far, it has not been possible to define a minimum concentration of sperm which must fulfil set motility criteria for the sample to be considered fertile. However, it is clear that fertile samples will contain at least some spermatozoa with a velocity $>25\mu$m/s and a lateral head displacement >4.5 but $<10\mu$m. The predictive value of motility measurements is increased if they are made after time has been allowed for capacitation in culture media, rather than soon after washing and resuspension in buffer, or even on sperm in seminal plasma. More work is needed to determine if this is related to capacitation or simply to the ability of the sperm to survive.

Some observers classify spermatozoa into those exhibiting rolling or yawing modes of progression. Rolling sperm progress in a spiral path about a nearly straight average axis of progression, the sperm rotating as it moves forward. Yawing sperm does not rotate but the head oscillates from side to side as the sperm moves forward leaving a characteristic zig-zag track on time-lapse photographs (Overstreet et al, 1979). Yawing and other unusual modes of progression may be an artifactual consequence of confining the sperm to a limited depth on the microscope slide but can be consistently induced by treatment of motile sperm populations with caffeine (Rees J. M., Ford, W.C.L., unpublished results). Rolling sperm predominate in fertile cases and most published analyses of sperm movement in relation to fertility exclude the yawing sperm.

Human sperm can be demembranated with Triton X100 and reactivated with ATP. This should allow the identification of defects in ATP generation or the control systems governing motility and fundamental defects in the structure or function of the flagellum. In a group of asthenospermic men, less demembranated sperm became activated by ATP than in fertile controls, suggesting that the flagellar cause of immotility predominated (Liu et al, 1987). Another future possibility is the use of computer based motility assessment to detect hyperactivated motility and to provide an index of capacitation (Robertson et al, 1987).

The measurement of ATP concentration in semen

Comhaire et al (1983) claimed that the concentration of ATP in semen is an excellent indicator of fertility. This is based on the assumption that ATP in whole semen may be an index of its concentration in viable spermatozoa. However, other authors found that the ATP concentration in human spermatozoa did not correlate with their motility (Levin et al, 1981), or fertilising ability (Chan and Wang, 1987). ATP had little additional predictive value once sperm numbers had been taken into account (Irvine and Aitken, 1985). We have demonstrated that the glycolytic rate and ATP concentration in spermatozoa from normal donors can vary over a wide range without affecting their motility. However, if metabolism is inhibited by placing an artificial constraint on ATP production, then a correlation between ATP and motility can be demonstrated when the ATP concentration falls below a critical level. This relationship is clearer if the ATP/ADP ratio rather than ATP concentration is used (Rees, J.M. and Ford, W.C.L., unpublished data). It may be possible to define a threshold for the ATP/ADP ratio in human spermatozoa. Failure to exceed the value would indicate a deficit in energy metabolism. In our view, ATP is unlikely to be of significant prognostic value despite continued claims to the contrary (Comhaire et al, 1987b). An unexpected observation related to ATP is that the concentration of the enzyme creatine phosphokinase in semen is inversely related to the sperm concentration (Huszar et al, 1988).

Tests of sperm viability

In many circumstances, it would be helpful to decide if spermatozoa were alive or not, eg. when scoring acrosome reactions or to decide if spermatozoa were immotile because of some defect in the motile apparatus or because they were simply dead. Traditionally, this test is done by staining with eosin or trypan blue when only spermatozoa with damaged plasma membranes stain red or blue respectively (see Mann & Lutwak-Mann, 1981). Two new methods have appeared recently. If spermatozoa are suspended in a hypotonic medium the intact sperm cells absorb water and swell whereas sperm with damaged membranes do not. The swollen sperm exhibit a characteristic "looped" or "hairpin" configuration of the tail which can easily be recognised (Jeyendran et al, 1984). This forms the basis of the "hypo-osmotic swelling test" or HOST. The other method employs the fluorescent DNA stain Hoechst 33258, which stains the nuclei of damaged cells. These exhibit a bright blue fluorescence under ultraviolet illumination (Cross et al, 1986). In our hands, both of these assays can detect changes in the damaged spermatozoa after they have been subjected to stress by high speed centrifugation or by heating, and the increase in damaged sperm numbers correlates well with the decline in the percentage of motile spermatozoa and the severity of stress (McLaughlin, E.A. and Ford, W.C.L., unpublished results).

Electron microscopy

Electron microscopy cannot strictly be described as a sperm function test but it provides the most definitive method to diagnose flagellar defects eg. Kartegeners syndrome or abnormal acrosome morphology. The use of the lectron microscope for this purpose has recently been reviewed (Zamboni, 1987). The greatest limitation with this technique is that only a small number of spermatozoa from each ejaculate can be examined and it is difficult to ensure that these form a representative sample.

Free oxygen radical production

In living cells molecular oxygen (O_2) can be reduced to the superoxide radical (O_2^-) by the leakage of electrons from the mitochondrial electron transport chain. Superoxide radicals can decompose to yield still more reactive free radical compounds including hydroxyl radicals ($OH^\bullet$): These radicals can damage cell structure in many ways but one of the most significant is lipid peroxidation. To protect themselves against the destructive effect of free oxygen radicals, cells contain superoxide dismutase which converts O_2^- to hydrogen peroxide and also contain catalase and glutathione peroxidase which decompose the hydrogen peroxide to water (see Chance et al, 1979). Phagocytes produce superoxide as part of the "killing" reaction directed against foreign cells. In this case superoxide is generated by a specific NADPH oxidase (Rossi, 1986).

Human sperm generate free oxygen radicals and the extent of lipid peroxidation which these cause correlates closely with the loss of sperm motility during prolonged incubation. The sperm contain superoxide dismutase and glutathione peroxidase required to detoxify superoxide (Alvarez et al, 1987). A burst of oxygen radical production by human spermatozoa can be stimulated by capacitating doses of the calcium ionophore A23187. In spermatozoa from a substantial number of infertile men, the rate of oxygen radical production made in this way is much greater than in "normal" spermatozoa. Elevated oxygen radical production also correlates very closely with poor performance in the hamster egg test. The A23187 stimulated oxygen radical production does not depend on mitochondrial respiration but has properties reminiscent of the NADPH oxidase of phagocytes (Aitken & Clarkson, 1987). These observations are very exciting because they represent the first identification of a biochemical cause for infertility in the spermatozoa of a large group of patients. A number of simple and reliable assays are available to measure free oxygen radical production and potential therapies exist (see Aitken, 1988).

The acrosome reaction

The acrosome reaction is one of the most prominent events in the fertilisation process and it would be desirable to be able to assess it with a simple and reliable assay. Unfortunately, it is not possible to decide whether or not the human sperm acrosome is intact by simple light microscopy. Until recently it has only been feasible to score it reliably by electron microscopy (eg. Stock & Fraser, 1987) and by a quite complex triple staining method (Talbot & Chacon, 1981). Recently, however, methods based on the binding of monoclonal antibodies, lectins, or chlorotetracycline to the acrosomal membranes have been developed (Cross et al, 1986; Mortimer et al, 1987; Lee et al, 1987; see Aitken, 1988). These methods require concomitant testing of sperm viability to ensure that only viable sperms are being counted as acrosome reacted. Although there is some way to go, they hold out the prospects of rapid and reliable scoring of the acrosome reaction. Once this is achieved assessment of the ability of sperm to undergo the acrosome reaction after suitable stimulation will be a very useful sperm function test, capable of demonstrating the sperm's ability to capacitate with fewer biological variability than the hamster egg test.

Zona binding assays.

When human eggs are stored in a suitable highly concentrated salt solution, the zona pellucida retains its ability to bind and to be penetrated by spermatozoa, but because the egg is no longer viable it loses the ability to harden following penetration by one sperm. Thus when such eggs are incubated with fertile sperm the perivitelline space will contain very many spermatozoa which can easily be seen and these stored ova provide a quantitative system to assess the ability of spermatozoa to bind to and penetrate the zona (Yanagimachi et al, 1979). Scoring the assay can be facilitated by staining the spermatozoa with Hoescht 33342, a fluorescent DNA stain (Boatman et al, 1988). Although this would appear to be a useful assay capable of measuring parameters of sperm function which cannot be determined with the HOPT (being zona free) it has not been extensively validated for its ability to assess human male fertility. This is probably a consequence of the difficulty of procuring sufficient human eggs.

Hamster oocyte penetration test (HOPT)

The hamster oocyte penetration test provides an index of fertility, and permits the chromosomes of the sperm to be isolated from the decondensed nucleus and examined (see Yanagimachi, 1984; Rogers, 1985; Aitken, 1986). The test demands that a wide range of sperm functions are intact. The sperm must be capable of capacitation, and of undergoing the acrosome reaction (because the zona has been removed, only acrosome reacted sperm can bind to the denuded eggs), it must also be able to fuse with the oolemma, be drawn into the egg cytoplasm and to decondense. However, success in the test is not closely correlated with motility (Aitken et al, 1985) and even immotile sperm from men with Kartegeners syndrome or sperm that lack the central ciliary doublet are capable of penetrating denuded hamster eggs (Aitken et al, 1983a; Morgan et al, 1986).

Sperm from normal fertile men penetrate 10 to 100 per cent of hamster ova. Results below 10 per cent are associated with sperm dysfunction (Karp et al, 1981; Aitken et al, 1982a). The outcome of the test has been shown to correlate with the duration of infertility as well as the frequency of pregnancy in prospective studies (Cohen et al, 1982; Aitken et al, 1984). It is of particular value in detecting subnormal sperm function in patients with normal findings on standard seminal analysis (Rogers et al, 1979; Aitken et al, 1982b). Most workers have shown good correlation between the results of HOPTs and human in vitro fertilisation rates (Margalioth et al, 1983; Ausmanas et al, 1985). However, there is controversy over the definition of an absolute lower limit of hamster egg penetration to assess couples with poor IVF prognosis. The matter is complicated by a relatively high false negative rate of 11 to 20 per cent (Wolf et al, 1983; Ausmanas et al, 1985).

The variability and false negative rates may be attributable to differences between individuals in both optimum time and conditions required for capacitation. Hence the number of acrosome reacted sperm available for reacting with the egg. Several techniques have been used to promote capacitation and to overcome these drawbacks. The prior incubation of spermatozoa in media in which calcium was replaced by strontium greatly enhanced the penetration rate (Mortimer, 1986; Mortimer et al, 1986). Capacitation could also be promoted by incubation of spermatozoa in hypertonic media or by adding the calcium ionophore A23187. The latter procedure gave excellent correlation with IVF results (Aitken et al, 1987; Aitken, 1988) and was able to determine the fertility of frozen semen used for AID (Irvine and Aitken 1986).

We have adopted the A23187 procedure in our laboratory and can confirm that it has the potential of giving consistently high penetration rates with fertile semen. However, the dose of A23187 is very critical and the quality of A23187 can vary between batches and with storage. A range of A23187 concentrations must be used in every assay or some quality control system to measure A23187 activity is required as otherwise false negative results will be encountered.

There are varying views on the application of the HOPT to assess male fertility. It is too expensive for routine use. It can give false results. Our view is that its primary use is quantitative but it lacks specificity. Human IVF provides specificity for the individual couple, but lacks quantitative value and is not readily repeatable. We therefore prefer to reserve the HOPT until after human IVF treatment has led to failure of fertilisation, to confirming suspected sperm dysfunction. In that sense we see human IVF as a valuable diagnostic test of sperm fertilising ability.

Assessment of sperm transport above cervical level

After leaving the cervical mucus, sperms must migrate through the uterine cavity and fallopian tubes to reach the definitive site of fertilisation in the ampulla. There is evidence that only a small number of sperms progress to this level (see above). Templeton and Mortimer (1982) described laparoscopic recovery of spermatozoa from the peritoneal cavity and fimbrial rinsings in a group of infertile women following insemination at mid-cycle. The presence or absence of spermatozoa showed a strong correlation with subsequent conception. Studies by Aitken et al (1983b) showed that sperm from ejaculates with high zona free hamster egg penetration rates never failed to reach the peritoneal cavity. Whilst laparoscopic sperm recovery is useful as a research method it does not lend itself to clinical application.

Summary of diagnostic criteria for male infertility

Despite the wide range of investigations available, there are still no reliable or absolute criteria for the diagnosis of male infertility. Our prospective studies comparing standard seminal analysis and the post-coital test have shown the latter to be of greater prognostic value whether applied to natural conception (Glazener et al, 1987), or in vitro fertilisation (Hull et al, 1987). Although more sophisticated techniques are now available for the investigation of sperm function, such as time lapse photography for motility assessment, computer assisted calculation of sperm swimming speed, zona free hamster egg penetration tests, and IVF itself, their cost and the time and expertise involved prevent their routine use in clinical practice. Even if several such tests were used and the results subjected to sophisticated analysis, their ability to distinguish between successful and unsuccessful ejaculates is only reliable in about 80 per cent of cases (Irvine and Aitken, 1986). Whether as a screening procedure before more detailed investigation or as a prognostic assessment of fertility, a properly standardised post-coital test, being both simple and cheap to perform, must remain vital in identifying sperm dysfunction. It should be supported if the result is negative or poor by crossed sperm-mucus invasion testing to confirm the sperm dysfunction. Further investigations for possible identifiable causes of sperm dysfunction should include antisperm antibody testing and the investigation of genital infection.

Treatment of male infertility

Therapeutic possibilities for the treatment of male infertility remain limited due to poor understanding of the underlying pathological mechanisms. Also the lack of reliable criteria for the definition of male infertility, makes interpretation of the results of treatment difficult. Many studies have not included control groups or taken account of factors affecting the female partner, and few have related cumulative conception rates specifically to duration of exposure.

The following examples illustrate the confusion and difficulty in interpreting much of the published literature on the "treatment" of "male infertility". In one of the earliest reports of apparently successful IVF treatment, Cohen et al (1984a) defined male infertility simply by the finding of oligozoospermia and then achieved good conception rates in those cases in which sperm recovery from culture medium was favourable. They rejected those men with unfavourable sperm recovery. It seems likely that the sperm recovery test distinguished between normal and abnormal sperm function, in other words between true and false "male infertility".

Kerin et al (1984) reported a small but controlled study of intrauterine insemination, with encouraging results. The diagnosis of "male infertility" was based largely on mild oligozoospermia. On the other hand, couples were excluded from the study if their SMCT (sperm-mucus contact test) was positive. That meant immobilisation of the sperm when semen and mucus were mixed. Thus sperm-mucus interaction was in fact normal in the couples treated, implying normal sperm function. The true diagnosis was therefore not male but unexplained infertility.

Wardle et al (1987) reviewed several reports in one journal including that of Kerin et al (1984) concerning intrauterine insemination for apparent male infertility. Conception rates per cycle were zero in three studies and by contrast 22 to 23 per cent in the other two, including Kerin's. From the results of investigations described in the reports, it was possible to revise the diagnoses based partly on sperm-mucus interaction, which when normal was taken to indicate normal sperm function. It appeared that the conception rates per cycle were 29 per cent in cases of cervical mucus disorder, 19 per cent in unexplained infertility, and zero when there was true sperm dysfunction (it was also zero in the remainder that could not be classified). The results seem convincing and illustrate that reports of treatment of male infertility are frequently not what they appear to be.

Specific treatments

A specific factor is identified in only a minority of infertile men, but even when apparently improved there may not neccessarily be any subsequent increase in pregnancy rates.

Varicocele has long been suggested to reduce fertility and surgical correction led to encouraging pregnancy rates in some uncontrolled studies (Dubin and Amelar, 1975; Abdelmassih et al, 1982), although others have failed to demonstrate any benefit (Nilsson et al, 1979). The only study using a control group reported no significant improvement in pregnancy rates in the partners of the surgically treated patients (Vermeulen and Vanderweghe, 1984). Similarly, in men with seminal antisperm antibodies, treatment with corticosteroids has led to reports of encouraging pregnancy rates (Hendry et al, 1981; Hargreave and Elton, 1982; Baker et al, 1983). A controlled trial has demonstrated no significant improvement in the pregnancy rates despite reduction of antibody levels (Coulson et al, 1986).

Antibiotic treatment of asymptomatic genital tract infection has been reported to improve sperm density, motility and morphology, reduce spontaneous agglutination and improve accessory gland function in several uncontrolled studies (see Megory et al, 1987). However, there are difficulties in establishing whether an infection is of significance in the absence of symptoms or a positive culture of a recognised pathogen. Microscopically there may be considerable difficulty in differentiating inflammatory cells from immature germinal cells, and a positive bacteriological culture may more frequently be due to contamination than to occult infection. Mycoplasma and chlamydia organisms are most frequently considered responsible. Baker et al (1984) undertook a double blind crossover controlled trial of empirical treatment with Erythromycin in a group of 78 men with asthenospermia and found no significant change in sperm motility or difference in pregnancy rates compared with a placebo. Toth et al (1983), in the only prospective controlled trial of treatment of mycoplasma infection, found a marked improvement in terms of the outcome of subsequent pregnancy rather than the chance of achieving pregnancy when doxycycline treatment was given to erradicate organisms in the male.

Empirical treatment

In the majority of cases male infertility is unexplained and numerous empirical treatments have been advocated (Schill, 1982). Hormonal treatments have long been used with the aim of stimulating spermatogenesis but interest is now focussed on artificial methods of facilitating fertilisation in vitro or in vivo.

Clomiphene citrate has antioestrogenic actions by competitively binding to oestrogen receptors. By neutralising negative feedback at the hypothalamic level it increases GnRH stimulation and gonadotropin secretion. Unfortunately, use of clomiphene citrate has not produced encouraging results in subfertile men, where either no alteration in seminal characteristics were demonstrated (Charny, 1979; Schellen, 1982), or, if improvements were found, there was not corresponding improvement in conception rates (Ronnberg, 1980). Clomiphene citrate has also been reported to produce shrinkage of seminiferous tubules and hyalinisation in sporadic cases. In daily dosages above 50 mg, it can suppress spermatogenesis (Heller et al, 1969).

Tamoxifen has similar antioestrogenic properties but with less intrinsic oestrogenic activity than clomiphene. It has negligible direct effect on the testes (Vermeulen and Comhaire, 1978). Studies of its effects in subfertile men have produced contradictory results, some showing improvement in seminal characteristics and pregnancy rates (Comhaire, 1976; Vermeulen and

Comhaire, 1978), whilst others report no significant change (Willis et al, 1977; Buvat et al, 1983). Any theoretical advantage over clomiphene citrate or beneficial effect on conception rates from its use in subfertile males remains to be proven.

Against this background it is clear that uncontrolled studies of empirical treatments should be interpreted with caution. Controlled trials to date have shown no benefit from suggested treatments such as kallikrein (Comhaire and Vermeulen, 1983), arginine (Pryor et al, 1978) and mesterolone (Aafjes et al, 1983).

Artificial insemination of husband's semen (AIH)

Intracervical insemination has a definite place in the treatment of disorders such as hypospadias and retrograde ejaculation. It is of no proven benefit in men with oligozoospermia (Nachtigall et al, 1979) or in couples with a failure of post-coital sperm-mucus penetration irrespective of sperm "count" (Glazener et al, 1987b).

Intrauterine insemination of sperms, washed and prepared in the same manner as for in vitro fertilisation, has been reported to improve pregnancy rates in some couples with oligoasthenoteratozoospermia (Toffle et al, 1985; Hoing et al, 1986; Yovich and Matson, 1986) but others have failed to confirm this (Hull et al, 1986). The interpretation of these reports is confused due to poor definition of the cause of infertility in some of the studies and the use of ovarian stimulation in others. Where sperm dysfunction has been clearly defined by poor sperm mucus interaction washed intrauterine AIH has been shown to be largely unsuccessful (Hewitt et al, 1985; Quagliarello and Arny, 1986; Wardle et al, 1987).

In vitro fertilisation

In vitro fertilisation requires a relatively small number of sperms for insemination compared with natural conception and therefore seems to offer attractive prospects for the treatment of male infertility. Success has been claimed by several centres (Cohen et al, 1984a; Yovich and Stanger, 1984; Cohen et al, 1985; De Kretser et al, 1985; Van Uem et al, 1985; Yates et al, 1986), but in all cases the criteria for defining male infertility have been based solely on standard seminal analysis, which is now clearly unreliable. Our studies have shown that in couples with a negative or poor PCT the fertilisation rate per oocyte is less than one third, and the rate per couple less than half that achieved in couples with tubal damage alone (Hull et al, 1984; Wardle et al, 1985). This suggests that sperms which are unable to penetrate and survive in pre-ovulatory cervical mucus are functionally deficient in features which are also required for fertilisation of the human oocyte. The implication that a negative PCT is generally indicative of sperm dysfunction rather than mucus hostility is supported by the work of Schats et al (1984) who demonstrated a clear correlation between sperm/mucus penetration in vitro and zona free hamster egg penetration.

Matson et al (1986) in a prospective study found the PCT to be of no prognostic value for IVF. However, the reliability of their PCT methodology remains uncertain, particularly ther criteria of mucus quality and the length of time after intercourse that the test was done. Any inadequacy in these respects would have been exaggerated by their failure to do more than one test. Other workers have confirmed a reduced incidence of oocyte fertilisation in patients with a poor PCT (Cohen et at, 1984b; Hewitt et al, 1985).

Both reports did not consider this a contradiction to IVF because pregnancies were nevertheless achieved. Although the pregnancy rate may be lower than for couples with other infertility problems undergoing IVF treatment, the results may well be an improvement on the chances of natural conception in patients with sperm dysfunction. Whether IVF treatment can be considered cost effective under these cicumstances remains to be seen.

Despite the reduced fertilisation and overall pregnancy rates in couples with negative or poor PCTs, IVF may be of value in confirming a diagnosis of sperm dysfunction and helping couples decide whether to accept donor insemination treatment, particularly when the husband does not have a severe seminal abnormality. Failure of fertilisation of mature oocytes under these circumstances would be a good indicator of the severity of sperm dysfunction in each individual couple. Specific semen collection and preparation methods are required to optimise the separation of active, normal sperms from the total ejaculate depending on the nature of the seminal abnormality present (Cohen et al, 1984c). Improvement of normal fertilisation rates due to more effective culture methods and a greater number of oocytes recovered would increase the confidence with which sperm dysfunction may be diagnosed.

In our own centre, the fertilisation rate of 71 per cent per "mature" oocyte in an appropriate optimal reference group with tubal infertility would give a confidence value of about 90 per cent if two oocytes failed to fertilise, 97 per cent if three oocytes failed, and greater than 99 per cent if four or more oocytes failed. Such an assessment may avoid the stress of treatments such as AIH which are unlikely to be successful under these circumstances (Hewitt et al, 1985; Glazener et al, 1987b) and would avoid unnecessary delay in either adoption application (where increasingly lower age restrictions are being imposed in many countries and where delay may therefore render a couple ineligible) or commencing AID treatment.

Artificial insemination of donor semen (AID)

In the absence of any treatment of proven value for sperm disorders AID is widely used to bypass the problem (Newall, 1976; Trounson et al, 1981; Albrecht et al, 1982). The growing demand for AID is exemplified by referral figures from the United Kingdom (Richardson, 1980) and France (Alfredsson et al, 1983).

With the recognition of the potential for human immunodeficiency virus (HIV) transmission by AID (Stewart et al, 1985), most centres are now restricted to using quarantined frozen semen for treatment. The fertilising potential of frozen thawed semen is reduced compared to that of fresh semen, depending on the cryoprotectant and freezing technique, but carefully controlled studies conclude that pregnancy rates are only slightly decreased (Steinberger and Smith, 1973; Stone, 1980; Richter et al, 1984).

Comparison of the pregnancy rates for couples receiving AID treatment with natural conception rates of presumed normal couples suggests that AID success rates are lower. However, direct comparison of such figures may not be appropriate as the populations being compared are different and there is considerable variation in reported fecundity rates with AID treatment from 11 to 13 per cent (Federation CECOS, 1982) to 30 per cent (Corson, 1980). The optimal fecundity rate with AID may even exceed that of the general population. Smith et al (1981), using accurately timed insemination with high quality semen in normally ovulating women who had no abnormality on full investigation, reported a fecundity rate of 51 per cent using fresh semen. Peek et al (1984) excluded confounding variables by comparing the fecundity rate in only those women who successfully conceived with AID and the rate in normal couples who conceived after stopping oral contraception. In both groups the rate at which fertile women became pregnant was the same, their fecundity varying from 20 to 22 per cent depending on parity.

AID pregnancy rates are lower in oligozoospermic patients than in those with azoospermia, presumably due to occult female factors (Albrecht et al, 1982; Emperaire et al, 1982; Foss and Hull, 1986). With the correction of any ovulatory disorder fecundability rates appear to be equivalent in oligozoospermic and azoospermic patients (Hammond et al, 1986). The emotional strain of the AID procedure may itself be the cause of such dysfunction (Czyba et al, 1978; Vere and Joyce, 1979). In addition, as oligospermic men are subfertile rather than infertile, failure to conceive may be due to additional occult female factors the longer the duration of subfertility. Undiagnosed tubal pathology (Aiman, 1982) and endometriosis (Jansen, 1986) have both been reported as examples of this. It may also explain the observation that the cumulative success rates of AID are significantly reduced in women over 30 years of age (Federation CECOS, 1982) when such pelvic pathology is perhaps more likely to occur.

Although AID is effective and an appropriate treatment for a large number of couples, there is little published data on its acceptability to patients. Apart from those who reject it on religious or moral grounds, there are others who may be unable to accept a diagnosis of irreversible infertility or that their chance of natural conception is extremely poor. Careful and sensitive counselling is essential for all those cases. In fact, about eight per cent of those who consent to AID subsequently stop treatment because of psychological or marital problems (Aiman, 1982). For them, adoption is the only other option. The number of babies available for adoption has decreased dramatically in the last 20 years in the United Kingdom, from 24,831 in 1968 to 2,621 in 1982. There are many reasons for this, the main being liberalisation of abortion laws, greater social acceptability of single parenthood, and effective and more readily available contraception. As a result, adoption authorities, of necessity, apply increasingly stringent criteria to limit the number of prospective adoptive parents.

Future developments

The development of micromanipulation techniques and improved culture methods for inducing human sperm capacitation may offer prospects of a radical change in the outlook for men with severe sperm dysfunction in the near future. Microinjection was first described by Uehara and Yanagimachi (1976) who injected single human sperms or sperm nuclei into the vitellus of mature hamster eggs which had been enzymatically denuded of their surrounding cumulus. Both fresh and freeze dried sperm were shown to be capable of nuclear swelling or male pronuclear formation in over half of cases thus treated.

Metka et al (1985) used microinjection of single spermatozoa into nine human oocytes and achieved a four-cell embryo and a pronuclear oocyte after using standard IVF preparation methods for the semen. Since that time, an improved method of semen preparation has been developed which enhances human sperm capacitation as demonstrated by the results of zona free hamster egg penetration tests (Mortimer et al, 1986). Using this method of semen preparation, Laws-King et al (1987) have described successful fertilisation of human oocytes after microinjection of single spermatozoa from normal donors beneath the zona pellucida. Five of seven mature oocytes manipulated within six to nine hours of recovery developed two pronuclei and two polar bodies. Electron-microscopy confirmed fertilisation. Three of these oocytes with two pronuclei one progressively cleaved to six cells.

Much work remains to be done before such techniques can be applied to the treatment of male infertility, in particular to determine whether functionally deficient spermatozoa are also genetically abnormal and whether they are capable of fertilisation when injected into the perivitelline space or the vitellus of the oocyte. Such treatment may raise serious ethical and moral issues. Nevertheless microinjection of spermatozoa has profound implications and may revolutionise the treatment of sperm dysfunction.

Table 12-1
Some measurements of human sperm motility

Criterion or procedure	*Group*	*Temperature °C*	*Medium*	*Velocity microns/sec*	*Lateral head displacement microns*	*Reference*
Normal sperm	pre-capacitation	37	BWW	22.8	—	Aitken et al 1982a
	post-capacitation			30.4	—	
Unexplained infertility	controls	37	BWW (post-cap)	30.4	—	Aitken et al 1982b
	unexplained			24.4	—	
Gossypol acetic acid (15 min exposure)	controls	37	BWW	39.0	—	Aitken et al 1983c
	50 μM			27.0	—	
	500 μM			22.0	—	
	1000 μM			4.0	—	
Normal sperm		RT	semen	29.5	5.4	Serres et al 1984
Normal sperm	after swim-up	37	Menezo's B2	28.0	5.5	Mortimer 1984 (photo method)
			BWW	29.0	5.9	
	after 7h incubation		Menezo's B2	39.0	5.7	
			BWW	34.0	6.5	
Normal sperm (fertile men)		37	semen	32.4	6.3	Aitken et al 1985
			BWW (3h)	43.8	6.4	

Table 12-1 (Continued)

Criterion or procedure	*Group*	*Temperature °C*	*Medium*	*Velocity microns/sec*	*Lateral head displacement microns*	*Reference*
IVF/HOPT	fertile	30	semen	34.2	—	Holt, Moore & Hillier 1985
	infertile			24.2	—	
Varicocoelectomy	control	RT	Hams F10	25.5	—	Burke 1987
	pre-op			12.8	—	
	post-op			27.7	—	
Iodoacetate	control	37	BWW (3h)	51.5	3.5	JM Rees & WCL Ford unpublished data
	20 μM			21.7	3.2	
Frozen/thawed semen	pc>10	37	BWW (pre-cap)	41.0	3.7	Ford, Rees, McLaughlin & Goddard 1988
	pc< 5			34.0	4.3	
	pc>10		BWW (post-cap)	43.0	4.0	
	pc< 5			23.0	3.3	

RT — *room temperature*
pc — *per cent chance of achieving a pregnancy/cycle of AID*
cap — *capacitation*

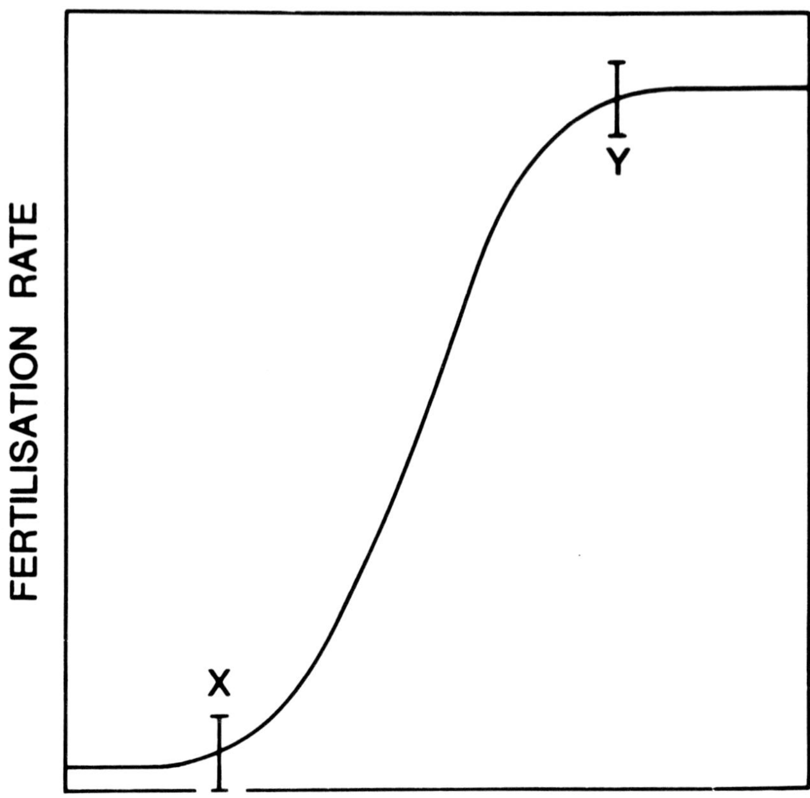

Figure 12-1

Stylised relationship between fertilisation (or conception) rates and sperm "counts", which follows a typical S-shaped biological response curve. Point X is the lower limit of sensitivity (bounded by confidence limits), representing the lowest sperm "count" to have achieved fertilisation (or pregnancy). Point Y is the upper limit of sensitivity, above which there is no further significant increase in the chance of fertilisation (or pregnancy). Fertilisation (or pregnancy) rates below point Y represent degrees of subfertility. Therefore point Y is the lower limit of normal, and can only be determined prospectively; whereas point X tends to be derived as the normal criteria from retrospective studies of partners of pregnant women.

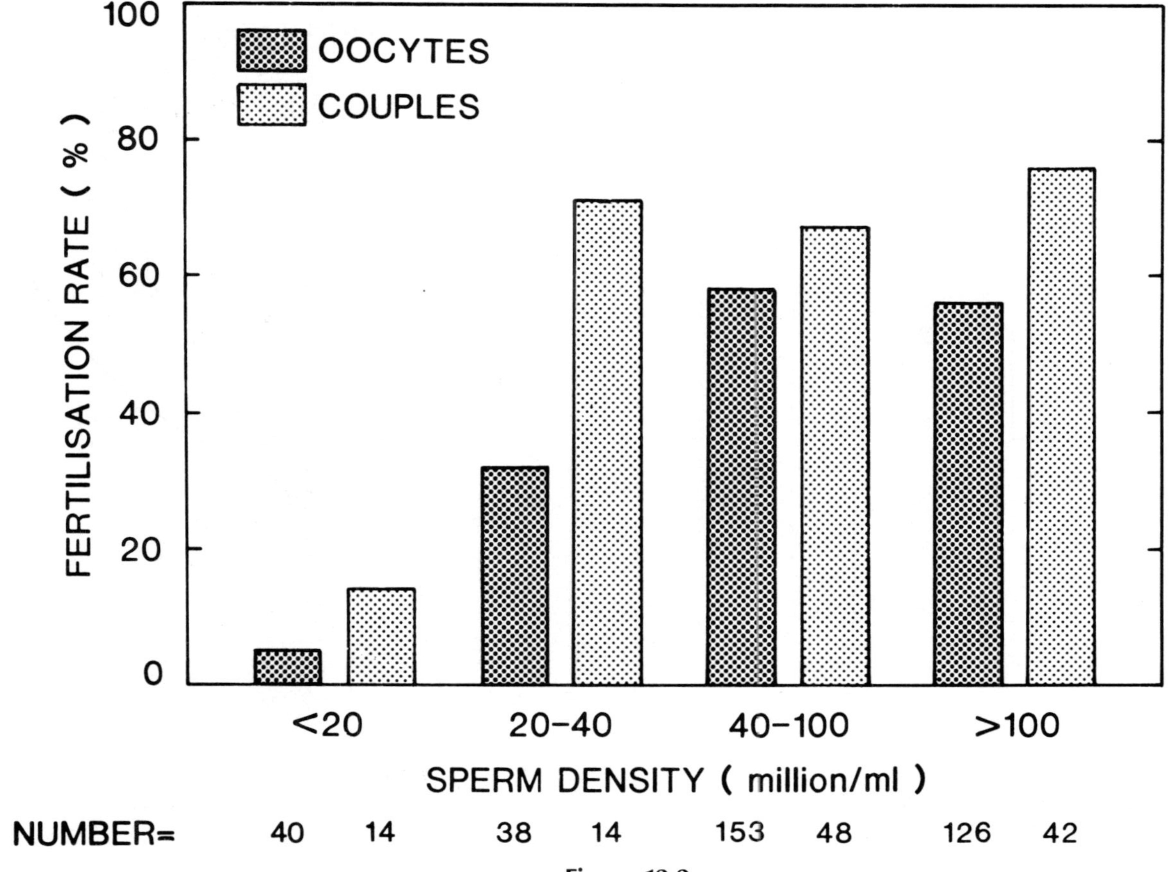

Figure 12-2
Fertilisation rates in vitro per mature oocyte related to sperm density in semen.

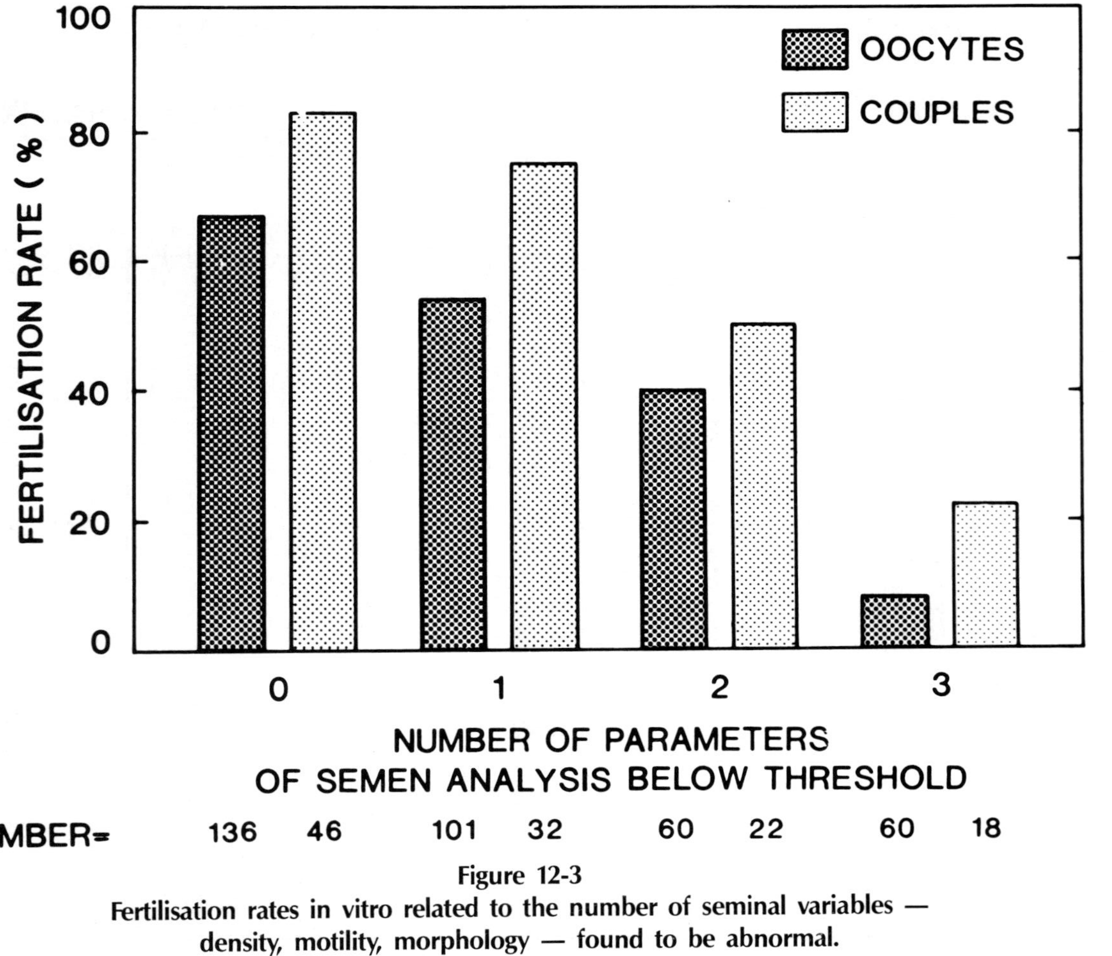

Figure 12-3
Fertilisation rates in vitro related to the number of seminal variables — density, motility, morphology — found to be abnormal.

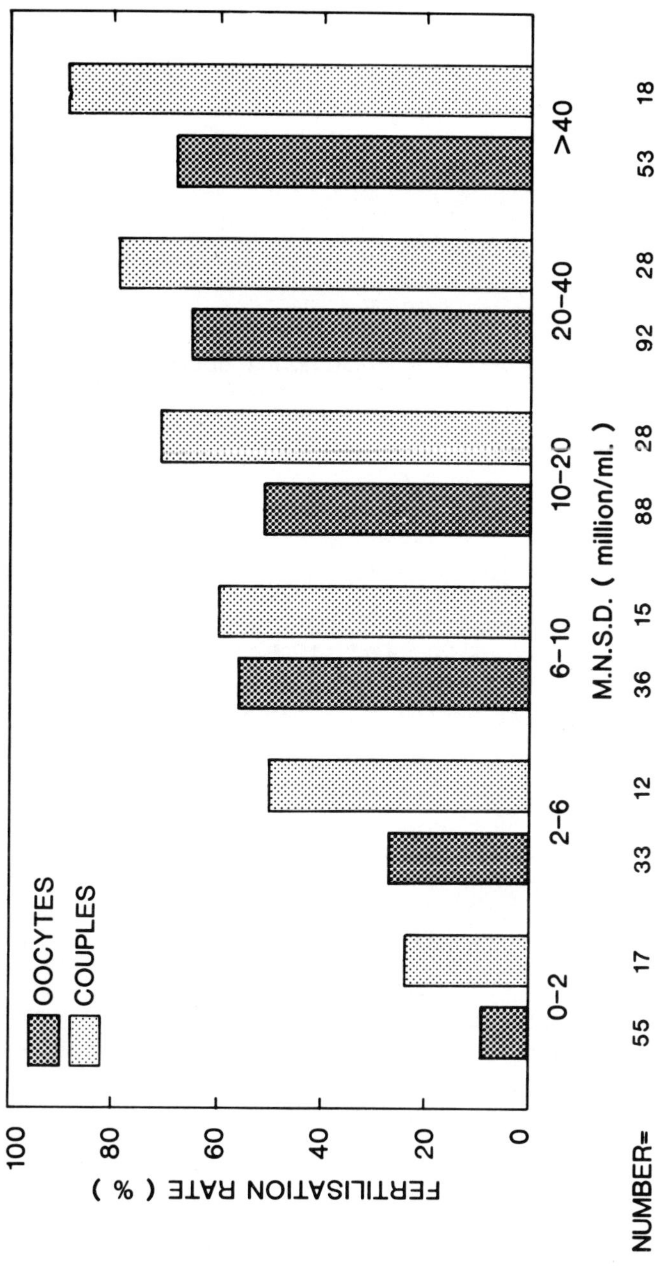

Figure 12-4
Fertilisation rates as in Figure 12-2 related to the motile normal sperm density (MNSD).

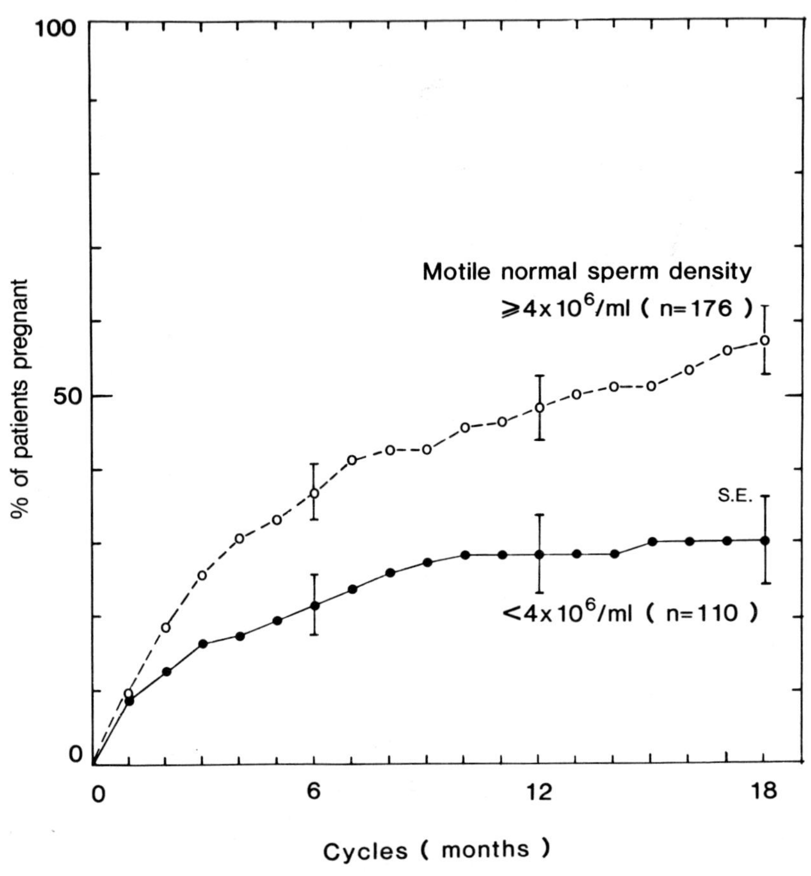

Figure 12-5
Cumulative conception rates in women with unexplained infertility related to the partner's motile normal sperm density about the derived critical value of 4 × 10^6/ml.

Source: Reproduced with permission from Glazener et al, 1987a.

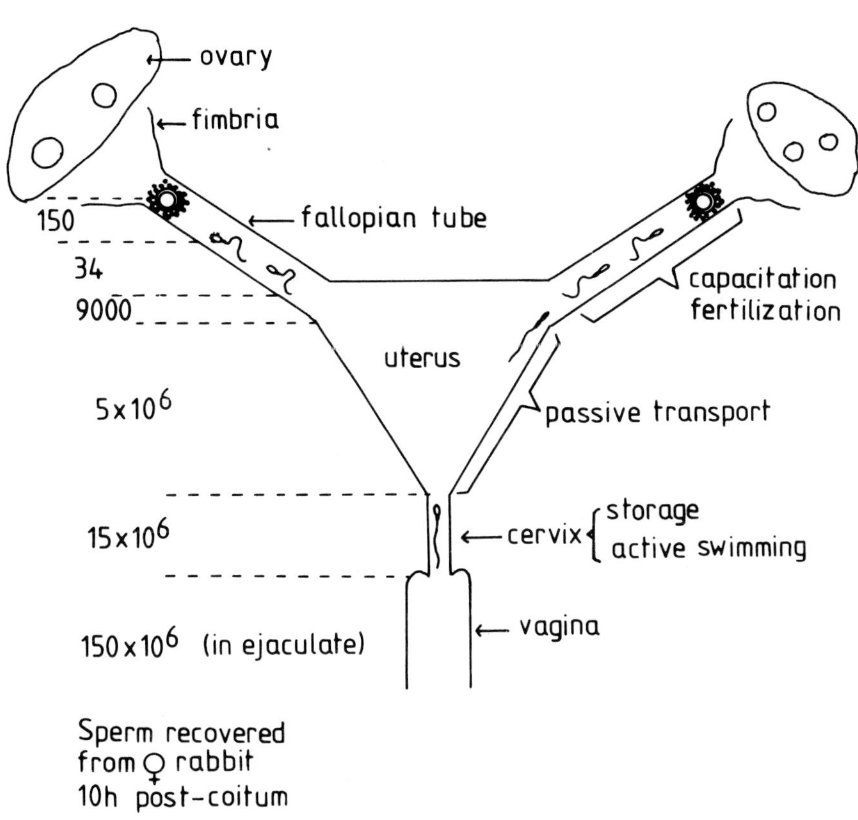

Figure 12-6
Sperm transport in the female reproductive tract depicted by the numbers of spermatozoa recovered at different sites in the rabbit 10 hours after coitus.

Source: From Overstreet and Cooper, 1978b.

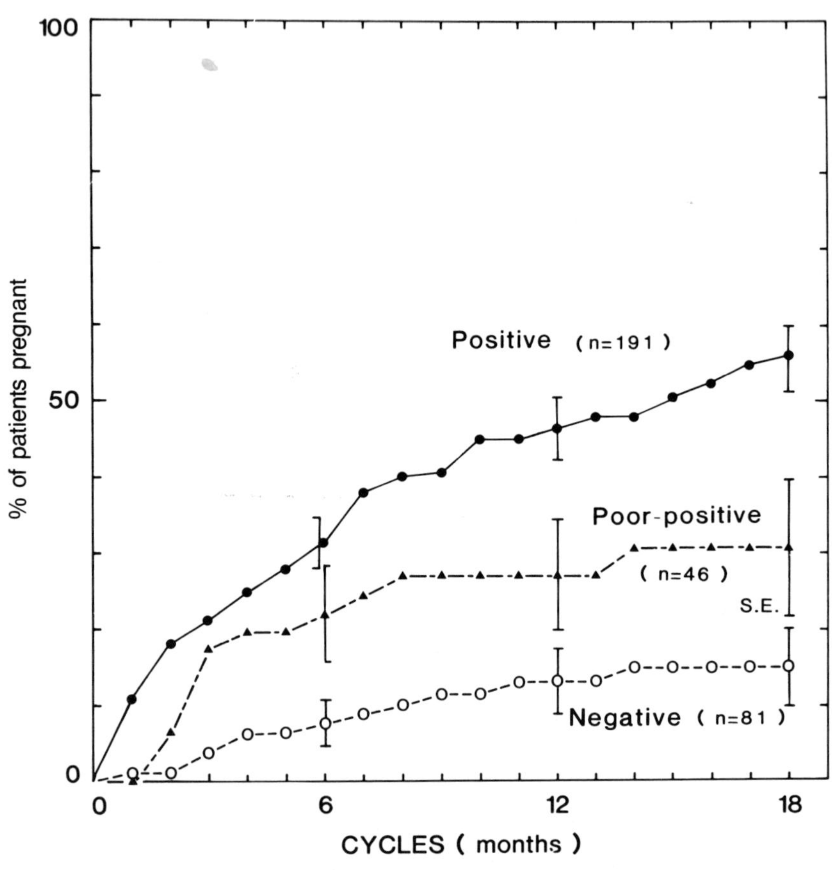

Figure 12-7

Cumulative conception rates as in Figure 12-5 related to the results of the PCT. A positive PCT implies the presence of forward progressing spermatozoa six to 18 hours after coitus, at least one such spermatozoon in every high power (×400) microscope field. Poor-positive means no more than one spermatozoon and none in some fields. Negative means lack of any normal forward-progressing spermatozoa in fully developed mucus in at least two separate cycles.

Source: Reproduced with permission from Glazener et al, 1987a.

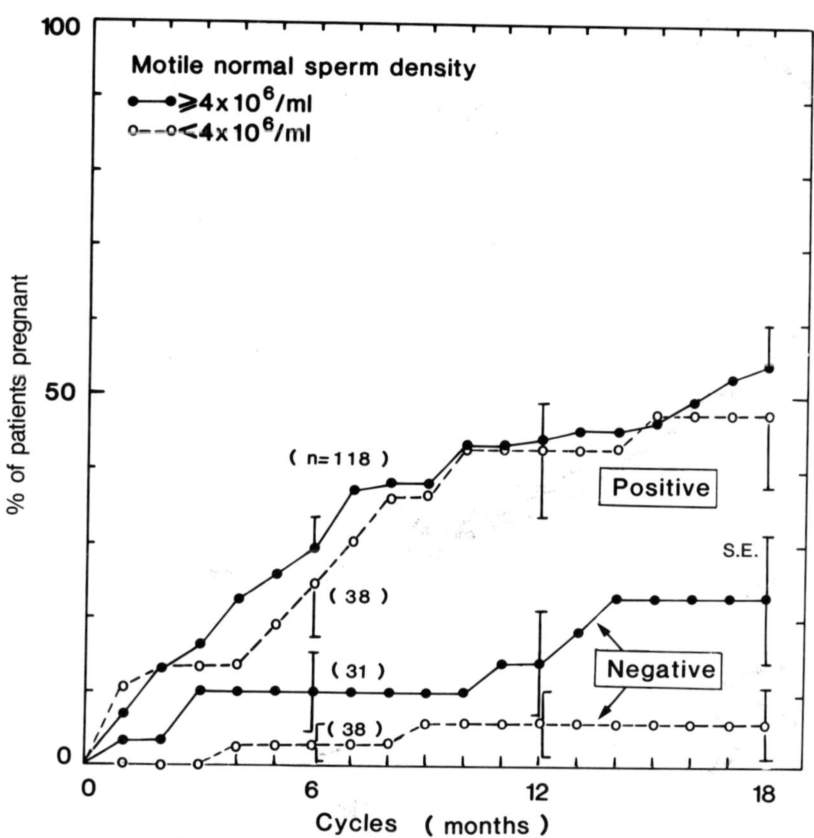

Figure 12-8
Cumulative conception rates as in Figures 12-5 and 12-7 comparing directly the results of seminal analysis and the PCT in the same couples.

Source: Reproduced with permission from Glazener et al, 1987a.)

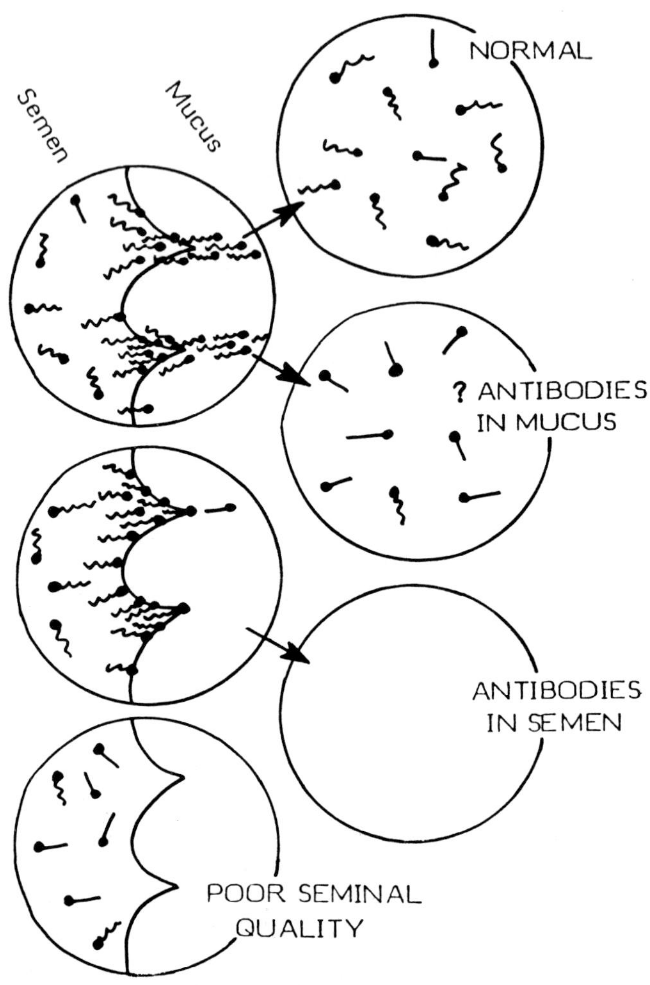

Figure 12-9
Diagrammatic illustration of normal and abnormal findings and the diagnostic implications of the sperm-mucus invasion test. Each circle represents a microscopic field, those on the left being at the sperm-mucus interface, those on the right deeper in the mucus. The diagnostic implications are from correlative studies by Glazener and Hull (1987).

References

Aafjes, J.H. and Van der Vivjer, J.C.M. Men with reduced fertility. *Dutch Journal of Medicine*, 1976; 120: 865.

Aafjes, J.H., Van der Vivjer, J. and Schenck, P.E. The duration of infertility: An important datum for the fertility prognosis of men with semen abnormalities. *Fertility and Sterility*, 1978; 30: 423.

Aafjes, J.H., Van der Vivjer, J.C., Brugman, F.W. and Schenck, P.E. Double blind crossover treatment with masterolone and placebo of subfertile oligosoospermic men: Value of testicular biopsy. *Andrologia*, 1983; 15: 531.

Abdelmassih, R., Fujisaki, S. and Fa'Undes, A. Prognosis of variocelectomy in the treatment of infertility, based on pre-surgery characteristics. *International Journal of Andrology*, 1982; 5: 452.

Acott, T.S. and Carr, D.W. Inhibition of bovine spermatozoa by cauda epididymal fluid II: Interaction of pH and a quiescence factor. *Biology of Reproduction*, 1984; 30: 926.

Ahlgren, M. Sperm transport to and survival in the human fallopian tubes. *Gynecol Invest*, 1975; 6: 206.

Alman, J. Factors affecting the success of donor insemination. *Fertility and Sterility*, 1982; 37: 94.

Aitken, R.J. (Ed), *The Zona Free Hamster Oocyte Penetration Test and the Diagnosis of Male Infertility*, International Journal of Andrology Supplement 6, 1986.

Aitken, R.J. Assessment of sperm function for IVF. *Human Reproduction*, 1988; 3: 89.

Aitken, R.J. and Clarkson, J.B. Cellular basis of defective sperm function and its association with the genesis of reactive oxygen species by human spermatozoa. *Journal of Reproduction and Fertility*, 1987; 81: 459.

Aitken, R.J., Best, F.S.M., Richardson, D.W., Djahanbakhch, O., Mortimer, D., Templeton, A.A. and Lees, M.M. An analysis of sperm function in cases of unexplained infertility: Conventional criteria, movement characteristics and fertilising capacity. *Fertility and Sterility*, 1982a; 38: 212.

Aitken, R.J., Best, F.S.M., Richardson, D.W., Djahanbakhch, O. and Lees, M.M. The correlates of fertilising capacity in normal fertile men. *Fertility and Sterility*, 1982b; 38: 68.

Aitken, R.J., Ross, A. and Lees, M.H. Analysis of sperm function in Kartageners syndrome. *Fertility and Sterility*, 1983a; 40: 696.

Aitken, R.J., Templeton, A., Schats, R., Best, F., Richardson, D., Djahanbakhch, O. and Lees, M.M. Methods for assessing the functional capacity of human spermatozoa: Their role in the selection of patients for in vitro fertilisation. In Beer, H.M. and Linder, H.R. (Eds), *Fertilisation of the Human Egg In Vitro*, Springer-Verlag, Berlin, 1983b, 147.

Aitken, R.J., Liu, J., Best, F.S.M. and Richardson, D.W. An analysis of the direct effect of gossypol on human spermatozoa. *International Journal of Andrology*, 1983c; 6: 157.

Aitken, R.J., Best, F.S.M., Warner, P. and Templeton, A. Prospective study of the relationship between semen quality and fertility in cases of unexplained infertility. *Journal of Andrology*, 1984; 5: 297.

Aitken, R.J., Sutton, M., Warner, P. and Richardson, D.W. Relationship between the movement characteristics of human spermatozoa and their ability to penetrate cervical mucus and zona free hamster oocyte. *Journal of Reproduction and Fertility*, 1985; 73: 441.

Aitken, R.J., Warner, P.E. and Reid, C. Factors influencing the success of sperm cervical mucus interaction in patients exhibiting unexplained infertility. *Journal of Andrology*, 1986; 7: 3.

Aitken, R.J., Thatcher, S., Glasier, A.F., Clarkson, J.S., Wu F.O.W. and Baird, D.T. Relative ability of modified versions of the hamster oocyte penetration test, incorporating hyperosmotic medium or the ionophore A23187 to predict IVF outcome. *Human Reproduction*, 1987; 2: 227.

Albrecht, E.H., Cramer, D. and Schiff, I. Factors influencing the success of artificial insemination. *Fertility and Sterility*, 1982; 37: 792.

Alfredeson, J.H., Gudmundason, S.P. and Snaedal, G. Artificial insemination by donor with frozen semen. *Obstetrical and Gynaecological Survey*, 1983; 38: 305.

Alvarez, J.G., Touchstone, J.C., Blasco and Storey, D.T. Spontaneous lipid peroxidation and production of hydrogen peroxide and superoxide in human spermatozoa: Superoxide dismutase as major enzyme protectant against oxygen toxicity. *Journal of Andrology*, 1987; 8: 338.

Ausmanas, M., Tureck, R.W., Blasco, L., Kopf, G.S., Ribas, J. and Mastroianni, L. Jr. The zona free hamster egg penetration assay as a prognostic indicator in a human in vitro fertilisation program. *Fertility and Sterility*, 1985; 43: 433.

Baker, H.W.G., Burger, H.G., De Kretser, D.M., Lording, D.W., McGowan, M.P. and Rennie, G.C. Factors affecting the variability of semen analysis results in infertile men. *International Journal of Andrology*, 1981; 4: 609.

Baker, H.W., Clarke, G.N., Hudson, B., McBain, J.C., McGowan, M.P. and Pepperall, R.J. Treatment of sperm auto-immunity in men. *Clinical Reproduction and Fertility*, 1983; 2: 55.

Baker, H.W.G., Straffon, W.G.E., McGowan, M.Fp., Burger, H., DeKretser, D.M. and Hudson, B. A controlled trial of the use of erythromycin for men with asthenospermia. *International Journal of Andrology*, 1984; 7: 383.

Bedford, J.M. Fertilisation in sperm cells and fertilisation. In Austin, C.R. and Short, R.V. (Eds), *Reproduction in Mammals*, Cambridge University Press, Cambridge, 1982, 128.

Benau, D.A. and Storey, B.T. Characterization of the mouse sperm plasma membrane zona binding site sensitive to trypsin inhibitors. *Biology of Reproduction*, 1987; 36: 282.

Bent, P.J. et al. Evidence for the activation of phospholipida during acrosome reaction of human spermatozoa elicited by Ca++ ionophore A23187. *Biochim Biophys Acta*, 1987; 919: 255.

Blasco, L. Clinical tests of sperm fertilizing ability. *Fertility and Sterility*, 1984; 41: 177.

Boatman, D.E., Andrews, J.C., Bainter, B.D. A quantitative assay for capacitation: Evaluation of multiple sperm penetration through the zona pellucida of salt stored hamster eggs. *Gamete Research*, 1988; 19: 19.

Bronson, R.A., Cooper, G.W. and Rosenfeld, D.L. Membrane-bound sperm-specific antibodies: Their role in infertility. In Vogel, H. and Jagiello, G. (Eds), *Bioregulators in Reproduction*, Academic Press, New York, 1981, 521.

Bronson, R.A., Cooper, G.W. and Rosenfeld, D.L. Correlation between regional specificity of antisperm antibodies to the spermatozoa surfaces and complement mediated sperm immobilisation. *American Journal of Reproductive Immunology and Microbiology*, 1982; 2: 222.

Bronson, R.A., Cooper, G.W. and Rosenfeld, D.L. Complement mediated effects of sperm head-directed human antibodies on the ability of human spermatozoa to penetrate zona free hamster eggs. *Fertility and Sterility*, 1983; 40: 91.

Brown, C.R. and Jones. Binding of zona pellucida proteins to a boar sperm polypeptide of Mr53000 and identification of zona mooieties. *Development*, 1987; 99: 333.

Burke, R.K. Sperm velocity, pre- and post-washing as a measure of the effects of varicocoelectomy and subsequent male fertility. *International Journal of Fertility*, 1987; 32: 213.

Buvat, J., Ardaens, K., Lemaire, A., Gauthier, A., Gosnault, J.P. and Buvat-Herbaut, M. Increased sperm count in 25 cases of idiopathic normogonadotrophic oligospermia following treatment with tamoxifen. *Fertility and Sterility*, 1983; 39: 700.

Carr, D.W. and Acott, T.S. Inhibition of bovine spermatozoa by cauda epididymal fluid: 1 Studies of a sperm motility quiescence factor. *Biology of Reproduction*, 1984; 30: 913.

Carr, D.W., Usselmann, M.C. and Acott, T.S. Effects of pH, lactate and visco elastic drag on sperm motility: A species comparison. *Biology of Reproduction*, 1985; 33: 588.

Chan S.Y.W. and Wang, C. Correlation between semen ATP and sperm fertilizing capacity. *Fertility and Sterility*, 1987; 47: 717.

Chance, B., Sies, H. and Boviris, A. Hydroperoxide metabolism in mammalian organs. *Physiology Review*, 1979; 59: 527.

Chantler, E. and Elstein, M. Structure and function of cervical mucus. *Seminars in Reproductive Endocrinology*, 1986; 4: 333.

Charny, C.W. Clomiphene therapy in male infertility: A negative report. *Fertility and Sterility*, 1979; 32: 551.

Cohen, J., Weber, R.F.A., Van der Vijver, J.C.M. and Zeilmaker, G.H. In vitro fertilising capacity of human spermatozoa with the use of zona free hamster ova: Interassay variation and prognostic value. *Fertility and Sterility*, 1982; 37: 565.

Cohen, J., Fehilly, C.B., Fishel, S.B., Edwards, R.G., Hewitt, J., Rowland, G., Steptoe, P.C. and Webster, J. Male infertility successfully treated by in vitro fertilisation. *Lancet*, 1984a; 1239.

Cohen, J., Hewitt, J. and Rowland, G.G. Application of in vitro fertilisation in cases of a poor post-coital test. *Lancet*, 1984b; ii: 583.

Cohen, J., Edwards, R.G., Fehilly, C.B., Fishell, S.B., Hewitt, J., Rowland, G., Steptoe, P.C., Webster, J. Treatment of male infertility by in vitro fertilisation: Factors affecting fertilisation and pregnancy. *European Journal of Fertility and Sterility*, 1984c; 15: 455.

Cohen, J., Edwards, R., Fehilly, C., Fishel, S., Hewitt, J., Purdy, J., Rowland, G., Steptoe, P., Webster, J. In vitro fertilisation: A treatment for male infertility. *Fertility and Sterility*, 1985; 43: 422.

Comhaire, F. Treatment of oligospermia with tamoxifen. *International Journal of Fertility*, 1976; 21: 232.

Comhaire, F.H. Simple model and empirical method for the estimation of spontaneous pregnancies in couples consulting for infertility. *International Journal of Andrology*, 1987; 10: 671.

Comhaire, F. and Vermeulen, L. Effect of high dose oral Kallikrein treatment in men with idiopathic subfertility: Evaluation by means of in vitro penetration test of zona free hamster ova. *International Journal of Andrology*, 1983; 6: 168.

Comhaire, F., Vermeulin, L., Ghedira, K., Mas, J., Irving, S. and Callipolitis, G. ATP in human semen: A quantitative estimate of fertility potential. *Fertility and Sterility*, 1983; 40: 500.

Comhaire, F.H., Hinting, A., Vermeulen, L., Schoonjans, F. and Goethals, I. Evaluation of the direct and indirect mixed antiglobulin reaction with latex particles for the diagnosis of immunological infertility. *International Journal of Andrology*, 1987a; ii: 37.

Comhaire, F.H., Vermeulen, L. and Schoonjans, F. Reassessment of the accuracy of traditional sperm characteristics and adenosine triphosphate (ATP) in estimating the fertilizing potential of human semen in vivo. *International Journal of Andrology*, 1987b; 10: 653.

Corselli, J. and Talbot, P. An in vitro technique to study penetration of hamster oocyte-cumulus complexes by using physiological numbers of sperm. *Gamete Research*, 1986; 13: 293.

Corson, L. Factors affecting donor artificial insemination success rates. *Fertility and Sterility*, 1980; 33: 415.

Coulson, C., Glazener, C.M.A., Sykes, J.A.C., McLaughlin, E.A., Lambert, P.A., Watt, E.M., Hinton, R.A. and Hull, M.G.R. Betamethasone treatment of male infertility due to antisperm antibodies in seminal plasma: A placebo controlled study. *Human Reproduction*, 1986; 1 (suppl 2): 2.

Cross, N.L., Morales, P., Overstreet, J.W. and Hanson, F.W. Two simple methods for detecting acrosome reacted human sperm. *Gamete Research*, 1986; 15: 213.

Cross, N.L., Merales, P., Overstreet, J.W. and Hanson, F.W. Induction of acrosome reactions by the human zona pellucida. *Journal of Andrology*, 1987; 8: 33.

Czyba, J.C., Cottinet, D. and Souchier, C. Disturbances in ovulation following artificial insemination with donors (AID). *Journal of Gynaecology, Obstetrics and Biol. Reproduction*, 1978; 7: 499.

Daunter, B., Chantler, E.N. and Elstein, M. Scanning electron microscopy of cervical mucus: Normal menstrual cycle and pregnancy. *British Journal of Obstetrics and Gynaecology*, 1976; 83: 738.

De Jonge, C., Rawlins, R.G., Zaneveld, L.J.D. Induction of human sperm acrosome reaction by human oocytes. *Journal of Andrology*, 1988; 9: 39.

De Kretser, D.M., Yates, C. and Kovacs, G.T. The use of IVF in the management of male infertility. In Wood, C. and Trouson, A. (Eds), *Clinics in Obstetrics and Gynaecology*, W.B. Saunders Company Limited, London, 1985, 12(iv): 767.

Dubin, L. and Amlelar, R.D. Varicocelectomy as therapy in male infertility: A study of 504 cases. *Fertility and Sterility*, 1975; 26: 217.

Emperaire, J.C, Gauzere-Soumireu, E. and Audebert, A.J.M. Female fertility and donor insemination. *Fertility and Sterility*, 1982; 37: 90.

Endo, Y., Mattei, P., Kopz, G.S. and Schultz, R.M. Effects of phorbol esters on mouse eggs, dissociation of sperm receptor activity from acrosome reaction inducing activity of the mouse zona pellucida protein ZP3. *Developmental Biology*, 1987; 574.

Federation CECOS, Schwartz, D. and Mayaux, M.J. Results of artifical insemination in 2193 nulliparous women with azoospermic husbands. *New England Journal of Medicine*, 1982; 306: 404.

Feneux, D., Serres, C. and Jouannet, P. Sliding spermatozoa: Dyskinesia responsible for human infertility? *Fertility and Sterility*, 1985; 44: 508.

Ford, W.C.L., Rees, J.M., McLaughlin, E.A. and Goddard, R.J. Estimation of the fertility of donors in our AID programme and its relationship to sperm function tests. Abstract E11, *5th European Workshop on Molecular and Cellular Endocrinology of the Testis*, 1988.

Fordney-Settlage, D. A review of cervical mucus and sperm interactions in humans. *International Journal of Fertility*, 1981; 26(3): 161.

Foss, G.L. and Hull, M.G.R. Results of donor insemination related to specific male infertility and unsuspected female infertility. *British Journal of Obstetrics and Gynaecology*, 1986; 93: 275.

Fraser, L.R. Mechanisms controlling mammallian fertilization. *Oxford Reg. Reprod. Biol.*, 1984; 6: 174.

Freund, M. Inter-relationships among the characteristics of human semen and factors affecting semen specimen quality. *Journal of Reproduction and Fertility*, 1962; 4: 143.

Frost, J. and Cummins, H.Z. Motility assay of human spermatozoa by photon correlation spectroscopy. *Science*, 1981; 212: 1520.

Gaddam-Rosse, P., Blandau, R.J. and Lee W.I. Sperm penetration into cervical mucus in vitro. 1. Comparative studies. *Fertility and Sterility*, 1980; 33: 636.

Glass, R.H. and Ericsson, R.J. Spontaneous cure of male infertility. *Fertility and Sterility*, 1979; 31: 305.

Glazener, C.M.A. and Hull, M.G.R. The sperm-mucus interface: Patterns of disorder in the diagnosis of specific causes of penetration failure related to fertility. *Human Reproduction*, 1987; 2: 673.

Glazener, C.M.A., Kelly, N.J., Weir, M.J.A., David, J.S.E., Cornes, J.S. and Hull, M.G.R. The diagnosis of male infertility: Prospective time specific study of conception rates related to seminal analysis and post-coital sperm-mucus penetration and survival in otherwise unexplained infertility. *Human Reproduction*, 1987a; 2: 665.

Glazener, C.M.A., Coulson, C., Lambert, P.A., Watt, E.M., Hinton, R.A., Kelly, N.J., and Hull, M.G.R. The value of artificial insemination of husband's semen in infertility due to failure of post-coital sperm-mucus penetration: Controlled trial of treatment. *British Journal of Obstetrics and Gynaecology*, 1987b; 94: 774.

Gottesman, I.S. and Bain, J. Subfertility and infertility in the male: A persistent dilemma. In Bain, J. and Hafez, E.S.E. (Eds), *Diagnostic Andrology*, Hartinus Nijhoff, Amsterdam, 1980, 79.

Gould, J.E., Overstreet, J.W. and Harrison, F.W. Assessment of human sperm function after recovery from the female reproductive tract. *Biology of Reproduction*, 1984; 31: 888.

Green, D.P.L. Mammalian sperm cannot penetrate the zona pellucida solely by force. *Experimental Cell Research*, 1987; 169: 31.

Hamilton, C.J.C.M., Evers, J.L.H. and De Haan, J. Ultrasound increases the prognostic value of the post-coital test. *Gynaecology and Obstetrics Investigation*, 1986; 21: 80.

Hammond, M.G., Jordan, S. and Sloan, C.S. Factors affecting pregnancy rates in a donor insemination program using frozen semen. *American Journal of Obstetrics and Gynecology*, 1986; 155: 480.

Hanson, F.W. and Overstreet, J.W. The interaction of human spermatozoa with cervical mucus in vivo. *American Journal of Obstetrics and Gynecology*, 1981; 140: 173.

Hargreave, T.B. Artificial insemination by donor. *British Medical Journal ii*, 1985; 613.

Hargreave, T.B. and Elton, R.A. Treatment with intermittent high dose methylprednisolone or intermittent betamethasone for antisperm antibodies: Preliminary communication. *Fertility and Sterility*, 1982; 38: 586.

Hargreave, T.B., Haxdon, M., Whitelas, J., Elton, R. and Chisholm, C.O. The significance of sperm agglutinating antibodies in men with infertile marriages. *British Journal of Urology*. 1980; 52: 566.

Harrison, R.F. The cervical factor — fact or fantasy? In Insler, V. and Bettendorf, G. (Eds), *The Uterine Cervix in Reproduction*, Georg Thieme, Stuttgart, 1977, 246.

Harrison, R.F. Pregnancy successes in the infertile couple. *International Journal of Fertility*, 1980; 25: 81.

Harrison, R.F. The diagnostic and therapeutic potential of the post-coital test. *Fertility and Sterility*, 1981 36: 71.

Heller, C.G., Rowley, M.J. and Heller, G.V. Clomiphene citrate: A correlation of its effects on sperm concentration and morphology, total gonadotropins, ICSH, estrogen and testosterone excretion and testicular cytology in normal men. *Journal of Clinical Endocrinology and Metabolism*, 1969; 29: 638.

Hendry, W.F., Stedronska, J., Parlow, J. and Hughes, L. The results of intermittent high dose steroid therapy for male infertility due to antisperm antibodies. *Fertility and Sterility*, 1981; 36: 351.

Heuchel, V., Schwartz, D. and Price, W. Within subject variability and the importance of abstinence period for sperm count, semen volume and prefreeze and post-thaw motility. *Andrologia*, 1981; 13: 479.

Hewitt, J., Cohen, J., Krishnaswamy, V., Fehilly, C.B., Steptoe, P.C. and Walters, D.E. Treatment of idiopathic infertility, cervical mucus hostility and male infertility: Artificial insemination with husband's semen or in vitro fertilisation? *Fertility and Sterility*, 1985; 44: 350.

Hoing, L.M., Devroey, P. and Van Steirtegham, A.C. Treatment of infertility because of oligo-asthenoteratospermia by transcervical intrauterine insemination of motile spermatozoa. *Fertility and Sterility*, 1986; 45: 388.

Holt, W.V., Moore, H.D.M. and Hillier, S.G. Computer assisted measurement of sperm swimming speed in human semen: Correlation of results with in vitro fertilisation assays. *Fertility and Sterility*, 1985; 44: 112.

Hotchkiss, R.S. Factors in stability and variability of semen specimens: Observations on 640 successive samples from 23 men. *Journal of Urology*, 1941; 45: 875.

Huhner, M. *Sterility in the Male and Female*, Rebman, New York, 1913.

Hull, M.E., Magyar, D.M., Vasquez, J.M., Hayes, M.F., and Moghissi, K.S. Experience of intrauterine insemination for cervical factor and oligospermia. *American Journal of Obstetrics and Gynecology*, 1986; 154: 1333.

Hull, M.G.R., Savage, P.E. and Bromham, D.R. The prognostic value of the post-coital test: A prospective study based on time specific conception rates. *British Journal of Obstetrics and Gynaecology*, 1982; 89: 299.

Hull, M.G.R. and Glazener, C.M.A. Male infertility and in vitro fertilisation. *Lancet*, 1984; ii: 231.

Hull, M.G.R., Joyce, D.N., McLeod, F.N., Ray, B.D. and McDermott, A. Human in vitro fertilisation, in vitro sperm penetration of cervical mucus and unexplained infertility. *Lancet*, 1984; ii: 245.

Hull, M.G.R., Glazener, C.M.A., Kelly, N.J., Con way, D.I., Foster, P.A., Hinton, R.A., Coulson, C., Lambert, P.A., Watt, E.M. and Desai, K.M. Population study of causes, treatment, and outcome of infertility. *British Medical Journal*, 1985; 291: 1693.

Hull, M.G.R., Glazener, C.M.A., Wardle, P.G., McLaughlin, E.A. and Sykes, J.A. Male infertility: Sperm penetration of mucus related to natural and in vitro fertility. In Ratman, S.S., Teoh E.S. and Anandakumar, C. (Eds), *Advances in Fertility and Sterility, Vol. 4. Infertility*, Parthenon, Carnforth, Lancs., 1987; 31.

Hunter, R.H.F. The timing of capacitation in mammalian spermatozoa: A reinterpretation. *Research in Reproduction*, 1987; 19: 3.

Huszar, G., Corrales, M. and Vique, L. Correlation between sperm creatine phosphokinase activity and sperm concentrations in normospermic and oligozoospermic men. *Gamete Research*, 1988; 19: 67.

Hyne, R.V. Bicarbonate and calcium dependent in duction of rapid guinea pig sperm acrosome reactions by monovalent ionophores. *Biology of Reproduction*, 1984; 31: 312.

Insler, V., Glezerman, M., Zeidel, L., Bernstein, D. and Misgar, N. Sperm storage in the human cervix: A quantitative study. *Fertility and Sterility*, 1980; 33: 288.

Irvine, D.S. and Aitken, R.J. Predictive value of in vitro sperm function tests in the context of an AID service. *Human Reproduction*, 1986; 1: 539.

Jansen, R.P.S. Minimal endometriosis and reduced fecundability: Prospective evidence from an artificial insemination by donor program. *Fertility and Sterility*, 1986; 46: 141.

Jeulin, C., Feneux, D., Serres, C., Jouannet, P., Guillet-Rosse, F., Belaisch-Allart, J., Frydman, R. and Testart, J. Sperm factors related to failure of human in vitro fertilisation. *Journal of Reproduction and Fertility*, 1986; 76: 735.

Jeyendran, R.S., Van der Ven, H.H., Perez-Pelaez, M., Crabo, B.G. and Zaneveld, L.J.D. Development of an assay to assess the functional integrities of the human sperm membrane and its relationship to other semen characteristics. *Journal of Reproduction and Fertility*, 1984; 70: 219.

Jonsson, B., Eneroth, P., Landgren, B.M. and Wikborn, C. Evaluation of in vitro sperm penetration testing of 176 infertile couples with the use of ejaculates and cervical mucus from donors. *Fertility and Sterility*, 1986; 45: 353.

Jouannet, P., Volodrine, B., Deguent, P., Serres, C. and David, G. Light scattering determination of various characteristic parameters of spermatozoan motility in a series of human sperm. *Andrologia*, 1987; 9: 36.

Joyce, C.L., Nuzzo, N.A., Wilson, L. and Zaneveld, L.J.D. Evidence for a role of cyclooxygenase (Prostaglandin synthetase) and prostaglandins in the sperm acrosome reaction and fertilization. *Journal of Andrology*, 1987; 8: 74.

Joyce, D.N. and Vassilopoulos, D. Sperm mucus interaction and artifical insemination. *Clinics in Obstetrics and Gynaecology*, 1981; 8: 587.

Kanwar, K.C., Yanagamachi, R. and Lopata, A. Effects of human seminal plasma on fertilising capacity of human spermatozoa. *Fertility and Sterility*, 1979; 31: 321.

Karp, L.E., Williamson, R.A., Noore, D.E., Shy, K.K., Plymate, S.R. and Smith, W.D. Sperm penetration assay: Useful test in evaluation of male infertility. *Obstetrics and Gynaecology*, 1981; 57: 620.

Katz, D.F. and Overstreet, J.W. Sperm motility assessment by videomicrography. *Fertility and Sterility*, 1981; 35: 188.

Katz, D.R. and Demestre, M.J. Thrust generation by mammalian spermatozoa against the zona pellucida. *Biophys. J.*, 1985; 47: 123.

Katz, D.F., Mills, R.N. and Pritchett, T.R. The movement of human spermatozoa in cervical mucus. *Journal of Reproduction and Fertility*, 1978; 53: 259.

Katz, D.F., Overstreet, J.W. and Hanson, F.W. A new quantitative test for sperm penetration into cervical mucus. *Fertility and Sterility*, 1980; 33: 179.

Katz, D.F., Frofeldt, B.T., Overstreet, J.W. and Hanson, F.W. Alteration of cervical mucus by vanguard human spermatozoa. *Journal of Reproduction and Fertility*, 1982; 65: 171.

Kerin, J.F.P., Kirby, C., Peek, J., Jeffrey, R., Warnes, G.M., Matthews, C.D. and Cox, L.W. Improved conception rate after intrauterine insemination of washed spermatozoa from men with poor semen quality. *Lancet*, 1984; i: 533.

Kovacs, G.T., Newman, G.B. and Henson, G.L. The post-coital test: What is normal? *British Medical Journal*, 1978; i: 818.

Kremer, J. *The In Vitro Spermatozoal Penetration Test*, Thesis, University of Groningen, 1968.

Kremer, J. Significance of progressively motile spermatozoa in the post-coital test for the fertility prognosis. In Insler, V. and Bettendorf, G. (Eds), *Advances in Diagnosis and Treatment of Infertility*, Elsevier/North Holland, Amsterdam, 1981, 229.

Kremer, J. and Jager, S. The sperm cervical mucus contact test: A preliminary report. *Fertility and Sterility*, 1976; 27: 335.

Kremer, J. and Jager, S. Characteristics of antispermatozoal antibodies responsible for the shaking phenomenon with special regard to immunoglobulin class and antigen-reactive sites. *International Journal of Andrology*, 1980; 3: 143.

Kremer, J. and Jager, S. Sperm-cervical mucus interaction, in particular in the presence of antispermatozoal antibodies. *Human Reproduction*, 1988; 3: 69.

Lambert, H. and Le, A.V. Possible involvement of a silylated component of the sperm plasma membrane in sperm zona interactions in the mouse. *Gamete Research*, 1984; 10: 153.

Lambert, H., Overstreet, J.W., Morales, P., Hanson, F.W., Yamagamachi, R. Sperm capacitation in the human female reproductive tract. *Fertility and Sterility*, 1985; 43: 325.

Laws-King, A., Trounson, A., Sathanathan, H. and Kola, I. Fertilisation of human oocytes by microinjection of a single spermatozoon under the zona pellucida. *Fertility and Sterility*, 1987; 48: 637.

Lee Ma, Tracco, G.S., Bechtol, K.B., Wummer, N., Kopf, G.S., Blascoh and Storey, B.T. Capacitation and acrosome reaction in human spermatozoa monitored by a chlorotetracycline fluorescence assay. *Fertility and Sterility*, 1987; 48: 649.

Levin, R.M., Shafer, J., Wein, A.J. and Greenberg, S.H. ATP concentration in human spermatozoa: Lack of correlation with sperm motility. *Andrologia*, 1981; 13: 441.

Levin, R.M., Latimore, J., Wein, A.J. and Van Arsdalen, K.N. Correlation of sperm count with frequency of ejaculation. *Fertility and Sterility*, 1986; 45: 732.

Liu D.Y., Jennings, M.G. and Baker, H.W.G. Correlation between defective motility (asthenospermia) and ATP reactivation of demembranated human spermatozoa. *Journal of Andrology*, 1987; 8: 349.

McBain, J.C. and Clarke, G.N. The role of acidity in cervical infertility. *Clinical Reproduction and Fertility*, 1986; 4: 178.

Macleod, J. and Gold, R.Z. The male factor in infertility II. Spermatozoa counts in 1000 men of known fertility and in 1000 cases of infertile marriage. *Journal of Urology*, 1951; 66: 436.

Macleod, J. and Gold, R.Z. The male factor in fertility and infertility IV. Semen quality and certain other factors in relation to ease of conception. *Fertility and Sterility*, 1953; 4: 10.

Macomber, D. and Sanders, M.B. The spermatozoa count: Its value in the diagnosis, prognosis and treatment of infertility. *New England Journal of Medicine*, 1929; 200: 981.

Makler, A. Use of the elaborated multiple exposure photography (MEP) method in routine sperm motility analysis and for research purposes. *Fertility and Sterility*, 1980; 33: 160.

Mandelbaum, S.L., Diamond, M.P. and De Cherney, A.M. Relationship of antisperm antibodies to oocyte fertilisation in in vitro fertilisation embryo transfer. *Fertility and Sterility*, 1987; 47: 644.

Mann, T. and Lutwak-Mann, C. *Male Reproductive Function and Semen*, Springer-Verlag, Berlin, 1981.

Margalioth, E.J., Navot, D., Laufer, N., Yosef, S.M., Rabinowitz, R., Yarkoni, S. and Shenker, J.G. Zona free hamster ovum penetration assay as a screening procedure for in vitro fertilisation. *Fertility and Sterility*, 1983; 40: 386.

Matson, P.L., Tuvik, A.J., O'Halloran, F., Yovich, J.L. The value of the postcoital test in predicting the fertilisation of human oocytes. *Journal of In Vitro Fertilisation and Embryo Transfer*, 1986; 3: 110.

Matthews, C.D., Makin, A.E. and Cox, L.W. Experience with in vitro sperm penetration testing in infertile and fertile couples. *Fertility and Sterility*, 1980; 33: 187.

Megory, E., Zuckerman, H., Shoham, S. and Lunenfeld, B. Infections and male fertility. *Obstetrical and Gynecological Survey*, 1987; 42: 283.

Meizel, S. and Turner, K.O. The effects of products and inhibitors of arachidonic acid metabolism on the hamster sperm acrosome reaction. *Journal of Experimental Zoology*, 1984; 231: 283.

Metka, M., Haromy, T., Huber, J. and Schurz, B. Artificial insemination using a micromanipulator. *Fertilitat*, 1985; 1: 41.

Miller, E.G. and Kurzrok. Biochemical studies of human semen III. Factors affecting migration of sperm through the cervix. *American Journal of Obstetrics and Gynecology*, 1932; 24: 19.

Milligan, M.P., Harris, S. and Dennis, K.J. Comparison of sperm velocity in fertile and infertile groups as measured by time lapse photography. *Fertility and Sterility*, 1980; 34: 509.

Moghissi, K.S. Postcoital test: Physiologic basis, technique and interpretation. *Fertility and Sterility*, 1976; 27: 117.

Morales, P., Cross, N.L., Overstreet, J.W. and Hanson, F.W. Initiation of human sperm binding to the human zona pellucida. *Journal of Andrology*, 1988; 9: 24.

Morgan, H., Stedronska, J., Hendry, W.E., Chamberlain, G.V.P. and Dewhurst, C.J. Sperm/cervical mucus crossed hostility testing and antisperm antibodies in the husband. *Lancet*, 1977; i: 1228.

Morgan, A.I., Guay, A.T. and Tulchinsku, D. Normal penetration of hamster ova by sperm with dyskinetic motility. *Fertility and Sterility*, 1986; 45: 735.

Mortimer, D. Sperm transport in the human female reproductive tract. *Oxford Reviews of Reproductive Biology*, 1983; 5: 30.

Mortimer, D. Comparison of the fertilizing ability of human spermatozoa pre-incubated in calcium and strontium-containing media. *Journal of Experimental Zoology*, 1986; 237: 21.

Mortimer, D., Courtol, A.M., Giovagrandi, V., Juclin, C. and David, G. Human sperm motility after migration into and incubation in synthetic media. *Gamete Research*, 1984; 9: 131.

Mortimer, D., Curtis, F.F. and Miller, R.G. Specific labelling by peanut agglutinum of the outer acrosomal membrane of the human spermatozoa. *Journal of Reproduction and Fertility*, 1987; 81: 127.

Mortimer, D., Curtis, E.F. and Dravland, J.E. The use of strontium-substituted media for capacitating human spermatozoa: An improved sperm preparation method for the zona free hamster egg penetration test. *Fertility and Sterility*, 1986; 46: 97.

Mortimer, D., Curtis, F.F. and Mitler, R.G. Specific labelling by peanut agglutinin of the outer acrosomal membrane of the human spermatozoon, *Journal of Reproduction and Fertility*, 1987; 81: 127.

Mrsny, R.J. and Meizel, S. Evidence suggesting a role for cyclic nucleotides in acrosome reactions in hamster sperm in vitro. *Journal of Experimental Zoology*, 1980; 211: 153.

Nachtigall, R.D., Faure, N. and Glass, R.H. Artificial insemination of husband's sperm. *Fertility and Sterility*, 1979; 32: 141.

Nagae, T., Yanagimachi, R., Srivastava, P.N. and Yanagamachi, H. Acrosome reaction in human spermatozoa. *Fertility and Sterility*, 1986; 45: 701.

Newall, R. AID, a review of 200 cases. *British Journal of Urology*, 1976; 58: 239.

Nilsson, S., Edvinsson, A. and Nilsson, B. Improvement of semen and pregnancy rate after ligation and division of the internal spermatic vein: Fact or fiction? *British Journal of Urology*. 1979; 51: 591.

Odelblad, E. Cervical factors. *Contributions in Gynaecology and Obstetrics*, 1978; 4: 132.

Odelblad, E. Sperm mucus interaction and cervical mucus penetration test. In Zatuchni, G.I., Goldsmith, A., Spiler, J.M. and Sciarra, J.J. (Eds), *Male Contraception: Advances and Future Prospects*, Harper and Row, Philadelphia, 1986, 134.

Overstreet, J.W. and Cooper, G.W. Sperm transport in the reproductive tract of the female rabbit: The rapid phase of transport. *Biology of Reproduction*, 1978a; 1: 101.

Overstreet, J.W. and Cooper, G.W. Sperm transport in the reproductive tract of the female rabbit II. The sustained phase of transport. *Biology of Reproduction*, 1978b; 19: 115.

Overstreet, J.W. and Katz, D.F. Semen analysis. *Urol. Clinc. N. America*, 1987; 14L: 441.

Overstreet, J.W., Katz, D.F., Hanson, F.W. and Fonesca, J.R. A simple inexpensive method for objective assessment of sperm movement characteristics. *Fertility and Sterility*, 1979; 31: 162.

Page, E.W. and Houlding, F. The clinical interpretation of 1000 semen analysis among applicants for sterility studies. *Fertility and Sterility*, 1951; 2: 140.

Peek, J.C., Godefrey, B. and Matthews, C.D. Estimation of fertility and fecundity in women receiving artificial insemination by donor semen and in normal fertile women. *British Journal of Obstetrics and Gynaecology*, 1984; 91: 1019.

Peek, J.C. and Matthews, C.D. The pH of cervical mucus, quality of semen and outcome of the post-coital test. *Clinical Reproduction and Fertility*, 1986; 4: 217.

Poland, M.L., Moghissi, K.S., Giblin, P.T., Ager, J.W. and Olson, J.M. Variation of semen measures within normal men. *Fertility and Sterility*, 1985; 44: 396.

Portuondo, J.A., Echanojauregui, A.D., Herran, C. and Agustin, A. Prognostic value of post-coital test in unexplained infertility. *International Journal of Fertility*, 1982; 27: 184.

Pryor, J.P., Blandy, J.P., Evans, P., De Santonge, D.M.C. and Underwood, M. Controlled clinical trial of arginine for infertile men with oligospermia. *British Journal of Urology*, 1978; 50: 47.

Pryor, J.P. Seminal analysis. In Hull, M.G.R. (Ed), *Clinics in Obstetrics and Gynaecology*, W.B. Saunders Company Limited, London, 1981, 8(iii): 571.

Quagliarello, J. and Arny, M. Intracervical versus intrauterine insemination: Correlation of outcome with antecedent post-coital testing. *Fertility and Sterility*, 1986; 46: 870.

Rehan, N.E., Sobrero, A.J. and Fertig, J. The semen of fertile men: Statistical analysis of 1300 men. *Fertility and Sterility*, 1975; 26: 492.

Richardson, D.W. AID and sperm banks in Great Britain. In David, G. Price, W. (Eds), *Human Artificial Insemination and Semen Preservation*, Plenum, New York, 1980.

Richter, M.A., Haning, R.V. Jr., Shapiro, S.S. Artificial donor insemination: Fresh versus frozen semen — the patient as her own control. *Fertility and Sterility*, 1984, 41: 277.

Robertson, L., Wolf, D.P. and Tash, J.S. Digital image analysis of capacitating human spermatozoa: Identification of subpopulations. *Biology of Reproduction*, 1987; 36 (supple 1): 61.

Rogers, B.J. The sperm penetration assay: Its usefulness reevaluated. *Fertility and Sterility*, 1985; 43: 821.

Rogers, B.J., Perreault, S.D., Bentwood, B.J., McCarville, C., Hale, R.W. and Soderdahl, D.W. Variability in the human hamster in vitro assay for fertility evaluation. *Fertility and Sterility*, 1983; 39: 204.

Rogers, B.J., Van Campen, H., Veno, M., Lambert, H., Bronson, R. and Hale, R. Analysis of human spermatozoal fertilising ability using zona free ova. *Fertility and Sterility*, 1979; 32: 664.

Ronnberg, L. The effect of clomiphene citrate on different sperm parameters and serum hormone levels in preselected infertile men: A controlled double blind crossover study. *International Journal of Andrology*, 1980; 3: 479.

Rossi, F. The O_2 forming NADPH oxidease of the phagocytes: Nature, mechanisms of activation and function. *Biochem. Biophys. Acta.*, 1986; 853: 65.

Rumke, P. and Hellinger, G. Autoantibodies against spermatozoa in sterile men. *American Journal of Clinical Pathology*, 1959; 32: 357.

Schats, R., Aitken, R.J., Templeton, A.A. and Djahanbakhch, O. The role of cervical mucus-semen interaction in infertility of unknown aetiology. *British Journal of Obstetrics and Gynaecology*, 1984; 91: 371.

Schellen, T.M. Clomiphene treatment in male infertility. *International Journal of Fertility*, 1982; 27: 136.

Schill, W.B. Medical treatment of idiopathic normogonadotrophic oligozoospermia. *International Journal of Andrology*, 1982; Suppl 5: 135.

Shulman, J.F. and Shulman, S. Methylprednisone treatment of immunologic infertility in the male. *Fertility and Sterility*, 1982; 38: 591.

Schwartz, D., Laplance, A., Jouannet, P. and David, G. Within-subject variability of human semen in regard to sperm count, volume, total number of spermatozoa and length of abstinence. *Journal of Reproduction and Fertility*, 1979; 57: 391.

Schwartz, D., Ducot, B., Auroux, M. and Collin, C. Within-subject variability of the percentage of morphologically abnormal spermatozoa among fertile men: Biological and measurement components. *Human Reproduction*, 1986; 1: 369.

Scott, J.Z., Nakamura, R.M., Mutch, J. and Davajan, V. The cervical factor in infertility: Diagnosis and treatment. *Fertility and Sterility*, 1977; 28: 1289.

Serres, C., Jouannet, P. and David, G. Influence of the flagellar wave development and propagation of the human sperm movement in seminal plasma. *Gamete Research*, 1984; 9: 183.

Sims, J.M. *Uterine surgery*, Wm Woods Company, New York, 1986.

Singer, S.L., Lambert, H., Overstreet, J.W., Hanson, F.W. and Yanagamachi, R. The kinetics of human sperm binding to the human zona pellucida and zona free hamster oocyte in vitro. *Gamete Research*, 1985; 12: 29.

Smith, K.D., Rodrigues-Rigau, L.J. and Steinberger, E. Relation between indices of semen analysis and pregnancy rate in infertile couples. *Fertility and Sterility*, 1977; 28: 1314.

Smith, K.D., Rodriguez-Rigau, L.J. and Steinberger, E. The influence of ovulatory dysfunction and timing of insemination on the success of artificial insemination donor (AID) with fresh or cyropreserved semen. *Fertility and Sterility*, 1981; 36: 496.

Smith, T.T., Koyanagi, F. and Yanagamachi, R. Distribution and number of spermatozoa in the oviduct of the golden hamster after natural mating and artificial insemination. *Biology of Reproduction*, 1987; 37: 225.

Soules, M.R., Moore, D.E., Spandoni, L.R. and Stenchever, M.A. The relationship between the post-coital test and the sperm penetration assay. *Fertility and Sterility*, 1982; 38: 384.

Spira, A. Epidemiology of human reproduction. *Human Reproduction*, 1986; 1: 111.

Steinberger, E. and Smith, K.D. Artificial insemination with fresh or frozen semen. *J.A.M.A.*, 1973; 223: 778.

Steinberger, E. and Rodriguez-Rigau, L.J. The infertile couple. *Journal of Andrology*, 1983; 4: 111.

Stewart, G.J., Cunningham, A.L., Driscoll, G.L., Tyler, J.P.P., Barr, J.A., Gold, J. and Lamont, B.J. Transmission of human T-cell lymphotrophic virus type III (HTLV-III) by artificial insemination by donor. *Lancet*, ii: 581.

Stock, C.E. and Fraser, L.R. The acrosome reaction in human sperm from men of proven fertility. *Human Reproduction*, 1987; 2: 109.

Stone, S.C. Complications and pitfalls of artificial insemination. *Clinical Obstetrics and Gynaecology*, 1980; 23: 667.

Stone, S.C. Peritoneal recovery of sperms in patients with infertility associated with inadequate cervical mucus. *Fertility and Sterility*, 1983; 40: 802.

Suarez, S.S. Sperm transport and motility in the mouse oviduct: Observations in situ. *Biology of Reproduction*, 1987; 36: 203.

Suarez, S.S. and Osman, R.A. Initiation of hyperactivated flagellar bending in mouse sperm within the female reproductive tract. *Biology of Reproduction*, 1987; 36: 1191.

Talbot, P. and Chacon, R.S. A triple stain technique for evaluating normal acrosome reactions of human sperm. *Journal of Experimental Zoology*, 1981; 215: 201.

Talbot, P. and Chacon, R.S. Ultrastructural observations on binding and membrane fusion between human sperm and zona pellucida-free hamster oocytes. *Fertility and Sterility*, 1982; 37: 240.

Templeton, A.A. and Mortimer, D. The development of a clinical test of sperm migration to the site of fertilisation. *Fertility and Sterility*, 1982; 37: 410.

Toffle, R.C., Nagel, T.C., Tagatz, G.E., Phansey, S.A., Okagaki, T. and Warin, C.A. Intrauterine insemination: The University of Minnesota experience. *Fertility and Sterility*, 1985; 43: 743.

Toth, A., Lesser, M.L., Brooks, C. and Labriola, D. Subsequent pregnancies among 161 couples treated for T-mycoplasma genital tract infection. *New England Journal of Medicine*, 1983; 308: 505.

Trounson, A.O., Matthews, C.D. and Kovacs, G.T. Artificial insemination by frozen donor semen: Results of multicentre Australian experience. *International Journal of Andrology*, 1981; 4: 227.

Turner, T.T. and Reich, G.W. Cauda epididymal sperm motility: A comparison among 5 species. *Biology of Reproduction*, 1985; 32: 120.

Usselman, M.C. and Cone, R.A. Rat Sperm are mechanically immobilised in the cauda epididymis by "Immobilin" a high molecular weight glycoprotein. *Biology of Reproduction*, 1983; 29: 1241.

Uehara, T. and Yanagamachi, R. Microsurgical injection of spermatozoa into hamster eggs with subsequent transformation of sperm nuclei into male pronuclei. *Biology of Reproduction*, 1976; 15: 467.

Van Uem, J.F.H.M., Burkman, L.J., Acosta, A.A., Veeck, L., Swanson, R.J., McDowell, J.S., Mayer, J., Bernardus, R.E., Ackerman, S. and Jones, H.W. Male factor evaluation in in vitro fertilisation: Norfolk experience. *Fertility and Sterility*, 1985; 44: 375.

Vere, M.F. and Joyce, D.N. Luteal function in patients seeking AID. *British Medical Journal*, 1979; ii: 100.

Vermeulen, A. and Comhaire, F. Hormonal effects of an antiestrogen: Tamoxifen in normal and in oligospermic men. *Fertility and Sterility*, 1978; 29: 320.

Vermeulen, A. and Vanderweghe, M. Improved fertility after varicocele correction: Fact or fiction? *Fertility and Sterility*, 1984; 42: 249.

Wardle, P.G., Mitchell, J.D., McLaughlin, E.A., Ray, B.D., McDermott, A. and Hull, M.G.R. Endometriosis and ovulatory disorder: Reduced fertilisation in-vitro compared with tubal and unexplained infertility. *Lancet*, 1985; ii: 236.

Wardle, P.G. Infertility studies using human in-vitro fertilisation. MD Thesis, University of Bristol, 1987.

Wardle, P.G., McLaughlin, E., Sykes, J.A. and Hull, M.G.R. Intrauterine insemination. *Lancet*, 1987; i: 270.

Wassarman, P.M. The biology and chemistry of fertilization. *Science*, 1987; 235: 553.

Willis, K.J., London, R.D., Bevis, M.A., Butt, W.R., Lynch, S.S. and Holder, G. Hormonal effects of tamoxifen in oligospermic men. *Journal of Endocrinology*, 1977; 73: 171.

Wolf, D.P., Sokoloske, J.E. and Quigley, M.M. Correlation of human in vitro fertilisation with the hamster egg bioassay. *Fertility and Sterility*, 1983; 40: 53.

Working, P.K. and Meizel, S. Correlation of increased intra-acrosomal pH with the hamster sperm acrosome reaction. *Journal of Experimental Zoology*, 1983; 227: 97.

World Health Organisation. Belsey, M.A., Eliason, R., Gallegos, A.J., Moghissi, K.S., Paulsen, C.A. and Prasad, M.R.N. (Eds), *Laboratory manual for the examination of human semen and semen-cervical mucus interactions*, Press Concern, Singapore, 1980.

Yanagimachi, R., Yanagimachi, H. and Rogers, B.J. The use of zona-free animal ova as a test system for the assessment of fertilising capacity of human spermotozoa. *Biology of Reproduction*, 1976; 15: 471.

Yanagimachi, R. Zona free hamster eggs: Their use in assessing fertilising capacity and examining chromosomes of human spermatozoa. *Gamete Research*, 1984; 10: 187.

Yanagimachi, R., Lopata, A., Odom, C.B., Bronson, R.A., Mahi, C.A. and Nicholson, G.L. Retention of biologic characteristics of zona pellucida in highly concentrated salt solutions. The use of salt stored eggs for assessing the fertilizing capacity of spermatozoa. *Fertility and Sterility*, 1979; 31: 562.

Yates, C.A., Trounson, A.O. and De Kretser, D.M. Fertilisation rates of male infertility patients in IVF. *Journal of In Vitro Fertilisation and Embryo Transfer*, 1986; 3: 154.

Yovich, J.L. and Stanger, J.D. Fertilisation rates of male infertility patients in IVF. *Journal of In Vitro Fertilisation and Embryo Transfer*, 1984; 3: 154.

Yovich, J.L. and Matson, P.L. Pregnancy rates after high intrauterine insemination of husband's spermatozoa or gamete intrafallopian transfer. *Lancet*, 1986; ii: 1287.

Zamboni, L. The ultrastructural pathology of the spermatozoon as a cause of infertility: The rate of electron microscopy in the evaluation of semen quality. *Fertility and Sterility*, 1987; 48: 711.

Zuckerman, Z., Rodriguez-Rigau, L.J., Smith, K.D. and Steinberger, E. Frequency distribution of sperm counts in fertile and infertile males. *Fertility and Sterility*, 1977; 28: 1310.

13
Immunological infertility

C. Chen

Introduction

Infertility may be due to a variety of causes, of which immunological factors probably play a role in about five per cent of cases. In the investigation of infertility there are a group of patients who show no apparent cause for their inability to conceive despite exhaustive tests. This is the group with so-called "idiopathic infertility" and accounts for 10 to 25 per cent of all cases of infertility (Behrman, 1965). Immunological incompatibility may play an etiological role in this category of patients.

Concept of immunological infertility

An understanding of the term immunological infertility is infertility which has an immunological basis; where the sperm becomes antigenic and provokes an immune reaction in the female or the male.

There is evidence from both animal and human studies for a likely association between immune reactivity to sperm and reduced fertility (Shulman, 1971a, 1971b; Rumke, 1974; Behrman, 1976). Whilst it may be tempting to attribute a causal relationship between immune factors and unexplained infertility, the same factors can also operate among patients with known organic causes of infertility. However, it is with the idiopathic group that clinical correlations can best be rationally assessed.

Following sexual intercourse, the deposition of sperm and other seminal products into the lower female genital tract may provoke an isoimmune response. The seminal material can provide the necessary antigenic stimulus for macrophage processing and presentation to the reticuloendothelial system, and eventually through the afferent limb of the immune response. The efferent pathways of isoimmunisation are both local (ie. genital tract) and systemic. The isoimmune response may be detected in the secretions of the genital tract (eg. cervical mucus) or in the blood (systemically). Therefore, both humoral and cell mediated immunity may be involved.

Autoimmunisation against male genital tract components can also occur. The testis is normally secluded immunologically by the so-called blood-testis barrier. Should this barrier be breached, autoimmunisation then develops. Clinical conditions such as mumps orchitis, epididymo-orchitis, prostatitis, seminal vesiculitis, testicular atrophy from trauma or infection, vasectomy, and even idiopathic situations, can lead to autoimmunity. The initial damage seems to be caused by the immune lymphocytes, followed by the appearance of cytotoxic antibodies, and complement. Subsequent disruption and blockage of the efferent duct systems lead to secondary immune damage within the seminiferous tubules. In its classic form, a full blown autoimmune allergic orchitis with disruption of testicular tissue, and resultant azoospermia occurs. Although the pathologic mechanisms described have largely been elucidated from animal studies, the actual situation in the human is somewhat unclear.

Pathogenic mechanisms

There is evidence obtained from various studies that suggest the role of immune factors in the pathogenesis of infertility (Beer & Neaves, 1978). Thus animals injected with sperm or testicular extracts become immunised against these antigens and subsequently become infertile.

The introduction of specific antigens (such as Salmonella typhosa lipopolysaccharide and T-4 coliphage) into the monkey vagina induces the formation of specific antibodies. These antibodies can be detected both in the blood (systematically) and locally (in the cervical mucus). This is a clear demonstration of local involvement of the genital tract in the manifestation of the immune response. When a homogenate of adult guinea pig testis is mixed with Freund's adjuvant, and then the whole injected into another male guinea pig, a bilateral immune aspermatogenesis is induced. There is degeneration of the seminiferous tubules, with the appearance of circulating antisperm antibodies. However, the injection of testicular homogenate from immature animals does not elicit such a response. This suggests that the sperm antigen is only present at or after the secondary spermatocyte stage. The use of purified testicular antigen produces the same effect, suggesting that the immunogenic properties reside in these antigens. The use of extracts from immature testes fails to induce an immune response because of the absence of the antigens which only appear when the animal matures.

Similar findings of aspermatogenesis can also be induced in men when Freund's adjuvant is injected into their testes. Circulating antisperm antibodies develop. Vasectomy has been found to induce antisperm antibodies, leading to a reduction in fertility when a reversal of the vasectomy is performed. Pregnancy rates after reanastomosis are significantly lower than anticipated from the patency rates. This may be explained by the presence of the circulating antisperm antibodies.

All the evidence cited above support the hypothesis that immunological factors can cause infertility. This is particularly true in the experimental animal. Coitus in the female, testicular damage, obstruction in the male by exposing the afferent limb of the immune response to seminal antigens that are foreign, could induce antibody formation with concurrent reduction of fertility. In the case of human infertility there has arisen an abundance of publications which are rich in controversy and the evidence is not entirely convincing.

Role of immunological mechanisms in infertility

The mechanism of sperm autoimmunity arising from genital tract disruption (such as testicular trauma, vasectomy) can be viewed as direct counterparts of the experimental animal models already discussed. What is unclear is how antisperm antibodies can occur in apparently healthy but infertile men. One explanation may be the occurence of occult genital tract infection. The blood-testis barrier may be breached, with the release of sperm antigens and subsequent immunisation. Genital tract obstruction from epididymo-orchitis can also result in circumvention of the physiological immunoregulatory mechanisms.

There is evidence for the existence of various immunological components necessary for mounting an immune reaction in the male genital tract. Thus secretory IgA and IgG are found in semen, probably arising from the rete testis and epididymis. Complement components are also present in semen. They complete the armamentarium for mediating antisperm reactions in the male genital tract. Seminal plasma which has both immunosuppresive and anticomplementary properties probably modulates some of these activities.

Infertility in the male could conceivably occur should sperm become agglutinated by agglutinating antibodies; or antisperm antibodies could immobilise the sperm or worse still, kill the sperm through cytotoxicity. The antibody could coat the sperm and adversely affect the sperm penetration of cervical mucus after intercourse. They could also neutralise such physiological events as sperm capacitation and even inhibit sperm-oocyte fusion. Sperm autoimmunity could produce disordered spermatogenesis resulting in oligo- and azoospermia; the autoimmune reaction being a potentiating factor following testicular or epididymal damage, or even genital tract obstruction.

Isoimmunity in the female may be antibody or cell mediated, and the response manifested largely locally rather than systemically. Local immunological activitiy is largely manifested at the cervical level with the uterine endometrium, fallopian tubes, and vagina making a minimal contribution. The antisperm antibodies are principally secretory IgA or IgG. Specific antibodies have also been detected in tubal secretion and even in follicular fluid.

The local antibodies can therefore disrupt the reproductive process in several ways. They may enhance the macrophage phagocytosis of sperm; they may kill sperm or immobilise them; they may entrap sperm within the cervical mucus or prevent sperm penetration in the mucus; or they may interfere with sperm capacitation, fertilisation, and even sperm selection.

Seminal plasma immunity

The role of seminal plasma antigens in the induction of infertility has received little attention. There is evidence of auto- or isoimmunisation to these antigens from studies in experimental animals. Thus, rabbits immunised against components of rabbit seminal plasma developed autoantibodies (Shulman, Riera and Yantorno, 1968). Li and Behrman (1970), in their studies on the immunisation of rabbits with human seminal plasma, found that the rabbit antisera obtained were capable of immobilising human sperm. A seminal plasma antigen called B_1 appeared responsible for the immobilisation phenomenon.

Although there are relatively extensive animal studies, there is a lack of information on human reactivity to seminal plasma antigens. One explanation may be a lack of sensitive investigatory tests. A further reason may be the antigenic complexity of seminal plasma. Low-titre antibody reactivity to human seminal plasma has been detected by Stevens, Fost and Balows (1965) using a haemagglutination technique. The reactions they observed were almost certainly due to naturally occurring serum blood group antibodies reacting with corresponding substances in seminal plasma.

Employing a technique involving the passive haemolysis reaction, Caretti (1974) found serum antibodies to human seminal plasma antigens among 33 per cent of women with unexplained infertility. Negative results were found in the unmarried or pregnant groups.

Using the technique of counterimmunoelectrophoresis, Chen and colleagues demonstrated the presence of antibodies to seminal plasma antigens among infertile women as well as in prostitutes (Chen and Simons, 1973, 1974; Chen et al, 1975). Further studies showed that the serum precipitating activity of seminal plasma was apparently produced by bacterial modification of native seminal plasma (Chen, Simons and Ratnam, 1977). The source of these bacteria was primarily the genitalia. Serum reactivity of these modified seminal plasma antigens was found in 86 per cent infertile and 63 per cent fertile patients.

Using a series of fractionation procedures, Chen and Simons (1977) were able to isolate a fraction from modified seminal plasma which contained antigenic activity directed against 16 per cent of women with no apparent cause for their infertility. No reactivity was obtained in the fertile subjects. They also found the frequency of positive reactions in women with subfertility who subsequently conceived (eight per cent) was significantly less than that among the non-pregnant groups (22 per cent). There is some evidence, based on animal immunisation studies, to suggest a possible association of these modified seminal plasma antigens with the intact sperm (Chen and Jones, 1979 unpublished observations).

Studies involving cell mediated immunity to seminal plasma components have been reported by Stites and Erickson (1975), Marcus, Freisheim and Herman (1977), and Lord, Sensabaugh and Stites (1977). Seminal plasma appears to suppress lymphocyte reactivity and may play a role in the suppression of local immunity against sperm following sexual intercourse in the female.

No discussion of seminal plasma immunity is complete without reference to anaphylactic reactions occurring rather dramatically among women immediately after coitus. These cases, although rarely reported, may perhaps be more often encountered with the local allergic variant.

The first case of allergy to human seminal plasma was reported by Halpern, Ky and Roberts (1966). The patient, who had no previous sexual exposure, immediately following coitus developed large erythematous, papular and pruritic rashes all over her body, with oedematous swelling of the lips, eyelids, tongue and pharynx. This was followed by severe asthmatic type dyspnoea, intense congestion of the mucous membranes, painful uterine cramps, and eventual loss of consciousness. These manifestations reached a peak 30 minutes after intercourse and eventually subsided 24 hours later. Most of the symptoms recurred with every coital act. The antigen responsible was identified as a small molecular weight glycoprotein, rich in sialic acid, and derived from seminal plasma. A high degree of atopic hypersensitivity was shown in the patient by skin reactions to human seminal plasma but not to that of animal origin. It was possible to transfer the hypersensitivity passively to man and monkey. The antibody responsible for these reactions was found to be reagin-like (IgE).

Similar cases were also described by Levine, Siraganian and Schenkein (1973), Frankland and Parish (1974), Mikkelsen et al (1975), and Siraganian,

Schenkein and Levine (1975). A case of bestiality in a woman involving a dog with sensitisation and anaphylaxis to dog semen was described by Holden and Sherline (1973). A milder form of seminal allergy occurring in four women in a family was observed by Chang (1976). The reaction was essentially a vulvovaginitis with stinging, burning, and pain in the vagina, persisting for 72 hours. Although the incidence of seminal sensitisation is apparently very low, it can possibly increase as a result of greater public and physician awareness. Treatment with Benadryl 50 mg given 30 minutes prior to intercourse is effective in mild cases. Prevention of contact with semen through the use of condoms seems to afford temporary relief. Desensitisation treatment with seminal fluid has given disappointing results.

Investigation of immunological infertility

A variety of tests have been developed for the detection of antisperm antibodies. But the antibodies they detect may or may not necessarily cause infertility. There is indeed some concern over the validity, interpretation, and standardisation of these tests. There is also considerable confusion about the clinical significance of the results obtained from some of these tests. These is especially with the detection of circulating antisperm antibodies. Hence there is a growing emphasis on the use of tests that detect local rather than systemic immunity to sperm.

Clinical presentation

Patients presenting with suspected immunological infertility generally give a history of an infertility problem of several years' duration. There are no overt clinical signs or symptoms associated with this type of infertility. Occasionally, incompatibility may be seen among patients who may have been fertile by a previous marriage. Couples presenting for investigation tend to complain of primary rather than secondary infertility and may be classed as "unexplained infertility". These patients should be thoroughly investigated and all organic causes excluded before their infertility can be considered "unexplained".

Thus, the husband's semen should meet the criteria of a normal spermiogram. There should be evidence of regular ovulation. The absence of pelvic pathology should be confirmed by laparoscopy. It is through the strict adherence to these criteria that the findings of immunological sperm tests can become more meaningful in terms of the persistence of the infertile state. Another type of clinical presentation of these infertile couples is the finding of repeatedly poor post-coital tests. Poor semen quality among infertile males is yet another reason for seeking further tests. The sperm density in these cases may be at hypo-, oligo- or azoospermic levels, with poor sperm motility, or even complete non-motility.

Indications for investigations

The indications which warrant investigation for antisperm immunity are therefore unexplained infertility, poor post-coital tests, and poor semen analysis. The value of investigating patients who already have organic causes is conjectural. Where the cause is a major one, the finding of an additional factor (viz. immunological) may be of academic interest. Where the cause is minor, there may be justification for proceeding with immunological testing.

Laboratory considerations

The investigation of immunological infertility is rather specialised, requiring appropriate laboratory facilities and personnel geared towards the satisfactory performance of the immunological tests. The staff should be adequately trained in the methodology of the tests as described by the WHO-sponsored international collaborative programme on antisperm antibody detection (Rose et al, 1976). This aspect merits attention in order that reliance may be placed on the results obtained. The interpretation of the clinical significance of these results may well depend on such technical considerations. Lack of uniformity in the performance of these tests in the past has led to confusion in interpreting results reported in many studies of antisperm antibodies.

Test materials for investigation

Serum from both partners should regularly be obtained for testing. In addition, the seminal fluid and cervical mucus (preferably obtained during the mid-ovulatory cycle) may also be investigated. As the volume of cervical mucus is normally small, some investigators have recommended the administration of oestrogens or the oral contraceptive pill to increase the amount of mucus produced. There is some reservation concerning the use of these drugs because of possible alterations in the properties of the mucus. However, those who regularly use them have apparently not encountered any adverse results.

Antisperm antibody tests

There are several tests available for the detection of antisperm antibodies in the serum and cervical mucus of both males and females. These tests can be categorised into groups based on the type of immune phenomenon observed, ie. agglutination, immobilisation, immunofluorescence, shaking, etc.

Sperm agglutination tests

The phenomenon of sperm agglutination involves basically two sets of sperm surface antigens which are located in the head and tail. Antibody activity directed against the head antigens and causing head-to-head agglutination are best revealed by the tube-slide agglutination test (TSAT) in which microscopic examination is required to detect the sperm agglutinates formed. At least 10 per cent or more of motile sperm should be agglutinated before a test can be considered positive. Antibody activity to the tail antigens are better demonstrated by the gelatin agglutination test (GAT) in which the sperm agglutinates are usually large enough to be seen by the naked eye as clumps suspended in the gelatin medium. The tray agglutination test (TAT) uses tissue typing trays as a variant of the technique. A test is positive where agglutination is seen in two or more consecutive dilutions.

There is variation in the incidence of positive sperm microagglutination tests in the serum of both infertile and fertile subjects. Several reasons may account for this. Sperm may agglutinate in the presence of bacteria, fungi, chemicals or even normal serum. Technical variations in quantitation and the omission of appropriate control experiments have tended to exaggerate the effect of these non-specific factors in many reports. Sperm microagglutination can also be induced by serum containing sex steroids of endogenous or exogenous origin. This activity has been found to reside in the steroid binding β-lipoprotein fraction. These findings may explain some of the confusion arising from studies involving pregnancy sera. Caution should therefore be exercised in the immunological and clinical interpretation of tests involving sperm microagglutination.

The observation of sperm macroagglutination as in the gelatin agglutination test has been used extensively in the investigation of infertile males. Its use in females has been limited because head-to-head agglutination, which appears to be mediated more commonly by antibodies developed in the female, is not readily detected by the gelatin method. By contrast, antibodies from males tend to produce tail-to-tail agglutination. The method requires careful control and interpretation under consistent laboratory conditions.

The antibodies involved in both micro- and macro-agglutination groups of tests are due to IgG and IgM antibodies.

The significance of serum antibody activity in relation to infertility may be appreciated from a study by Shulman, Jackson and Stone (1976) involving 150 couples almost all of whom were cases of "unexplained infertility". Employing the gelatin agglutination test, 23 per cent of the women and 20 per cent of the men gave positive results. With the tube-slide test, 16 per cent of the female and five per cent of the male sera were positive. It should therefore be noted that positive sera are often positive by one test and not the other, and only occasionally are positive by both. Therefore both tests should be used in any investigation of sperm agglutination.

Additional supporting evidence for the clinical importance of sperm agglutinins has been given by Rumke and Hellinga (1959). Using the gelatin agglutination test they found an incidence of 3.3 per cent positive among 2105 infertile males. To reduce the frequency of false positives they disregarded those results where the antibody titres were below 1:32. Using this criterion, none of their control fertile subjects were positive. The presence of high serum antibody titres in males has been found to be associated with decreased sperm penetrability of cervical mucus (Rumke and Hellinga, 1959; Fjallbrant, 1968).

Sperm immobilisation tests (SIT)

The phenomenon of complement dependent sperm immobilisation forms the basis of a simple yet reproducible test for antisperm antibodies. The interaction of antibodies with sperm antigens in the presence of complement causes disruption of the sperm membrane. This results in loss of sperm motility and eventual cell death. The effects can be observed microscopically and, if necessary, with the aid of dye which can be seen to enter the sperm. Sperm immobilising activity has been shown to reside in both the IgG and IgM fractions of positive sera. Sera with sperm immobilising activity usually show sperm agglutinating activity, but the converse is not true.

Several sperm immobilisation procedures have been devised but most are based on the original method of Isojima (1968). Where a large number of sera is to be tested, the adaptation of a microtechnique using tissue typing trays provides ease of titration (Husted and Hjort, 1975). A test is considered positive when more than 50 per cent reduction in motility (compared with the control) is obtained.

The sperm immobilisation test provides the most reliable method of detecting humoral antisperm activity and has a good correlation with infertility. It is the method of choice for screening females for serum antibodies. However, it appears to exhibit a relatively low titre of reactivity in male subjects.

The incidence and clinical significance of sperm immobilisation has been reported by Isojima et al (1972). In a study of 74 women with "unexplained infertility", 19 per cent were positive for sperm immobilisation. None of the controls gave a reaction.

Sperm immunofluorescence tests

The indirect immunofluorescent antibody technique is the most suitable immunofluorescent procedure for the study of antisperm antibodies (Jones and Ing, 1975). The earlier use of unfixed sperm was not satisfactory. Fixation of sperm smears by methanol and refinements in technique have led this test into popular use for the investigation of immunological infertility. Serum from both males and females may be studied. There are, however, a number of difficulties associated with this technique. Some of the problems encountered are: background fluorescence and unevenness of staining; variation in the staining patterns because of semen quality; and heterogeneity of staining, in which up to 30 per cent of the sperm may fail to exhibit a predominant pattern. The source of fluorescent conjugates and non-specific staining are additional factors to be considered.

Weak staining reactions of uncertain significance are often seen with undiluted serum. Positive results should only be reported on titres greater than 1:16. Non-specific staining patterns are commonly seen over the equatorial segment, neck and mid-piece. However, immune reactions mainly involve the acrosome and tail. Both IgM and IgG antibodies are responsible for acrosomal staining, whereas staining of the main tail piece appears to be exclusively due to IgG. Staining of the tail end-piece is occasionally seen and is due to IgM antibodies.

It must be emphasised that the staining patterns obtained on methanol fixed sperm involve subsurface antigens which are probably of less importance than the surface antigens in the induction of antibodies with potential clinical significance. This is borne out by the generally poor correlation of immunofluorescence test results with infertility. In addition, there is also poor correlation with results from immobilisation and agglutination tests. Sperm immunofluorescence is therefore not recommended for routine testing.

Testing for antibodies in cervical mucus

The cervix is the most accessible and important site of local immunity in the female genital tract. Local isoimmunity to sperm can also operate at higher levels, such as the uterus, fallopian tubes and ovaries, since sperm immobilising antibodies have been detected in follicular fluid. Studies of cervical mucus have been neglected largely because of logistic difficulties in its collection and use. There is, however, a trend towards greater emphasis in the investigation of local immunity rather than systemic immunity. This has arisen from the realisation that sperm antibodies may be produced locally and be present in the cervical mucus in the absence of detectable serum levels.

Cervical mucus is best collected at mid-cycle. Various techniques have been used to prepare the mucus prior to antisperm antibody testing. They include, ultracentrifugation, liquefaction with bromelin, and extraction in buffer, followed by centrifugation. The mucus extract can then be used for tests involving sperm agglutination, immobilisation and immunofluorescence. Test for sperm immobilisation can be suitably performed on a microscale using tissue typing trays (Isojima and Koyama, Chen and Jones, 1981).

Tests involving sperm immobilisation and cytotoxicity correlate best with infertility. Both the indirect immunofluorescence test and sperm micro-agglutination test have not given as good a correlation. Parish, Carron Brown and Richards (1967) described three of 48 infertile females with complement dependent cytotoxic sperm antibody. Soffer et al (1976), in a study of 11 couples with negative post-coital tests found positive sperm immobilisation in the cervical mucus from six of them. Sudo, Shulman and Stone (1977) detected sperm agglutinating antibodies in the mucus of three per cent of 450 infertile women.

Testing for antibodies in seminal plasma

Sperm antibodies may appear in seminal plasma when they are present in relatively high titre in serum (Rumke and Hellinga, 1959; Friberg, 1974). When higher titres are detected in seminal plasma, there is probably local production of antibodies, although transudation of IgG antibodies from serum may also occur. The direct identification of seminal antibodies is of uncertain value since serum titres can usually be used to predict the likely local situation. Husted (1975) claims that when sperm aglutinating titres reach a level of 1:64 in serum, the ejaculated semen shows spontaneous sperm agglutination.

The sperm cervical mucus contact test (SCMC)

This is a test involving both partners. It may be performed either by mixing sperm and cervical mucus on a microscope slide or by putting a drop of sperm onto mucus spread over a slide. Kremer and Jager (1976) first introduced this test which demonstrates the presence of local antibodies in either partner. The antibodies presumably belong to the secretory IgA class. It is hypothesised that following attachment of antibody to the sperm, the Fc fragment of the IgA molecule adheres to the glycoprotein micelles of cervical mucus.

In a positive test the sperm undergo characteristic shaking movements which can be seen microscopically. In the Kremer hypothesis, antibodies derived from seminal plasma will attach mainly to the sperm tail and, after coitus, subsequently bind to the cervical mucus by their Fc fragment. On the other hand, if the antibodies are derived from cervical mucus, they adhere by their Fc piece to the cervical micelles and subsequently bind to the sperm head via their Fab fragments following intercourse. A positive test is defined as one in which more than 25 per cent of the sperms demonstrate shaking movements.

As a variation of the test, the husband's sperm may be tested against donor cervical mucus, donor sperm against the wife's mucus, and donor sperm against donor mucus. Using this crossed hostility test, it is possible to identify whether the sperm or the cervical mucus is primarily at fault. A good indication for the use of this test is the finding of a consistently poor post-coital test. One clear advantage in its performance is the identification of the partner who has sperm antibodies. It stands to reason that condom therapy (see below) cannot improve the situation if antibodies are already present in the husband's semen. Kremer, Jager and Kuiken (1977) found a good correlation of the test with poor post-coital test results in 32 infertile women studies. There was also similar correlation between the test and the presence of sperm agglutinins in the serum, semen, and cervical mucus of the infertile couples investigated. In another report, Morgan et al (1977) concluded that the test, taken with the post-coital test, could provide a useful screen for immunological causes of infertility and an accurate assessment of the clinical relevance of sperm antibody tests.

Immunobead test (IBT)

More recently, additional tests have been introduced with improvements in sensitivity and quantitation (Jager et al, 1978; Bronson et al, 1982; Clarke et al, 1985). The immunobead test is one such test and uses polyacrylamide beads which are coated with anti-immunoglobulin. Exposure of these beads to sperm with suspected bound antibodies will shown bead attachment (direct test). The indirect test uses sperm which must first be exposed to serum suspected of having antisperm antibodies. At least 50 per cent of sperm should show bead attachment before the test can be said to be positive.

Enzyme linked immunosorbent assay (ELIZA)

The ELIZA sperm assay uses sperm or its extract to coat microtitre wells which are then used for detecting sperm antibodies in semen or cervical mucus. An anti-Ig enzyme conjugate and an enzyme substrate are added successively. A position colour reaction occurs which can be quantitated in an autoreader.

The diagnosis of immunological infertility

The diagnosis of immunological infertility is largely based on laboratory findings. Some clinical features and abnormal routine laboratory tests may serve as pointers to the possible presence of the condition. Thus, prolonged unexplained infertility, persistently negative post-coital tests in the absence of clinical lesions, and poor semen quality, merit further investigation.

In the assessment of immunological infertility, tests should be conducted on the blood, semen and cervical mucus of the partners involved. In general, the results of sperm agglutination tests probably do not correlate as well as those of sperm immobilisation, in relation to the infertile state. Demonstration of sperm immunofluorescence may well be of academic interest. Greater emphasis should be given to tests demonstrating local rather than sytemic immunity, for it is in the local genital tract that immunological damage is expected to occur. Although homologous immunity to seminal plasma antigens is of recent interest, for the sake of completeness, it may be useful to include this aspect in the investigation of the infertile couple. The final conclusion that an immunological factor may be present in any couple being investigated must depend on careful consideration of all available test results.

Treatment

On the whole, the treatment of sperm iso- or autoimmunisation is still far from satisfactory. Pregnancies have been reported following the use of various therapeutic regimens. Some of the reports have been anecdotal in nature and in others careful control studies have not been included, so that the results obtained may not necessarily be valid. Some workers have adopted purely empirical treatments so that overall the results of therapy remain variable and somewhat confusing.

Treatment of the female

Condom therapy

Among a variety of therapeutic procedures available, condom therapy (occlusive therapy) has perhaps been the most frequently prescribed. It was first introduced by Franklin and Dukes in 1964 and was based on the concept that the prevention of continuous exposure of the female to sperm, through the use of condoms, should result in a decline in sperm antibody levels. A six month period of condom usage was popularly recommended in anticipation of a satisfactory fall in sperm antibody activity. Thereafter, unprotected intercourse was resumed in the hope of a pregnancy. However, six months may not necessarily be sufficient time to produce a satisfactory fall in antibody levels. It is indeed erroneous to entertain such a concept because of the possibility of individual variation in response. Thus, the desired decrease in sperm antibody level may occur in six months, or in nine or even 12 months. In some cases it may not occur at all. What is more relevant is the need for tracking of the antibody levels. Blood, and if possible, cervical mucus, should be tested every three months or oftener until the desired response is obtained.

The results of condom treatment have been variable. Dukes and Franklin (1968) persuaded 29 couples to restrict intercourse to the use of condoms. Their sperm agglutinating antibody titres declined markedly and in 25 of them activity was no longer detectable. After resumption of unprotected sexual intercourse 20 women became pregnant. Ansbacher, Yeung and Behrman (1973), in a study of 26 women with sperm agglutinating antibodies, found a decrease in antibody activity in 19, and 10 subsequently became pregnant, giving a pregnancy rate of 53 per cent. The remaining seven continued to show high antibody titres and only one became pregnant. All these reports were based on sperm agglutination tests. In patients monitored by sperm immobilising antibody tests, the results have been less convincing. Isojima (1969) reported little success in his series. There was also no observable fall in the titre of antibody activity. In studies where both sperm agglutinating and sperm immobilising activity has occasionally fallen or disappeared, the gelatin or tube-slide agglutination titres have fluctuated. In these cases, pregnancies have resulted following resumption of unprotected coitus. In other cases, both the immobilising and agglutinating activity have fluctuated and no pregnancy resulted (Kay, 1977).

Immunosuppression

The use of immunosuppression is based on the assumption that circulating antibody production may be reduced by the use of corticosteroids. Very high doses require to be administered in order to achieve adequate suppression. There are several regimens available. One employs methylprednisolone in a dose of 96mg daily for a week (Shulman et al, 1978). Serum, semen and cervical mucus samples are tested for antibody activity at weekly intervals. A fall in activity is expected to occur. If pregnancy does not ensue, the course of medication is repeated. Where there is no fall in antibody levels, treatment is discontinued. Shulman reported a success rate of 14 per cent using the regimen in seven women, one of whom became pregnant (Shulman et al, 1978). The assessment of the value of this type of treatment awaits the outcome of properly controlled trials.

Intrauterine insemination

Based on the finding that sperm antibodies in cervical mucus attach to sperm, resulting in non-progressive shaking movements, Kremer, Jager and Kuiken (1977) suggested overcoming this cervical barrier by performing insemination directly into the uterine cavity. Before the actual insemination, as much as possible of the cervical mucus is removed by aspiration. This may prevent accidental introduction of mucus into the uterine cavity. The insemination should be continued over a period of six months. Kremer, Jager and Kuiken (1977), in a study of 20 females, achieved four (20 per cent) conceptions. This technique has given variable results. If local immunity is present, antibodies should be expected to be present at all levels of the female genital tract so that insemination above the cervical level need not necessarily prove helpful.

Other modalities of therapy

Pre-ovulatory oestrogens have been administered to increase the quantity and quality of cervical mucus in the hope of diluting the concentration of antisperm antibodies at the cervix. There appears to be some improvement in sperm and cervical mucus interaction with this treatment.

Antibiotic therapy has also been prescribed to women on the hypothesis that antisperm activity may be enhanced because of the adjuvant effects of genital infection. Elimination of the infection may therefore give beneficial results.

In vitro fertilisation (IVF) is being offered as an option to couples with sperm immunity. The results of IVF therapy show a reduced rate of fertilisation. The pregnancy rates are also disappointingly poor, suggesting peri-implantation loss and embryo mortality in the presence of antisperm antibodies.

Treatment of the male

In the male, treatment by hormonal suppression of spermatogenesis, immunosuppresion, sperm washing, and antibiotics have all be tried.

Hormonal therapy

Based on the hypothesis that sperm agglutinating antibodies may be formed as a result of sperm resorption, suppression of spermatogenesis for a prolonged period should result in a fall in antibody production. Testosterone in a dose of 250mg fortnightly was used by Schoysman (1970) in the treatment of 17 infertile males who had sperm agglutinating titres in excess of 1:64. A fall in titre was observed in 14 of them after six months of therapy and five (35.5 per cent) became fertile. This regimen was not successful in the hands of Rumke et al (1973). In a study of 12 patients who developed temporary azoospermia induced by the treatment, only four patients responded by a fall in antibody titre. However, despite the reappearance of these antibodies, two became fertile subsequently. In the light of these studies, hormonal suppression of spermatogenesis is probably not justified.

Immunosuppression

The administration of ACTH or corticosteroids in an attempt to suppress immunity to sperm has been tried. Rumke (1968) used ACTH and corticosteroids in moderate doses for two months and obtained no reduction in the serum antibody titres or in the frequency of occurrence of autoagglutination of sperm in his infertile males. However, encouraging results have been reported to justify further investigation into this area.

Bassili and El-Alfi (1970) treated 18 of their infertile male patients with prednisolone in a dose of 40mg daily for a fortnight, then tailing off the drug over a nine week period. An increase in sperm count was observed in nine of them, one of whom eventually fathered a child. Shulman et al (1977), using the regimen of methylprednisolone at 96mg/day for seven days, treated 18 infertile men, four of whom became fertile, giving a success rate of 22 per cent. In one of the men, the sperm antibody levels in both his serum and seminal plasma fell over a period of three weeks and the wife conceived. Hendry, Morgan and Stedronska (1977) prescribed prednisolone at 15mg a day for 17 male patients for six months, five of whom showed an improvement in sperm count and one pregnancy resulted. In another group of 17 males given methylprednisolone at 96mg per day for seven days, the sperm antibody titre also fell and one pregnancy resulted. On the whole, there is some potential benefit with the use of corticosteroids whether given in high, medium, or low doses, either continuously or intermittently (Hargreave & Elton, 1982).

Sperm washing insemination method

The basis of this procedure is to attempt the removal of antibody present in seminal plasma by washing and subsequently inseminating the wife with the washed sperm. The regimen described by Shulman et al (1977) involves the centrifugation at 2000 rpm for five minutes of spouse semen diluted fourfold in a sterile four per cent solution of human serum albumin. Centri-ugation is repeated three times and the final sperm pellet resuspended in 0.5ml of the albumin medium for subsequent intrauterine insemination. Among seven couples treated in this fashion, one pregnancy resulted.

Artificial insemination by donor

Where other forms of treatment have failed, AID may be the only option remaining. Overall, the results appear acceptable, provided the female partner is fertile.

References

Ansbacher, R., Yeung, K.K. and Behrman, S.J. Clinical significance of sperm antibodies in infertile couples. *Fertility and Sterility*, 1973; 24: 305.

Bassili, F. and El-Alfi, O.S. Immunological aspermatogenesis in man. I. Blastoid transformation of lymphocytes in response to seminal antigen in cases of non-obstructive azoospermia *Journal of Reproduction and Fertility*, 1970; 21: 23.

Beer A.E. and Neaves, W.B. Antigenic status of semen from the viewpoints of the female and male. *Fertility and Sterility*, 1978; 29: 3.

Behrman, S.J. Agglutinins, antibodies and immune reactions. *Clinical Obstetrics and Gynecology*, 1965; 8: 91.

Behrman, S.J. The immunologic role of the female genital tract in reproduction. *Andrologia*, (Supplement No 1), 1976; 8: 69.

Bronson R., Cooper G. and Rosenfeld D. Detection of sperm-specific antibodies on the spermatozoan surface by immunobead binding. *Archives of Andrology*, 1982; 9: 61.

Carretti, N. The passive haemolysis reaction for the identification of antiseminal plasma antibodies in the serum of women with unexplained sterility. In *Immunology in Obstetrics and Gynaecology*, ICS No 327, Excerpta Medica, 1974, 71.

Chang T.W. Familial allergic seminal vulvo-vaginitis. *American Journal of Obstetrics and Gynecology*, 1976; 126: 422.

Chen, C. and Jones, W.R. Application of a sperm microimmobilisation test for cervical mucus in the investigation of immunological infertility. *Fertility and Sterility*, 1981; 35: 542.

Chen, C. and Simons, M.J. Rapid detection of antibodies to seminal fluid by counterimmunoelectrophoresis. In *International Congress of Immunology in Obstetrics and Gynaecology*, ICS no. 281, Excerpta Medica, Amsterdam, 1973, 8.

Chen, C. and Simons, M.J. Counterimmunoelectrophoresis — rapid method for the detection of antibodies to seminal plasma. IRCS. *Journal of International Research Communications, Medical Science*, 1974; 2: 1647.

Chen, C. and Simons, M.J. Modified seminal plasma antigens. Further characterisation of antigenic activity. In Boettcher, B. (Ed), *Immunological Influence on Human Fertility*, Academic Press, Sydney, 1977; 263.

Chen, C., Simons, M.J., Ratnam, S.S. and Rajan, V.S. Occurence of antibody to seminal plasma among prostitutes. *Proceedings of the Tenth Singapore-Malaya Congress of Medicine*, Academy of Medicine, Singapore, 1975; 10: 368.

Chen, C., Simons, M.J. and Ratnam, S.S. Immunity to modified seminal plasma antigens associated with subfertility. *Acta Obstetricica et Gynecologica Scandinavica*, 1977; 56: 515.

Clarke G.M., Elliot P.J. and Smaila C. Detection of sperm antibodies in semen using the immunobead test. *American Journal of Reproductive Immunology and Microbiology*, 1985; 7: 118.

Dukes, C.D. and Franklin, R.R. Sperm agglutinins and human infertility: female. *Fertility and Sterility*, 1968; 19: 263.

Fjallbrant, B. Sperm antibodies and sterility in men. *Acta Obstetricia et Gynecologica Scandinavica*, 47, (Supplement 4), 1968.

Frankland, A.W. and Parish, W.E. Anaphylactic sensitivity to human seminal fluid. *Clinical Allergy*, 1974; 4: 249.

Franklin R. and Dukes C.D. Antispermatozoal antibody and unexplained infertility. *American Journal of Obstetrics and Gynecology*, 1964; 89: 6.

Friberg, J. Clinical and immunological studies on spermagglutinating antibodies in semen and seminal fluid. *Acta Obstetricia et Gynecologica Scandinavica*, (Supplement 36), 1874.

Halpern, B.M., Ky, T. and Roberts, B. Clinical and immunological study of an exceptional case of reaginic type sensitisation to human seminal fluid. *Immunology*, 1966; 12: 247.

Hargreave T.B. and Elton R.A. Treatment with high dose methyl prednisolone or intermittent betamethasone for antisperm antibodies: preliminary communication. *Fertility and Sterility*, 1982; 38: 568.

Hendry, W.F., Morgan H., and Stedronska, J. The clinical significance of antisperm antibodies in male subfertility. *British Journal of Urology*, 1977; 49: 757.

Holden, T.E. and Sherline, D. Bestiality, with sensitisation and anaphylactic reaction. *Obstetrics and Gynaecology*, 1973; 42: 138.

Husted, S. Sperm antibodies in men from infertile couples. *International Journal of Fertility*, 1975; 20: 133.

Husted, S. and Hjort, T., Microtechnique for simultaneous determination of immobilising and cytotoxic sperm antibodies: Methodological and Clinical studies. *Clinical and Experimental Immunology*, 1975; 22: 256.

Isojima, S. Relationship between antibodies to spermatozoa and sterility in females. In Edwards, R.G. (Ed), *Immunology and Reproduction,* International Planned Parenthood Federation, London, 1969, 267.

Isojima, S. and Koyama, K. Microtechnique of sperm immobilisation test. In Bratanov, K.,

Vulchanov, V.H., Dikov, V. Somlev, B., and Kozhouharova (Eds), *Immunology of Reproduction*, Proceedings of the Third International Symposium, Academy of Sciences, Soifa, 1974, 215.

Isojima, S., Li T.S. and Ashitaka, Y. Immunologic analysis of sperm-immobilising factor found in sera of women with unexplained infertility. *American Journal of Obstetics and Gynecology*, 1968; 101: 677.

Isojima, S., Tsuchiya, K., Koyama, K., Tanaka C., Nakka O. and Adachi, H. Further studies on sperm immobilising antibody found in sera of unexplained cases of sterility in women. *American Journal of Obstetrics and Gynecology*, 1972; 112: 199.

Jager J., Kremer J. and van Slochteren-Draaisma T. A simple method of screening for anti-sperm antibodies in the human male. Detection of spermatozoal surface IgG with mixed anti-globulin reaction carried out in untreated fresh human semen. *International Journal of Fertility*, 1978; 23: 12.

Jones, W.R. and Ing, R.M.Y. An immunofluorescent study of sperm isoimmunisation in infertile women. *Journal of Obstetrics and Gynaecology of the British Commonwealth*, 1974; 81: 385.

Kay, D.J. Clinical significance of antibodies to antigens of the reproductive tract. In Boettcher, B. (Ed), *Immunological Influence on Human Fertility*, Academic Press, Sydney, 1977; 119.

Kremer, J. and Jager, S. The sperm-cervical mucus contact test: a preliminary report. *Fertility and Sterility*, 1976; 27: 335.

Kremer, J., Jager, S. and Kuiken, J The clinical significance of antibodies to spermatozoa. In Boettcher, B. (Ed), *Immunological Influence of Human Fertility*, Academic Press, Sydney, 1977; 47.

Levine, B.B., Siraganian, R.P. and Schenkein, I. Allergy to human seminal plasma. *New England Journal of Medicine*, 1973; 288: 894.

Li T.S. and Behrman, S.J. The sperm- and seminal plasma-specific antigens of human semen. *Fertility and Sterility*, 1970; 21: 565.

Lord, E.M., Sensabaugh, G.F. and Stites, D.P. Immunosuppressive activity of human seminal plasma. I. Inhibition of in vitro lymphocyte activation. *Journal of Immunology*, 1977; 118: 1704.

Marcus, Z., Freisheim, J. and Herman, J.H. In vitro cell mediated immunity (CMI) to human seminal plasma fractions. *Federation Proceedings*; Federation of American Societies for Experimental Biology, 1977; 36: 371.

Mikkelsen, E.J., Henderson, L.L., Leiferman, K.M. and Gleich, G.J. Allergy to human seminal fluid. *Annals of Allergy*, 1975; 34: 239.

Morgan, H., Hendry, W.F., Stedronska, J. and Chamberlain, G.V.P. Sperm/cervical mucus crossed hostility testing and antisperm antibodies in the husband. *Lancet*, 1977; 1228.

Parish, W.E., Carron-Brown, J.A. and Richards, C.P. The detection of antibodies to spermatozoa and to blood group antigens in cervical mucus. *Journal of Reproduction and Fertility*, 1967; 13: 469.

Rose, N.R., Hjort, T., Rumke, P, Harper, M.J.K. and Vyazov, O. Techniques for detection of iso- and autoantibodies to human spermatozoa. *Clinical and Experimental Immunology*, 1976; 23: 175.

Rumke, P. Sperm agglutinating autoantibodies in relation to male infertility. *Proceedings of the Royal Society of Medicine*, 1968; 61: 275.

Rumke, P. Autoantibodies against spermatozoa in infertile men. *Journal of Reproduction and Fertility*, (Supplement) 1974; 21: 169.

Rumke, P. and Hellinga, G. Autoantibodies against spermatozoa in sterile men. *American Journal of Clinical Pathology*, 1959; 32: 357.

Rumke, P., van Amstel N., Messer, E.N. and Bezemer, P.D. Prognosis of men with auto-spermagglutinins in the serum and unsuccessful treatment with testosterone. In Bratonov,

K., Edwards. R.G., Vulchanov, V.H., Dikov V. and Somlev, B. (Eds), *Immunology of Reproduction*, Bulgarian Academy of Sciences, Sofia, 1973; 319.

Schoysman, R. Treatment of male infertility due to autoagglutination of spermatozoa. In Halbrecht, I. (Eds), *Proceedings VIth World Conference of Fertility and Sterility*, Israel Academic Press, Tel-Aviv, 1970; 112.

Shulman, S. Immunity and infertility: A review. *Contraception*, 1971a; 4: 135.

Shulman, S. Antigenicity and autoimmunity in sexual reproduction: A review. *Clinical and Experimental Immunology*, 1971b; 9: 267.

Shulman, S., Davis, P., Lade, P. and Reyniak, J.V. Immune infertility and new approaches to treatment. In Boettcher, B. (Eds), *Immunological Influence on Human Fertility*, Academic Press, Sydney, 1977; 281.

Shulman, S., Harlin, B., Davis P. and Reyniak, J.V. Immune infertility and new approaches to treatment. *Fertility and Sterility*, 1978; 29: 309.

Shulman, S., Jackson H. and Stone M. Antibodies to spermatozoa, VI. Comparative studies of sperm agglutinating activity in groups of infertile and fertile women. *American Journal of Obstetrics and Gynecology*, 1976; 123: 139.

Shulman, S., Riera, C. and Yantorno, C. Studies on organ specificity XIX. Antigenic specificity of seminal plasma and the formation of autoantibodies. *Journal of Immunology*, 1968, 100: 682.

Soffer. Y., Marcus, Z.H., Bukovsky, I. and Caspo, E. Immunological factors and post-coital test in unexplained infertility. *International Journal of Fertility*, 1976; 21: 89.

Siraganian, R.P., Schenkein, I. and Levine, B.B. Immunologic studies of a patient with seminal allergy. *Clinical Immunopathology*, 1975; 4: 59.

Stevens, K.M., Fost, C.A. and Balows, A. Circulating antibodies to human seminal plasma in man. *Journal of Reproduction and Fertility*, 1965; 10: 137.

Stites, D.P. and Erickson, R.P. Suppressive effect of seminal plasma on lymphocyte activation. *Nature*, 1975; 235: 727.

Sudo, N., Shulman, S. and Stone, M. Antibodies to spermatozoa. IX. Spermagglutination phenomenon in cervical mucus in vitro: a possible cause of infertility. *American Journal of Obstetrics and Gynecology*, 1977; 129: 360.

14
Antisperm antibodies in infertility

Tigris T.Y. Lee, M.C. Hsu and Y.S. Yang

Introduction

Unexplained infertility accounts for more than one quarter (27.2 per cent) of the infertile female partners investigated (Cook, 1986), although our study showed 18.5 per cent.

Immunological causes have always been thought to play a role. There is some evidence to show that antisperm antibodies can impede spermatozoal transport through the female reproductive tract (Menge et al, 1982) and impair the ability of human spermatozoa to interact with oocytes (Hass et al, 1985; Bronson et al, 1982).

Recent advances in antisperm monoclonal antibody development, molecular biology, and immunohistochemical studies have given further insight into the significance and possible mechanisms by which the antisperm antibody affects human fertility.

Historical background

The first experimental study of immunity to sperm antigens was in the animal and was published independently by Landsteiner (1899) and Metchnikoff (1899). Since then, an extensive literature has accumulated concerning experimental immunisation in animals.

The relationship between sperm autoimmunity and infertility was provided by the pioneering work of Rumke (1954) and Wilson (1954). Sperm agglutinating autoantibodies were demonstrated in the sera of infertile men by these two researchers. Wilson drew further attention to the fact that there was poor sperm penetration and a rapid loss of sperm motility of sperm from these men when exposed to cervical mucus, both in vivo and in vitro. Franklin and Dukes (1964) later demonstrated sperm agglutinating antibodies in the sera of women with unexplained infertility. Experiments by Katsh (1959) and Edwards (1964) revealed that immunity to sperm induced by intraperitoneal inoculation of female guinea pigs and mice with sperm of homologous or heterologous species impaired reproductive performance. A detailed description of the animal model for studying autoimmune aspermatogenic orchitis, also called experimental allergic orchitis, has been given by Voisin et al (1974).

Huang, Tung and Yanagimachi (1981), Menge and Black (1979), and Bronson, Cooper and Rosenfeld (1983) have shown that antisperm antibodies may be involved in sperm-egg interactions in both animal and human. Autoantibodies from vasectomized guinea pigs have inhibitory effects on the acrosome reaction, sperm-zona binding, and sperm-ovum fusion (Huang, Tung and Yanagimachi, 1981). Antisperm antibodies lower the penetrability of human sperm through zona free hamster ova (Menge and Black, 1979; Bronson, Cooper and Rosenfeld, 1983). Antisperm antibodies also inhibit sperm attachment and penetration of human zona pellucida (Bronson, Cooper and Rosenfeld, 1982a; Tsukuis et al, 1986) as well as fertilisation (Clarke et al, 1985). Antibodies may also interfere with early embryonic development and/or implantation (Naz, Saxe and Menge, 1983).

Autoimmunity to sperm in the male

Mature sperm possesses a variety of unique organ specific and tissue specific antigens which are not present during fetal life. During spermatogenesis, sperm cells acquire new antigens that are not recognised as self by the individual (Romrell and O'Rand, 1978). These antigens are capable of eliciting an immune response in situations when they gain access to the host's immune system.

The blood-testis barrier provided by the Sertoli cell tight junction prevents the immune system from recognising sperm antigens under normal circumstances. However, with prostatic infection, trauma to the testis, or a breach of the male reproductive tract, such as in vasectomy, these antigens escape and stimulate an immune response. Indeed, vasectomy is a common cause of such sensitisation. Circulating sperm antibodies may be encountered in 30–50 per cent of men who undergo this operation (Alexander and Anderson, 1979).

The presence of these antibodies in reproductive tract secretion, obtained at the time of vasovasostomy, has correlated with an impaired chance of subsequent fertility (Gupta et al, 1975; Hjort and Meinertz, 1988). It is still unclear what triggers antisperm antibody formation in men who do not have a history of trauma, infection or any demonstrable organic lesion in the reproductive tract. Antisperm antibodies can theoretically be found in three compartments: directly on the sperm, in seminal plasma, and in the blood.

The two major classes of antisperm antibodies are IgG and IgA. IgG is a systemic immunoglobulin that is secreted in a variety of tissues and fluid compartments. IgA, on the other hand, is a secretory antibody whose production may be locally mediated. Significant levels of IgM do not reach the reproductive tract fluid in the male and it is unlikely that IgM antibodies contribute to infertility in the male. The degree of fertility impairment, however, seems to depend partially on the serum titer, and the degree of transfer of antibodies to the seminal fluid. The fluid contains less than one per cent of circulating IgG, one to two per cent of circulating IgA and virtually no IgM under normal circumstances (Rumke, 1974). It was thought that circulating antisperm antibodies occur by transudation through the prostate. The prostate gland is capable of mounting a local immune response following antigenic stimulation (Rumke, 1974).

Isoimmunisation to sperm in the female

The female reproductive tract is not an immunologically privileged site. Bacterial toxins, cell wall fragments, virus particles, and fungus, when placed in the vagina will elicit a measurable systemic and local antibody response, confirming the sensitivity of the female reproductive tract to antigens. Sperm contains proteins which are foreign to the woman. The introduction of sperm through coitus into the female genital tract may provoke an isoimmune response. The uterine cervix is the major site of secretory immunologic activity in the female genital tract; while the endometrium and fallopian tubes may participate to a lesser extent; the vagina is probably inactive. The sperm antigens thus introduced are processed by macrophages and then presented to the reticuloendothelial system. The efferent pathways are both systemic and local and involve humoral antibody formation and cell mediated immunity.

The cervix is adequately equipped with plasma cells, and cervical mucus contains immunoglobulins, some of which are locally secreted. Secretory immunoglobulin A(SIgA), serum immunoglobulin A(IgA), and immunoglobulin G(IgG) are all found in cervical mucus. Immuno-globulin and C3 complement levels in cervical mucus vary during the menstrual cycle, tending to be lowest at the time of ovulation. The overall antibody concentration in cervical mucus and tubal secretions during the woman's cycle may be roughly estimated at 10 per cent of the level in circulation. Shortly before or at the time of ovulation, these levels decrease to about one to two per cent of the serum level (Schumacher and Yang, 1977; Schumacher, 1980).

Tests for the detection of sperm-reactive antibodies

A bewildering variety of tests for antisperm antibodies have been devised. These have variable sensitivity and specificity. It is not possible to give a complete description of the various techniques available, but merely to summarise the principles on which they are based and discuss some of their advantages, disadvantages and difficulties.

Sperm agglutination tests

In sperm agglutination tests, agglutination of sperm is observed following exposure of sperm to serum in variable titers. The gelatin agglutination tests (GAT) of Kibrick, Belding and Merrill (1952) is widely used, especially for studies of the male. Agglutination is observed macroscopically by the appearance of white floccules in the suspending medium held in narrow test tubes.

The tail-to-tail sperm agglutination occurs in the GAT, whereas head-to-head agglutination is better seen in the microagglutination test, and is due more commonly to antibodies developed in the female. The micro-agglutination test for sperm antibody is determined by microscopic analysis. The tray agglutination test (TAT) described by Friberg (1974), is performed in a tissue typing tray, whereas the tube-slide agglutination test (TSAT) of Franklin and Dukes (1964) is performed on a microscope slide and detects mainly head-to-head agglutination, and to a lesser extent, tail-to-tail agglutination. In all these assays, there is a fairly high occurrence of false positive result, due to non-specific agglutination by microbial agents, fungi, chemicals, steroids, and even homologous serum.

Sperm immobilisation test

The sperm immobilisation test was introduced by Isojima, Li and Ashitaka (1968). Complement dependent sperm immobilisation forms the basis of a simple reproducible tests for sperm antibodies. The interaction of antibody molecules with sperm antigens activates the complement system and disrupts the permeability and integrity of the cell membrane of the sperm acrosome and midpiece. The ultimate effect on the sperm is seen microscopically as a loss of motility followed by cell death. The test can detect IgG or IgM antibody activity in the sera of males and females. The major problem of the test is the source of complement with good activity and without nonspecific toxicity. It is one of the tests in which there are essentially no false positive reactions.

Enzyme-Linked Immunosorbent Assay (ELISA)

The ELISA method (Zanchetta, Busolo and Mastrogiacomo, 1982) utilises an antiglobulin to which an enzyme has been covalently linked. The antiglobulin may bind to surface bound antisperm antibodies. A substrate for the enzyme is then added, and its product is measured colorimctrically. The test utilises sperm membrane extracts coated onto microtiter wells and used as antibody targets. The fixation techniques used may lead to denaturation of sperm antigens or membrane damage, resulting in both false positive and false negative results. However, the test offers an advantage in providing a quantitative index and is also immunoglobulin specific.

Immunofluorescence

Indirect immunofluorescent tests, reviewed by Hass and Beer (1986), commonly employ either air drying or methanol fixation of sperm, which can lead to disruption of the plasma membrane and exposure of internal sperm antigens, so a high incidence of false positive results may be encountered.

Detection of immunoglobulins on the sperm surface

The detection of surface bound antibodies provides the best indicator of biologically significant antisperm antibodies. The mixed agglutination reaction (MAR) has been used by Jager, Kremer and Van Slochteren-Draaisma, (1978). A washed suspension of Rh-positive human red blood cells (RBCs) sensitised with a human IgG anti-Rh antibody is mixed with drops of semen to be tested and a xenogenous (eg. rabbit) anti-human IgG antiserum. If spermatozoa in the ejaculate is antibody bound, it will form mixed agglutinates wih the RBCs in the presence of the antisperm antibodies.

The radiolabelled antiglobulin tests developed by Hass, Cines and Schreiber (1980) provide another quantitative assessment of antibody binding to the sperm surface and is highly reliable and reproducible. The immunobead test (Telang, Reyniak and Shulman, 1978) allows direct detection of immunoglobulins on the surface of living sperm. Sperm in suspension is mixed with a suspension of immunobeads which are micron sized polyacrylamide spheres to which rabbit anti-human antibodies have been linked. Sperm which have antibodies bound adhere to the immunobeads on contact. The pattern of binding of the beads allows determination of (1) the sperm surface antigenic sites, (2) the proportion of sperm in the ejaculate which are antibody bound, and (3) the antibody isotype (IgA, IgG, or IgM). The MAR, radiolabelled antiglobulin test, and the immunobead test, can also be used indirectly using the patient's serum and donor sperm.

The major problem in the diagnosis of antisperm antibodies is the selection of appropriate testing methodologies. It is quite clear that many of the techniques that have been employed for the diagnosis of antisperm antibodies lack the sensitivity and/or specificity to be of clinical value.

The main indications for antisperm antibody testing are sperm agglutination in the ejaculate, repeated poor postcoital tests (PCT), and unexplained infertility. Sperm agglutination in the ejaculate can be non-specific. The absence of sperm agglutination in a semen sample does not exclude the presence of antisperm antibodies.

Incidence of antisperm antibodies

The incidence of antisperm antibodies in infertile couples varies considerably, depending on the tests used, the patient population, criteria of diagnosis, and local or systemic immunity. Since immunity to sperm is not an all-or-none phenomenon, sperm antibodies are a relative, rather than an absolute cause of infertility. Sperm antibodies may reduce, but not totally prevent, the occurrence of pregnancy (Bronson, Cooper and Rosenfeld, 1984) The standardisation of interpretation of tests is difficult. Antibodies in reproductive tract secretions may be transudated from the blood or secreted locally by submucosal plasma cells within the reproductive tract (Uehling, 1979; Murdoch, Buckley and Fox, 1982). Given these two potential sources of immunoglobulins, antisperm antibodies can be present in serum, yet undetectable in semen or female reproductive tract secretions. Local immunity to sperm has also been demonstrated in the absence of detectable humoral antibodies both in men (Bronson, Cooper and Rosenfeld, 1982) and in women (Menge et al, 1982).

Most of the previous studies have attempted to detect the presence of sperm antibodies in the sera of infertile couples. Sperm agglutinating or immobilising antibodies have been reported in seven to 17 per cent infertile women, the percentage varying with type of test performed and the population screened (Beer and Neaves, 1978; Jones, 1974). A higher incidence of antisperm antibodies in the sera of both men and women with unexplained infertility has been reported by Jones (1974). Beer and Neaves (1978) observed that 14 to 40 per cent of couples with unexplained infertility have immunological factors. In general, higher positive rates of antisperm antibodies were observed in the sera of couples with poor postcoital tests. In Bronson's series using the indirect immunobead test, 24 per cent of males and 35 per cent of females with infertility were positive for antibodies (Bronson, Cooper and Rosenfeld, 1984).

In our study, we investigated antisperm antibodies among 56 infertile couples with unexplained infertility, and who also had repeated poor post-coital tests. Twenty fertile couples served as controls. We used the ELISA (Jer, Jerusalem) and the immunobead test (Bio-Rad Richmond CA, USA) for the detection of antisperm antibodies in the sera, seminal plasma, and cervical mucus. The results are shown in Tables 14-1 and 14-2.

For the ELISA method, a titer of 1:32 or greater was defined as positive. In the female (Table 14-1), 25 per cent of sera and 22 per cent of cervical mucus were found to have antisperm antibodies, as compared with five per cent in the control fertile females. The occurrence of antisperm antibodies in the sera of infertile females was significantly higher than those of fertile females ($p < 0.05$). In the male, 20 per cent of sera and nine per cent of seminal plasma were positive by ELISA, whereas only five per cent of the sera of the fertile male controls were positive.

Semen samples having at least 50 per cent antibody bound sperm were defined as positive for the immunobead test. Fourteen out of the 56 infertile males showed a positive result. The class of immunoglobulin in these 14 patients with positive immunobead tests was mainly IgG and/or IgA (Table 14-2).

Clinical significance of antisperm antibodies in the female partner

The occurrence of antisperm antibodies in sera of infertile women (Menge, 1980) varies between five and 30 per cent by the sperm agglutination test, and two and 16 per cent by the sperm immobilisation test. Unexplained infertility of three years or longer had lower pregnancy rates with positive tests compared with those with negative tests. Some investigators (Rumke et al, 1984; Menge et al, 1982) have commented that the probability of pregnancy was much lower when the immobilisation titer was four or greater, or when the agglutination titer was 16 or higher. Sperm immobilisation was more significant than sperm microagglutination in terms of pregnancy rates. If pregnancy did occur, the time interval between the test and pregnancy was much longer in women who had higher antibody titers than in those with lower serum titers (Rumke et al, 1984).

Antisperm antibodies in cervical mucus seems more relevant to infertility, as they may interfere with sperm penetration. Since the first report of Parish, Carron-Brown and Richards (1967) on antisperm activity in female cervical mucus, there has been increasing evidence of a local antibody response to sperm. The incidence of local sperm agglutinating antibodies varies from three to nine per cent and of immobilising antibodies from eight to 32 per cent (Jones, 1974). This incidence is higher compared with that in sera.

As antisperm antibodies in serum do not correlate with that in cervical mucus, it is necessary to test both serum and cervical mucus. There is good correlation betwen antisperm antibodies in cervical mucus and the degree of disturbed migration of sperm through cervical mucus (Menge et al, 1982). Repeated negative postcoital tests performed one or two days before or on the day of ovulation in the presence of good seminal and mucus quality are an indication of disturbed sperm-mucus interaction, which may indicate the existence of antisperm antibodies.

Mathur et al (1984) demonstrated that sperm motility in the postcoital test has a predictive value of 72 per cent for male autoimmunity and 57 per cent for female isoimmunity in the presence of normal cervical mucus and in the absence of infection. The oscillating movement of sperm in cervical mucus called the "shaking phenomenon" by Kremer and Jager, has served as the basis of their sperm-cervical mucus contact test (SCMC) test (Kremer and Jager, 1976). A positive test suggests antisperm antibodies in either semen or cervical mucus (or both). It was originally hypothesised that the phenomenon was mediated by "stickness" of the Fc fragment of the IgA antibody to the glycoprotein micelles of cervical mucus. However, it now appears that the "shaking" phenomenon can be mediated by F(ab')2 fragments of antisperm antibodies in both IgA and IgG classes (Haas, 1983). The SCMC test is a valuable test for local antibodies and is suitable for crossover testing, using normal donor sperm and donor cervical mucus.

Clinical significance of antisperm antibodies in the male partner

The first study on the incidence of sperm agglutinating antibodies was performed on sera from infertile and fertile men by Rumke and Hellinga (1959). Similar studies have since been carried out by others. A positive sperm agglutination test was found in three to 13 per cent of infertile men, compared with two per cent fertile controls. The sperm immobilisation test, however, was positive only in the sera of two to three per cent of infertile males, with none in the fertile controls (Rumke et al, 1974). The titer of these antibodies appears to correlate with the prognosis for fertility. According to Rumke and associates (1974), a low titer ($<$ 1:32) may not be significant, whereas a high titer ($>$ 1:1024) seems to correlate with infertility.

In their study involving a follow up of 254 men over 16 years, none with high titers succeeded in impregnating their wives. Although conception may occur occasionally in men with agglutination titers varying between 1:64 and 1:512, titers of 1:32 or higher are considered to be clinically significant.

Immunoglobulin concentrations are normally very low in seminal plasma (one to two per cent) of circulating immunoglobulins. High titers of sperm agglutinating or sperm immobilising activity in serum may also lead to these antibodies appearing in seminal plasma. A proportion of men with autoimmunity to sperm may also have surface bound antisperm antibody. We investigated the effects of autoimmunity on sperm-cervical mucus interaction by testing which partner's locally produced antibodies related to poor postcoital tests. We also performed a crossover SCMC test using healthy donor sperm and normal cervical mucus in our study of infertile couples with poor postcoital tests.

Table 14-3 shows the results of our SCMC in 47 couples having surface bound antisperm antibody. Most of the men (12/14) who had surface bound antisperm antibodies exhibited the "shaking phenomenon" in the SCMC test in the presence of good normal cervical mucus. These results suggest that couples whose SCMC test gives the shaking phenomenon should be evaluated for surface bound antisperm antibody in the partner's semen.

In a recent study, Avyaliotis et al (1985) found a correlation between the presence of antibody bound sperm and the prospects of conceiving over a six to 46 month period. The pregnancy rate for those couples with autoimmunity to sperm as the sole definable factor leading to infertility was only 15 per cent, when more than half of the sperm were antibody bound. A significantly higher chance of pregnancy occurred (67 per cent) in those where less than half of their sperm had bound antibodies. These sperm surface bound antibodies seem to affect fertility adversely.

Treatment for immunity to sperm in the female

Many authors have used a variety of therapeutic approaches for the treatment of isoimmunity to sperm, with disappointing results. One of the earliest regimens used was the condom, also termed occlusive treatment. Earlier publication claimed a high degree of success after condom usage of six months. The hypothesis was that the woman's sensitivity to sperm would have diminished following such non-exposure to sperm. Several studies have reported pregnancy rates varying greatly from 11 to 56 per cent (Haas, 1983; Schwimmer, Ustay and Behrman, 1967). Unfortunately, the majority of these studies failed to show a significant decrease in titers of antisperm antibodies in either serum or cervical mucus, besides lacking adequate controls.

Immunosuppression with steroid medication was the next therapeutic recourse. The results seem to be equivocal and unclear. Steroids can produce some unpleasant side effects. The risk-benefit ratio may be unfavourable for the treatment of women with antisperm antibodies. In those with antisperm antibodies in their cervical mucus, intrauterine insemination with their husband's sperm after sperm washing has been advocated (Schwimmer, Ustay and Behrman, 1967). This approach attempts to bypass the mucus-antibody barrier and may be appropriate therapy if the postcoital test is poor. However, the theoretical possibility of inducing an immune response to sperm in the female partner following repeated intrauterine inseminations should be considered.

The phenomenon of cyclical changes in antisperm antibody levels in cervical mucus and oviductal secretions is documented. This provides the basis of administering high doses of estrogen or human menopausal gonadotropin to women during the proliferative phase of their menstrual cycle in an attempt to increase genital mucus production with resultant dilution of these antibodies.

In vitro fertilisation may be another therapeutic approach for antisperm antibodies. Recently, Matson et al (1986) observed that women with antisperm antibodies in their sera had fertilisation of their oocytes in vitro and pregnancies following embryo transfer when donor serum was used as the culture medium supplement. Daitoh et al (1987) also reported successful pregnancies by IVF-ET in infertile women with sperm immobilising antibodies when donor sera were used. A pregnancy after zygote intrafallopian transfer (ZIFT) in a woman with antisperm antibodies in her serum was reported by Devroey et al (1986).

Treatment for immunity to sperm in the male

The use of corticosteroids for suppressing the immune response in men with significant levels of antisperm antibodies seems logical. Unfortunately, there are no proper controlled studies to demonstrate its efficacy in men following therapy. Nevertheless, it is clear that an appropriate regimen of immunosuppression should lead to a decrease in antisperm antibody, especially when high cyclic doses of corticosteroid therapy are used. There are a variety of regimens for the use of corticosteroids in the treatment of antisperm antibodies. Both the timing and dosage of the therapy are empirical.

Shulman and Shulman (1982), using methylprednisolone 96mg per day on days 21–28 of the wife's menstrual cycle, reported an overall pregnancy rate of 44 per cent in 71 patients treated. Hendry et al (1981), using methyl-prednisolone (Medrol), 32mg, thrice a day, on days 21–28 of the wife's cycle, achieved a pregnancy rate of 31 per cent in 45 patients. Mathur et al (1981), using prednisone, 15mg daily for 3–26 weeks obtained an overall pregnancy rate of 36 per cent in 25 patients. Recently, Alexander (1983) compared the pregnancy rates in men treated with a seven-day course of 60mg prednisone per day versus an untreated group. Forty-five per cent of couples achieved a pregnancy within four months of treatment, compared with 12 per cent for their control subjects. There is no established superior regimen. Serious side effects such as aseptic hip necrosis, gastrointestinal problems, as well as less serious but unpleasant side effects have been reported. A reevaluation of the risk-benefit ratio of the high dosage therapy may be required.

Sperm washing and intrauterine insemination have not been successful for the treatment of men with surface bound antisperm antibodies. The affinity of antibodies for antigens on the sperm surface defy simple sperm washing to remove them. There is no clear evidence of a therapeutic benefit from these methods.

The successful fertilisation of human oocytes requires penetration of the zona pellucida. Bronson et al (1984) utilised salt-stored human oocytes and showed that IgA and IgG antibodies effectively inhibited the attachment of sperm to the zona. Clarke et al (1985a) demonstrated poor fertilisation rates in a group of men with high levels of both IgG and IgA antisperm antibodies detected by the direct immunobead test in his IVF programme. We also investigated the effect of surface bound antisperm antibodies detected in our IVF programme with the immunobead test. Three men had IgG and IgA antibody bound sperm. Five out of 18 mature oocytes from their spouses after insemination in IVF were fertilised (28 per cent) compared with 82 per cent without antisperm antibody. Junk et al (1986) presented evidence that the combination of IgA and IgG together in semem resulted in a significantly reduced fertilisation rate. There may be some benefit in removing the cumulus oophorus cells before insemination, or even the direct microinjection of sperm into the perivitelline space of the oocyte in the treatment of these cases (Lasalle, Courto and Testart, 1985).

Conclusion

Although evidence is accumulating in favour of antisperm antibodies affecting reproductive function adversely and causing infertility, the etiology remains unresolved. Infertile couples with unexplained infertility or with poor postcoital tests require tests for antisperm antibodies. The isolation and characterisation of sperm antigens in the future may assist the classification and identification of specificities of antisperm antibodies. Despite advances in diagnostic technology, treatment remains unsatisfactory. However, recently developed procedures, such as IVF-ET, pronuclear stage transfer (PROST) or ZIFT, and micromanipulation may offer hope for those couples suffering from immunological infertility.

Acknowledgement

The authors thank Ms M.J. Tsai for preparing this manuscript.

Table 14-1
Results of ELISA for antisperm antibodies in sperm, seminal plasma and cervical mucus of 56 infertile couples and 20 fertile couples

	IgG	*IgA*	*IgG+IgA*	*IgM*	*Total*	%
Infertile female						
Serum	7	4	2	1	14	25.0**
Cervical mucus*	3	4	1	0	8	22.2
Fertile female						
Serum	1	0	0	0	1	5.0
Infertile male						
Serum	5	4	1	1	11	19.6
Seminal plasma	2	3	0	0	5	9.0
Fertile male						
Serum	1	0	0	0	1	5.0

* *36 samples*
** *$p<0.05$ as compared with fertile female.*

Table 14-2
Results of immunobead test for 56 couples with unexplained infertility and poor postcoital tests

	IgG	*IgA*	*IgG+IgA*	*IgM*	*Total*	*(%)*
No. of patients with positive tests	7	4	2	1	14	(25)

Table 14-3
Results of sperm-cervical mucus contact test (SCMC)

Sperm surface bound antibodies	*SCMC (semen quality/mucus quality)*			
	G/G	*B/G*	*G/B*	*B/B*
No. of patients tested	0	22	16	9
Ig G(+)	0	6	0	1
Ig A(+)	0	3	1	0
Ig G(+) & Ig A(+)	0	2	0	0
Ig M(+)	0	1	0	0

G: good quality
B : bad quality

References

Alexander, N.J. Pregnancy rates in patients treated for antisperm antibodies with prednisolone. *International Journal of Fertility,* 1983; 28: 63.

Alexander, N.J. and Anderson, D.J. Vasectomy: Consequences of autoimmunity to sperm antigens. *Fertility and Sterility,* 1979; 32: 253.

Avyaliotis, B., Bronson, R., Rosenfeld, D. and Cooper, G. Conception rates in couples where autoimmune to sperm is detected. *Fertility and Sterility,* 1985; 43: 739.

Beer, A.E. and Neaves, W.B. Antigenic status of semen from the viewpoints of the female and male. *Fertility and Sterility,* 1978; 29: 3.

Bronson, R.A., Cooper, G.W. and Rosenfeld, D.L. Sperm-specific iso-antibodies and auto-antibodies inhibit the binding of human sperm to the human zona pellucida. *Fertility and Sterility,* 1982; 38: 724.

Bronson, R.A., Cooper, G.W. and Rosenfeld, D. Use of freeze thawed sonicated human sperm as an in vitro immunoabsorbent. *American Journal of Reproductive Immunology,* 1982; 2: 161.

Bronson, R.A., Cooper, G.W. and Rosenfeld, D.L. Complement mediated effects of sperm head directed human antibodies on the ability of human spermatozoa to penetrate zona free hamster eggs. *Fertility and Sterility,* 1983; 40: 91.

Bronson, R.A., Cooper, G.W. and Rosenfeld, D. Sperm antibodies: Their role in infertility. *Fertility and Sterility,* 1984; 42: 171.

Clarke, G.N., Lopata, A., McBaine, J.C., Baker, H.W.G. and Johnston, W.I.H. Effect of sperm antibodies in male on human in vitro fertilization. *American Journal of Reproductive Immunology,* 1985; 8: 62.

Clarke, G.N., McBain, J.C., Lopata, A. and Johnston, W.I.H. In vitro fertilization results for women with sperm antibodies in plasma and follicular fluid. *American Journal of Reproductive Immunology,* 1985; 8: 130.

Cook, I.D. Investigation of the subfertile couple: Results from the female partner. *Proceedings of 12th World Congress on Fertility and Steriliry,* Singapore, 1986.

Daitoh, T., Morik, Ueda, T., Shitsukawa, K., Furumoto, H., Bandoh, R.M., Azuma, K., Irahara, M., Yamano, S., Kamada, M. and Aono, T. Blocking effect of sera with sperm immobilizing antibody on human fertilization in vitro and successful treatment by IVF-ET with replaced serum. Abstract, *VI World Congress on Human Reproduction*, Tokyo, 1987, 25.

Devroey, P., Braeckmans, P., Smitz, J., Van Waes Berghe, L., Wisanto, A. and Van Sterirteghem, A. Pregnancy after translaparoscopic zygote intrafallopian transfer in a patient with serum antibodies. *Lancet*, 1986; 1: 1329.

Edwards, R.G. Immunological control of fertility in female mice. *Nature*, 1964; 203: 50.

Franklin, R.R. and Dukes, C.D. Antispermatozoal antibody and unexplained infertility. *American Journal of Obstetrics and Gynecology*, 1964; 89: 6.

Friberg, J. A simple and sensitive micromethod for demonstration of sperm agglutinating activity in serum from infertile men and women.*Acta Obsterica et Gynaecologica Scandinavia*, 1974; 36: 21.

Gupta, I., Dhawan, S., Goel, G.D. and Saha, K. Low fertility rate in vavovasostomized male and its possible immunologic mechanism. *International Journal of Fertility*, 1975; 20: 183.

Haas, G.G. Immunologic infertility: Which approaches are best. *Contemporary Obstetrics and Gynaecology*, 1983; 22: 141.

Hass, G. and Beer, A. Immunologic influences on reproductive biology: Sperm gametogenesis and maturation in the male and female genital tracts. *Fertility and Sterility*, 1986; 46: 753.

Hass, G.G., Cines, D.B. and Schreiber, A.D. Immunologic infertility: Identification of patients with antisperm antibody. *New England Journal of Medicine*, 1980; 303: 722.

Hendry, E.F., Stedronske, J., Parslow, J. and Hughes, L. The result of intermittent high dose steroid therapy for male infertility due to antisperm antibodies. *Fertility and Sterility*, 1981; 36: 351.

Hjort, T. and Meinertz, H. Antisperm antibodies and immune subfertility. *Human Reproduction*, 1988; 3: 59.

Huang, T.T.F., Tung, K.S.K. and Yanagimachi, R. Autoantibodies from vasectomised guinea pigs inhibit fertilization in vitro. *Science*, 1981; 213: 1267.

Isojima, S., Li, T.S. and Ashitaka, Y. Immonological analysis of sperm immobilizing factor found in sera of women with unexplained infertility. *American Journal of Obstetrics and Gynecology*, 1968; 101: 677.

Jager, S., Kremer, J. and Van Slochteren Draaisma, T. A simple method of screening for antisperm antibodies in the human male: Detection of spermatozoan surface IgG with the direct mixed agglutination reaction carried out on untreated fresh human semen. *International Journal of Fertility*, 1978; 23: 12.

Jones, W.R. The use of antibodies developed by infertile women to identify relevant antigens. In Diczfalusy, E. and Diczfalsy, A. (Eds), *Karolinska Symposia on Research Methods in Reproductive Endocrinology: Immunological Approach to Infertility*, Karolinska Institute, Stockholm, 1974, 376.

Junk, S.M., Maston, P.L., Yovich, J.M., Boostman, B. and Yovich, J.L. The fertilization of human oocytes by spermatozoa from men with antispermatozoal antibodies in semen. *Journal of in Vitro Fertilisation and Embryo Transfer*, 1986; 3: 350.

Katsh, S. Infertility in female guinea pigs induced by injection of homologous sperm. *American Journal of Obstetrics and Gynecology*, 1959; 78: 276.

Kibrick, S., Belding, D.L. and Merrill, B. Methods for detection of antibodies against mammalian spermatozoa: A gelatin agglutination test. *Fertility and Sterility*, 1952; 3: 430.

Kremer, J. and Jager, S. The sperm-cervical mucus contact test: A preliminary report. *Fertility and Sterility*, 1976; 27: 335.

Landsteiner, K. Iur kenntnis der spezifisch auf blutkorperchen wirkende sera. *Zentbl Bakt*, 1899; 25: 546.

Lasalle, B., Courto, A.M. and Testart, J. Fertilization of hamster oocyte by injection of human sperm in the perivitelline space. In Testar, J. and Frydman, R. (Eds), *Human In Vitro Fertilization*, Elsevier, Amsterdam, 1985, 209.

Mathur, S., Baker, E.R., Williamson, H.O., Derrick, R.C., Teague, K.J. and Fudenbery, H.H. Clinical significance of sperm antibodies in infertility. *Fertility and Sterility*, 1981; 36: 486.

Mathur, S., Williamson, H.O., Baker, M.E., Rust, P.F., Holtz, G.L. and Fudenberg, H.H. Sperm motility on postcoital testing correlates with male autoimmunity to sperm. *Fertility and Sterility*, 1984; 41: 81.

Matson, P.L., Junk, S.M., Yovich, J.M. and Yovich, J.L. The fertilizing capacity of spermatozoa from men with antispermatozoal antibodies in semen is determined by the class of antibody present. In *Proceedings of 12th World Congress on Fertility and Sterility*, Singapore, 1986.

Menge, A.C. Clinical immunologic infertility: Diagnostic measures, incidence of antisperm antibodies, fertility and mechanisms. In Dhindsa, D.S. and Schumacher, G.F.B. (Eds), *Immunological Aspects of Infertility and Fertility Regulation*, Elsevier, New York, 1980, 205.

Menge, A.C. and Black, C.S. Effects of zona free hamster ova. *Fertility and Sterility*, 1979; 32: 214.

Menge, A.C., Medley, N.E., Margione, C.M. and Dietrid, J.W. The incidence and influence of antisperm antibodies in infertile human couples on sperm cervical mucus interaction and subsequent fertility. *Fertility and Sterility*, 1982; 38: 439.

Metchnikoff, E. Etudes sur la resorption des cellules. *Annles Institut Pasteur*, 1899; 13: 737.

Murdoch, A.J.M., Buckley. C.H. and Fox, H. Hormonal control of the secretory immune system of the human uterine cervix. *Journal of Reproductive Immunology*, 1982; 4: 23.

Naz, R.K., Saxe, J.M. and Menge, A.C. Inhibition of fertility in rabbits by monoclonal antibodies against sperm. *Biology of Reproduction*, 1983; 28: 249.

Parish, W.E., Carron-Brown, J.A. and Richards, C.B. The detection of antibodies to spermatozoa and blood group antigens in cervical mucus. *Journal of Reproduction and Fertility*, 1967; 13: 469.

Romrell, L.J. and O'Rand, M.G. Capping and ultrastructural localisation of sperm surface isoantigens during spermatogenesis. *Developmental Biology*, 1978; 63: 76.

Rumke, P. The presence of sperm antibodie in the serum of two patients. *Vox Sang*, 1954; 4: 135.

Rumke, P. The origin of immunoglobulins in semen. *Clin Exp Immunology*, 1974; 17: 287.

Rumke, P. and Hellinga, G. Autoantibodies against spermatozoa in sterile men. *American Journal of Clinical Pathology*, 1959; 32: 357.

Rumke, P., Renckens, C.N.M., Bezemer, R.D. and Amstel, N.V. Prognosis of fertility in women with unexplained infertility and sperm agglutinins in the serum. *Fertility and Sterility*, 1984; 42: 561.

Rumke, P., Van Amstel, N., Messer, E.N. and Bezemer, P.D. Prognosis of fertility of men with sperm agglutinins in serum. *Fertility and Sterility*, 1974; 25: 393.

Schumacher, G.F.B. Humoral immune factors in the female reproductive tract and their changes during the cycle. In Dhindsa, D.S. and Schumacher, G.F.B. (Eds), *Immunological Aspects of Infertility and Fertility Regulation*, Elsevier/North Holland, New York, 1980, p93.

Schumacher, G.F.B. and Yang S.L. Cyclic changes of immunoglobulins and specific antibodies in human and rhesus monkey cervical mucus. In Insler, V. and Bettendorf, G. *The Uterine Cervix in Reproduction*, Georg Thieme, Stuttgart, 1977, 187.

Schwimmer, W.B., Ustay, K.A. and Behrman, S.J. An evaluation of immunologic factors of infertility. *Fertility and Sterility*, 1967; 18: 167.

Shulman, J.F. and Shulman, S. Methylprednisolone treatment of immunologic infertility in the male. *Fertility and Sterility*, 1982; 38: 591.

Telang, M., Reyniak, J.V. and Shulman, S. Antibodies to spermatozoa VIII: Correlation of sperm antibody activity with postcoital tests in infertile couples. *International Journal of Fertility*, 1978; 23: 200.

Tsukuis, Noda, Y., Yano, J., Fukuda, A. and Mori, T. Inhibition of sperm penetration through human zona pellucida by antisperm antibodies. *Fertility and Sterility*, 1986; 46: 92.

Uehling, D.T. Secretory IgA in seminal fluid. *Fertility and Sterility*, 1971; 22: 769.

Voisin, G.A., Toullet, F. and D'Almeida, M. Characterisation of spermatozoal auto-, iso-, and allo-antigens. In Diczfalusy, E. (Ed), *Immunological Approaches to Infertility Control*, Karolinska Institues, Stockholm, 1974, 173.

Wilson, L. Sperm agglutinins in human semen and blood. *Proceedings of Soc Exp Biol Med*, 1954; 85: 652.

Zanchetta, R., Busolo, F. and Mastrogiacomo, I. The enzyme-linked immunosorbent assay for detection of the antispermatozoan antibodies. *Fertility and Sterility*, 1982; 38: 730.

15
Artificial insemination by donor

P.C. Ho and M.S.W. Kwan

Introduction

Since the first successful performance of artificial insemination with donor semen (AID) by Pancoast in 1884, considerable advances have taken place in the practice of AID worldwide. The discovery of the cryoprotective effect of glycerol in the preservation of spermatozoa (Polge et al, 1949) has made sperm storage a distinct possibility. The first pregnancy obtained using cryopreserved sperm was with the dry ice method, reported by Bunge et al in 1953. Subsequently, in 1963, Sherman described the use of liquid nitrogen vapour to freeze sperm. Pregnancies were subsequently achieved using this technique (Perloff et al, 1964). Developments in cryopreservation techniques have led to the establishment of sperm banks and it has become feasible to provide AID as a service on a larger organised scale. With the liberalisation of abortion in many countries, the number of children available for adoption has come increasingly more difficult in recent years. Hence, there is an increase demand for AID. However, the report of transmission of the human immunodeficiency virus (HIV) and the acquired immunodeficiency syndrome following AID has caused a setback (Stewart et al, 1985). The practice of AID with emphasis on its clinical aspects will be reviewed and discussed. Interested readers may wish to refer to monographs for detailed discussion on other aspects of AID (Brudenell et al, 1976; Richardson et al, 1979; David & Price, 1980; American Fertility Society, 1986).

Indications

The most common indication for AID is azoospermia. Patients whose spouses have oligozoospermia, asthenozoospermia and teratozoospermia may have the potential for pregnancy and AID is indicated after the couple has tried unsuccessfully to conceive over a reasonable period of time and where other methods of therapy have failed. Less common indications for AID include noncorrectable ejaculatory dysfunction, hereditary or genetic disorder of the husband eg. Tay-Sachs disease, Huntington's disease, haemophilia or chromosomal anomalies. Severe Rh-isoimmunisation of the wife when the husband is RH-positive also constitutes a valid indication for AID using semen from Rh-negative donors. In some countries, AID may also be performed for unmarried women. This is a controversial matter and is not universally acceptable.

Assessment of recipient couples

The male partner of an infertile marriage should be thoroughly investigated to exclude the possibility of any correctable disorders before resorting to AID. Medical or surgical treatment should be offered where indicated. The female partner should be evaluated to exclude co-existing infertility factors. Tubal patency should be tested especially in patients where their history or physical findings are suggestive of tubal problems. In some programmes, tubal patency tests are obligatory after three cycles of failed AID.

In our programme, which was established in 1981, hysterosalpingogram is performed before AID. Our Hong Kong sperm bank is the result of a collaborative effort between the Family Planning Association and the Hong Kong University Department of Obstetrics and Gynaecology. Where there is a history suggestive of pelvic inflammatory disease or endometriosis, or if the hysterosalpingogram suggests any abnormality, laparoscopy is required to be performed. Ovulation status should be assessed by means of basal body temperature charts, mid-luteal plasma progesterone assay, or late-luteal endometrial biopsy. The preovulatory cervical mucus should also be examined. Any co-existing infertility factors should be corrected before AID. The rubella titer should be measured and vaccination offered if the test is negative. Serologic tests for syphilis, Hepatitis B antigen, HIV and cytomegalovirus should also be performed. Cervical cultures should be tested for gonorrhoea and chlamydial infection. The health of the recipient should also be evaluated to ensure that there is no contraindication to pregnancy. The physical characteristics of the couple such as race, height, eye colour, body build and hair colour are noted for donor matching.

The couple should be interviewed and counselled on the implications of AID, the question of confidentiality, as well as the legal aspects. During the interview, the couple's relationship and their feelings on AID should be assessed. The couple should have a stable relationship and be emotionally stable. Written consent should also be obtained.

Recruitment and screening of donors

Donors can be recruited from various sources, including medical students, husbands of obstetric patients, pre-vasectomy patients, or the general public. The choice depends on the local situation. In some centres, medical students comprise the main source of donors. In Hong Kong, we have difficulty in recruiting donors among medical students; our donors come mainly from the general public through mass media advertisement. Many centres pay donors a token sum of money to cover both travelling expenses and partial loss of income because of time spent at the AID clinic. All the donors must be screened for their fertility and freedom from infections or hereditary diseases. Guidelines for the screening and selection of donors have already been published by the American Fertility Society (1986b).

It is probably advisable to screen donor semen samples before proceeding with extensive donor screening. Acceptable criteria for screening the samples are: volume > 2 ml; sperm count > 50 million per ml; motility > 60 per cent and normal morphology > 70 per cent. Analysis of data from our AID programme which uses frozen semen shows that even with strict criteria for selecting donor semen samples, pregnancy rates may not be substantially increased (Wong et al, 1988).

In donor screening for genetic diseases, a detailed history, including a family history, should be obtained. The donor should be below 50 years of age, be free of any malformation, such as cleft lip, cleft palate, spina bifida, congenital heart malformation, congenital hip dislocation, clubfoot or hypospadias, any nontrivial mendelian disorder (such as albinism, haemophilia, haemoglobin disorder, hereditary hypercholesterolaemia, neurofibromatosis, or tuberous sclerosis), any familial disease with a known or reliably indicated major genetic component (such as asthma, juvenile diabetes mellitus, epileptic disorder, hypertension etc.) or an autosomal recessive gene for any disease known to be prevalent in the donor's ethnic background for which heterozygosity can be detected (eg. thalassaemia in Mediterranean or Chinese populations or sickle cell disease in blacks). A complete sexual history should also be obtained and donors excluded who have had homosexual contacts since 1978. Those who are known intravenous drug users, or who have sexual partners who are in the acquired immunodeficiency syndrome at risk groups, or who have multiple sexual partners, or demonstrate any evidence or past history of sexually transmitted diseases should be excluded.

A physical examination should be performed and any urethral discharge, genital warts, or genital ulcers excluded. The physical characteristics of the donors are recorded for prospective matching of recipient couples. The legal implications of AID require to be explained and a written consent obtained. Serological tests such as VDRL, hepatitis B surface antigen and core antibody, to HIV, and cytomegalovirus should be performed. Additional investigations may be indicated where thalassaemia is prevalent in the local population, necessitating routine screening for the haemoglobin pattern of the donors. There is controversy over the need for karyotyping for all semen donors. The incidence of chromosomal abnormality in a phenotypically normal donor population is small and routine karyotyping is not cost effective. We therefore do not routinely karyotype our donors.

A period of surveillance of the donors is recommended to seek evidence of manifestations of sexually transmitted diseases. Contributing donors should also be rescreened every six months. A final screen should be repeated, if possible, 60 days following cessation of the donor status. Where frozen semen is used, the samples should be held in quarantine until these screening procedures have been completed. Recipient couples should also be followed up for any development of sexually transmitted diseases. The number of pregnancies conceived by any single donor should be recorded. It is judicious to restrict the use of any individual donor to 10 pregnancies obtained. Strict anonymity of the donors should be maintained. The donors should only be identified by code numbers.

Fresh versus frozen semen

AID may be performed with either fresh or frozen sperm. Pregnancy rates using fresh semen appear better than those using frozen semen (Table 15-1). However, comparison of results between published reports is difficult because of differences in the criteria for selecting donors and recipients, the methods employed in timing ovulation the technique of insemination, and the calculation of pregnancy rates. Indeed, some comparative studies have failed to show any significant differences in pregnancy rates between fresh and frozen semen (Trounson et al, 1979; Iddenden et al, 1985; Hammond et al, 1986). Improvement in cryopreservation techniques may have contributed as well.

The use of frozen semen has several advantages. Frozen semen is more economical to use because semen from one ejaculate can be aliquoted and used for several inseminations and the patient can be inseminated on two or more occasions using the same donor. The organisation of the AID service is consequently simpler. Semen can be stored in a bank and donors need not be called upon daily. Semen banks can also be organised at a regional or national level to cater for multiple AID clinics. Matching the donor with the recipient is also more convenient, with little risk of the recipient accosting the donor. Semen when stored frozen can await the results of bacteriological and serological screening tests to exclude infection. We therefore believe that the advantages of using frozen semen far outweigh those of fresh semen.

Cryopreservation of semen

Various techniques of cryopreservation of human semen have already been surveyed previously (Richardson, 1976; Read, 1979). In principle, cryopreservation of human spermatozoa involves the admixture of semen with a cryoprotective medium, followed by a short period of equilibration, then cooling and eventual storage. The most popular cryoprotective agent is glycerol. It exerts its cryoprotective effect by virtue of its high electrolyte binding and hydrophilic properties. It probably combines with the water moities associated with the hydrated proteins of spermatozoa, thereby stabilising their structure during the freezing process. Glycerol reduces the formation of ice crystals and the damaging effects of dehydration arising from intracellular concentration of electrolytes, with possible disruption of cellular macromolecules. Glycerol also aids in maintaining the cell volume. The cryoprotective medium used in our programme is as described by Richardson (1976). It is added slowly to the semen sample to be frozen, thoroughly mixed, and equilibrated for two to five minutes. The mixture is then dispensed into coded ampoules or plastic straws, sealed, and cooled.

The cooling process can be achieved with programmable freezers. Alternative methods include suspension of the semen mixture in nitrogen vapour for about 30 minutes, or freezing in a −70 °C refrigerator, before storing the samples in liquid nitrogen (Richardson, 1976; Ing, 1982). In our programme, we use the Linde Portable Biological Freezing System (CRFC-2 and CRCI). The semen is cooled at a rate of −4.5 °C per minute from 20 °C (room temperature) to −18 °C and then to −80 °C at a rate of −40 °C per minute before storage in liquid nitrogen. Stored in this fashion, there is no loss of sperm motility even after three years, although some samples show reduced motility when stored for longer (Smith and Steinberger, 1973). Most workers thaw in water baths at either +20 °C or +37 °C. The thawing rate does not appear to affect post-thaw motility (Sherman, 1963).

Insemination

AID must be performed close to ovulation to achieve optimum results. This is particularly relevant when frozen semen is used because thawed sperm has a decreased motility life span (Keel and Black, 1980). Studies have shown that optimal pregnancy rates are obtained when inseminations are performed both on the day of the LH peak and the following day (Matthews, 1979). Several methods are available for assessing ovulation: the menstrual history, basal body temperature chart (BBT), cervical mucus score, pelvic ultrasonography, and plasma and urinary luteinizing hormone (LH) assays. Basal body temperature charts can be difficult to interpret in terms of the time of ovulation. Pelvic ultrasonography requires both facilities and expertise. Because of the varying sizes of preovulatory follicles, this approach precludes its use as a single parameter for the prediction of ovulation (Queenan et al, 1980). Plasma LH by radioimmunoassay is accurate as a method of predicting ovulation (World Health Organization, 1980). The disadvantage lies in the need for frequent venepunctures and a radioimmunoassay laboratory. More recently, a simple haemagglutination test (Higonavis) and an enzyme immunoassay kit technique (Ovustick, Monoclonal Antibodies Inc.; Right Day, Leeco Diagnostics Inc.) have been developed for the assay of LH in the urine. These tests are simple to perform and results are available within 45 minutes to two hours.

We compared the usefulness of BBT charts, the cervical mucus score, and the Higonavis assay in our programme, using the plasma LH radioimmunoassay is a reference (Ho et al, 1985). Our cervical mucus scoring system was modified from Insler (1972), and shown in Table 15-2. We found that the BBT nadir could not be identified from 18 per cent of the charts. The day of the peak cervical mucus score coincided with that of the plasma LH peak among 63 per cent of cycles (Figure 15-1) and it occurred within 24 hours of the plasma LH peak in over 95 per cent of cycles. The urinary LH peak occurred one day after the blood LH peak in 50 per cent of cycles. The urinary LH peak also occurred within 24 hours of the plasma LH peak in over 95 per cent of cycles. The BBT nadir coincided with the plasma LH peak in only 28.6 per cent. Since there was variation between the peak cervical mucus score and the peak urine LH level, the peaks could only be identified after the cervical mucus score and urinary LH levels began to fall. It is clearly necessary to determine the critical values of these parameters indicating impending ovulation. Our data showed that the critical level for cervical mucus score was eight or greater, while the critical level for Higonavis was 100 iu/1 or more. The cervical mucus score first reached the level of eight or more within 24 hours of the plasma LH peak in 90 per cent of the cycles, while the urinary LH first reached the level of 100 iu/1 within 24 hours of the plasma LH peak in all the cycles studied. Therefore, both methods were quite accurate in predicting the time of ovulation.

We subsequently extended our study and compared the Higonavis assay with the Ovustick test and found that both gave comparable results. They detected the LH surge in 94 per cent of the cycles, 90 per cent of which occurred within 24 hours of the plasma LH peak. Transient false positive LH rises occurred in six per cent of cycles with the Higonavis assay but not with the Ovustick test (Poon et al, 1986). Although these urinary LH assay kits give acceptable results and are simple to use, they tend to be costly. The cervical mucus score is easy to perform, being reasonably accurate, and inexpensive. For our programme, we predict ovulation from the previous menstrual history and BBT charts. We then ask the patient to attend our clinic about two days before the expected day of ovulation for assessment of the cervical mucus score. Insemination is performed when the score is > 8 and repeated daily until a definite rise in BBT or a concomitant fall in the cervical mucus score occurs. We use urinary LH assays only for patients where the cervical mucus is poor. A survey performed in Australia showed that the success among AID centres is similar whether cervical mucus score or plasma LH radioimmunoassay were used (Trounson et al, 1981).

The most common approaches for insemination are intracervical or pericervical. The volume of semen used is about 0.5 ml. Insemination is performed with a 1 ml syringe. In our programme, we use an insemination device specially designed for frozen semen stored in straws (Instruments De Medicine Viterinaire, France). An additional approach is intrauterine insemination but this may result in uterine cramps and even infection. This method is not used regularly except where problems such as hostile cervical mucus exist. Following insemination, the patient usually rests in the recumbent position for about 15 minutes.

Pregnancy rates

The pregnancy rates obtained by researchers have been expressed in a variety of ways, making comparison of results difficult. For meaningful comparison, the cumulative pregnancy rates calculated by life-table analysis, and the monthly fecundability rate are the most useful (Cramer et al, 1979). Pregnancy rates from large studies worldwide were summarised in Table 15-1. Their cumulative pregnancy rates ranged from 44 per cent to 76 per cent over six cycles and 68 per cent to 87 per cent for 12 cycles. These results suggest that AID is an effective form of infertility treatment. The cumulative pregnancy rates continue to increase for up to 12 cycles. Therefore, AID treatment should be continued for at least 12 cycles. If the patient does not conceive by the 12th cycle, she should be reassessed. In some AID centres, gamete intrafallopian transfer or in vitro fertilisation and embryo transfer are offered. There are number of factors that may affect the pregnancy rates. The age of the recipient is one. Earlier studies show that the pregnancy rates decrease after the age of 35 (Glezerman, 1981; Foss 1982; Virro and Shewchuk, 1984). Our AID data show that pregnancy rates in fact start to fall after the age of 30 (Wong et al, 1988). The presence of other associated infertility factors also adversely affect the results of AID (Sulewski et al, 1978; Aiman, 1982; Hammond et al, 1986). Treatment with clomiphene citrate has not given pregnancy rates better than those without (Wong et al, 1988). This may be explained by inadequacy of the luteal phase or the antio-estrogenic effect of the drug, resulting in poor cervical mucus. Pregnancy rates bear an inverse relationship with the duration of infertility (Glezerman, 1981). They are also lower in patients with poor cervical mucus (Edvinsson et al, 1983; Wong et al, 1988). Patients in the lower socioeconomic class and also those who lack support from the spouse have a lower pregnancy rate and a higher dropout rate (Glezerman, 1981).

The presence of male factor problem seems to influence AID pregnancy rates. Patients whose partners have oligozoospermia have lower pregnancy rates compared with those having azoospermia (Formigli et al, 1985; Hammond et al, 1986).

Potential problems

Possible problems associated with AID include (1) transmission of infection, (2) transmision of genetic disease, (3) inadvertent consanguinous marriage, (4) harmful effect on the family relationship. Transmission of infection and genetic disease can be minimised by careful screening and selection of donors. The risk of infection can be further minimised through the use of frozen semen. Since children conceived by AID do not know their genetic fathers, there is a potential risk of inadvertent consanguinous marriges among these children. The chance of this occurring is dependent upon the number of children derived from the donor and the number of people in the potential breeding pool. It has been estimated that in a breeding pool of 20,000, the chance of inadvertent consanguinous marriages is less than 0.00004 per cent when the number of AID children derived from a donor is 10 (Danks, 1980).

Therefore in a much larger population, the risk will be extremely small. This can be further minimised by limiting the number of pregnancies from any single donor (Warnock Committee, 1984; American Fertility Society, 1986). There is no evidence to suggest that AID can lead to marital breakdown. Children conceived by AID using frozen semen develop well, with intelligence quotients higher than average (Iizuka, 1987). On the whole, complications following AID are few. AID is therefore a safe and effective form of infertility treatment.

Legal and ethical aspects

The legal status of AID varies from country to country. In many, there is no law governing AID or the status of the AID child, the legal status of the donor or the recipient. This may lead to potential problems should marital disharmony arise or the donor seeks a claim against the AID child. There is a need for legislation to clarify these concerns so that the rights of the various parties involved may be protected. The ethical aspects of AID have been considered by working parties in various countries. The reader may wish to refer to the literature for details (American Fertility Society, 1986a; Warnock Committee, 1984).

Table 15-1
Review of AID results using fresh or frozen semen

Authors	*No. of insemination cycles*	*Type of semen*	*Pregnancy rate per cycle (%)*	*Cumulative pregnancy rates (%)*			
				3 months	*6 months*	*9 months*	*12 months*
David et al, 1980 (France)	5255	frozen	9.8	28.6	46.9	58.0	67.9
Trounson et al 1981 (Australia)	5461	frozen	—	34.6	49.8	57.3	64.0
Glezerman, 1981 (Israel)	1162	fresh	19.7	59.3	75.8	82.3	86.8
Kwan et al, 1987 (Hong Kong)	984	frozen	10.0	30.0	47.4	59.0	—

Table 15-2
Cervical mucus score

	0	*1*	*2*	*3*
Cervical dilatation	Closed	<2mm	2–3mm	>3mm
Amount of mucus	Nil	<0.2ml	0.2–0.5m	>0.5ml
Spinnbarkeit	1–2cm	3–10cm	11–19cm	>19cm
Ferning	None	Linear	Partial	Complete

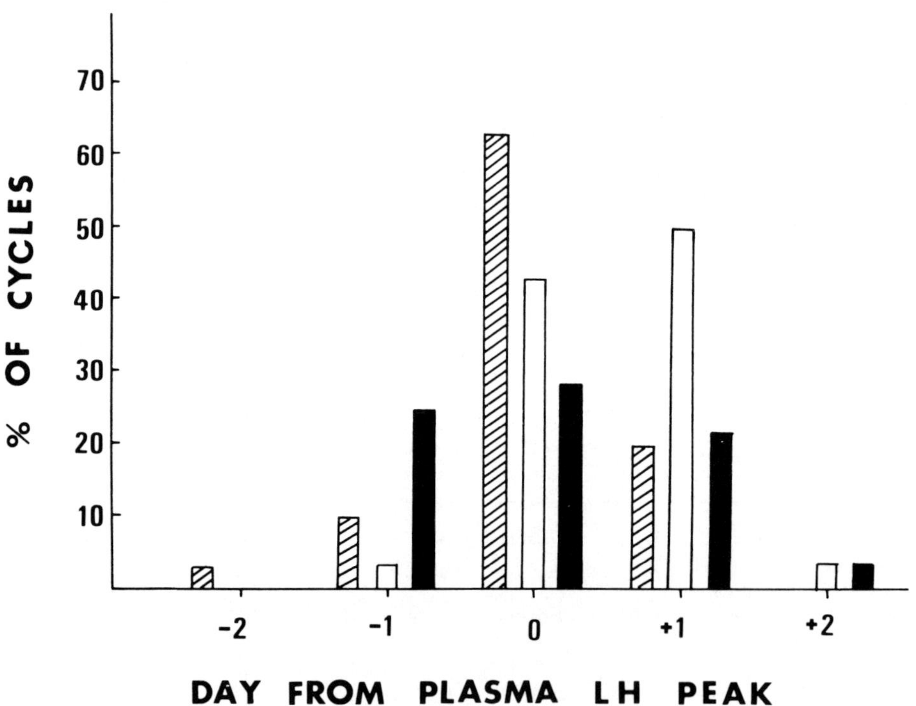

Figure 15-1
Timing of cervical mucus score peak (▨), urinary LH peak (□) and BBT nadir (■) in relation to the plasma LH peak (Day 0).

References

Aiman, J. Factors affecting the success of donor insemination. *Fertility and Sterility*, 1982; 37: 94.

American Fertility Society. Ethical considerations of the new reproductive technologies. *Fertility and Sterility*, 1986a; 46 (supplement 1): 1.

American Fertility Society. New guidelines for the use of semen donor insemination, 1986. *Fertility and Sterility*, 1986b; 46 (supplement 2): 95S.

Brudenell, M., McLaren, A., Short, R.V. and Symonds, E.M. *Artificial Insemination*, Royal College of Obstetricians and Gynaecologists, London, 1976.

Bunge, R.G. and Sherman, J.K. Fertilizing capacity of frozen human spermatozoa. *Nature*, 1953; 172: 767.

Cramer, D.W., Walker, A.M. and Schiff, I. Statistical methods in evaluating the outcome of infertility therapy. *Fertility and Sterility*, 1979; 32: 80.

Danks, D.M. Genetic considerations. In Wood, C., Leeton, J. and Kovacs, G. (Eds), *Artificial Insemination by Donor*, Brown Prior Anderson, Melbourne, 1980, 94.

David, G. and Price, W. *Artificial Insemination and Semen Preservation*, Plenum, New York, 1980.

Edvinsson, A., Bergman, P., Steen, Y. and Nilsson, S. Characteristics of donor semen and cervical mucus at the time of conception. *Fertility and Sterility*, 1983; 39: 327.

Formigili, L., Formigli, G. and Gottardi, L. Artificial insemination by donor results in relation to husband's semen. *Archives of Andrology*, 1985; 14: 209.

Foss, G.L. Artificial insemination by donor: A review of 12 years' experience. *Journal of Biosocial Science*, 1982; 14: 253.

Glezerman, M. Two hundred and seventy cases of artificial donor insemination: Management and results. *Fertility and Sterility*, 1981; 35: 180.

Hammond, M.G., Jordan, S. and Sloan, C.S. Factors affecting pregnancy rates in a donor insemination program using frozen semen. *American Journal of Obstetrics and Gynecology*, 1986; 155: 480.

Ho P.C., Kwan, M., Chan S.Y.W., Chan P.H. and Tang L.C.H. Rapid urinary LH assay for prediction of ovulation. *Australian and New Zealand Journal of Obstetrics and Gynaecology*, 1985; 25: 230.

Iddenden, D.A., Sallam, H.N. and Collins, W.P. A prospective randomized study comparing fresh semen and cryopreserved semen for artificial insemination by donor. *International Journal of Fertility*, 1985; 30: 54.

Iizuka, R. Follow up study of AID children born from cryopreserved semen, and recent progress of sperm cyropreservation. Abstract, *XI Asian and Oceanic Congress of Obstetrics and Gynaecology*, Hongkong, 1987, 57.

Ing R.M.Y. A simplified liquid nitrogen vapour method for the cryopreservation of human semen. *Clinical Reproduction and Fertility*, 1982; 1: 137.

Keel, B.A. and Black, J.B. Reduced motility longevity in thawed human spermatozoa. *Archives of Andrology*, 1980; 4: 213.

Kwan M.S.W., Wong A.W.Y., Ho P.C. and Ma H.K. Artificial insemination by donor semen. *Journal of the Hong Kong Medical Association*, 1987; 39: 96.

Matthews, C.D., Broom, T.J., Crawshaw, K.M., Hopkins, R.E., Kerin, J.F.P. and Svigos, J.M. The influence of insemination timing and semen characteristics on the efficiency of a donor insemination program. *Fertility and Sterility*, 1979; 31: 45.

Perloff, W.H. Conception with human spermatozoa frozen by nitrogen vapour techniques. *Fertility and Sterility*, 1964; 15: 501.

Polge, C., Smith, A.V. and Parkes, A.S. Revival of spermatozoa after vitrification and dehydration of low temperature. *Nature,* 1949; 164: 666.

Poon I.M.L., Ho P.C., Chan S.Y.W. and Wang, C. Comparison of Higonavis with Ovustick in the prediction of ovulation. Abstracts, *12th World Congress on Fertility and Sterility,* Vol 1, Singapore, 1986, 55.

Queenan, J.F., O'Brien, G.D., Bains, L.M., Simpson, J., Collins, W.P. and Campbell, S. Ultrasound scanning of ovaries to detect ovulation in women. *Fertility and Sterility,* 1980; 34: 99.

Read, M.D. The relationship between methods of freezing human semen and successful AID. In Richardson, D., Joyce, D. and Symonds, E.M. (Eds), *Frozen Human Semen,* Royal College of Obstetricians and Gynaecologists, London, 1979, 89.

Richardson, D.W. Techniques of sperm storage. In Brudenell, M., McLaren, A., Short, R. and Symonds, M. (Eds), *Artificial Insemination,* Royal College of Obstetricians and Gynaecologists, London, 1976, 97.

Richardson, D., Joyce, D. and Symonds, M. *Frozen human semen,* Royal College of Obstetricians and Gynaecologists, London, 1979.

Sherman, J.K. Improved methods of preservation of human spermatozoa by freezing and freeze drying. *Fertility and Sterility,* 1963; 14: 49.

Smith, K.D. and Steinberger, E. Survival of spermatozoa in a human sperm bank. *Journal of the American Medical Association,* 1973; 223: 774.

Stewart, G.J., Tyler, J.P.P., Cunningham, A.L., Barr, J.A., Driscoll, G.L., Gold, J. and Lamont, B.J. Transmission of human T-lymphotropic virus type III (HLTV III) by artificial insemination by donor. *Lancet,* 1985; 2: 581.

Sulewski, J.M., Eisenberg, F. and Stenger, V.G. A longitudinal analysis of artificial insemination with donor semen. *Fertility and Sterility,* 1978; 5: 527.

Trounson, A.O., Mahadevan, M., Wood, J. and Leeton, J.F. Studies on the deep freezing and artificial insemination of human semen. In Richardson, D., Joyce, D.N. and Symonds, E.M. (Eds), *Frozen Human Semen,* Royal College of Obstetricians and Gynaecologists, London, 1979, 173.

Trounson, A.O., Matthews, C.D., Kovacs, G.T., Spiers, A., Steigrad, S.J., Saunders, D.M., Jones, W.R. and Fuller, S. Artificial insemination by frozen donor semen: Results of multicentre Australian experience. *International Journal of Andrology,* 1981; 4: 227.

Virro, M.R. and Shewchuk, A.B. Pregnancy outcome in 242 conceptions after artificial insemination with donor sperm and effects of maternal age on the prognosis for successful pregnancy. *American Journal of Obstetrics and Gynecology,* 1984; 148: 518.

Warnock Committee. *Report of the Committee of Inquiry into Human Fertilisation and Embryology,* Department of Health and Social Security, London, 1984.

Wong A.W.Y., Ho P.C., Kwan, M. and Ma H.K. Factors affecting the success of artificial insemination by frozen donor semen. *International Journal of Fertility,* 1988; in press.

World Health Organisation. Temporal relationships between ovulation and defined changes in the concentration of plasma estradiol-17, lutenizing hormone, follicle stimulating hormone, and progesterone. I probit analysis. *American Journal of Obstetrics and Gynecology,* 1980; 138: 383.

16
Diagnostic and operative hysteroscopy

P.J. Taylor and R.K. Goswamy

Introduction

Since the introduction of laparoscopy, the intrapelvic anatomy, particularly the fallopian tubes, has been the subject of intense endoscopic scrutiny. Visualisation of the uterine cavity has been somewhat neglected. With the introduction of more effective uterine distension media and better instruments for uterine visualisation, this part of the lower female genital tract is now accessible. Diagnostic, and in certain cases, operative procedures can be carried out.

For the reader interested in the various types of hysteroscope and details of hysteroscopic technique, a number of excellent reviews are available (Valle and Sciarra, 1979; Hamou and Taylor, 1982; Taylor and Gomel, 1986). All personal observations described in this chapter were made with the panoramic hysteroscope or the Hamou microcolpohysteroscope (MCH) (Karl Storz GMB Tuttlingen FDR). It is the purpose of this chapter to discuss the place of diagnostic and therapeutic hysteroscopy in the female partner of a couple experiencing infertility or habitual abortion. The timing of hysteroscopy in the overall evaluation of such patients, the complementary role of hysteroscopy and hysterosalpingography and the hysteroscopic findings will be described both from the point of view of their appearance and their significance. Hysteroscopic operative procedures will also be described.

Timing

Infertility

All endoscopic procedures are invasive and as such should be one of the later investigations performed. Despite sophisticated methods of investigation, the history is still of paramount importance, and it is on the basis of the history that at the first visit women patients can be divided into those who are apparently ovulatory and those who are apparently anovulatory.

The apparently ovulatory woman

A regular menstrual cycle, particularly if accompanied with cramps, premenstrual symptoms and mid-cycle pain is clinically suggestive that ovulation is taking place. That such is the case should be confirmed by use of the basal body temperature graph and measurements of serum progesterone values where appropriate. Detailed ultrasonographic and endocrine evaluation of the quality of ovulation should be one of the last investigations and employed only when no other obvious cause of infertility has been demonstrated. While ovulation is being confirmed, two properly collected semen samples should be analysed and the nature of the sperm/cervical interaction determined.

If there is no historical reason to believe that the tubes or uterus are damaged, and the patient is less than 35 years of age, any apparently detected male or cervical factor should be treated for six months prior to evaluation of the uterus and fallopian tubes. If such a trial of treatment has failed, or prior to such treatment, if the woman is of advanced reproductive age or has a history suspicious of uterine or tubal lesions, the lower genital tract should be evaluated initially by hysterosalpingography.

The anovulatory patient

The patient who is clinically anovulatory must be evaluated fully using standard endocrinological techniques. Hysteroscopy in such patients is usually restricted to those in whom a diagnosis of Asherman's syndrome (Asherman, 1948) is suspected. such a diagnosis should be entertained if the patient has become amenorrheic following any form of curretage, particularly to complete an abortion or if she fails to show withdrawal bleeding to an oestrogen-progesterone challenge. The patient with Asherman's syndrom will have normal levels of gonadotrophins and prolactin and no evidence of other endocrinopathy. While in most instances we favour hysterosalpingography as a preliminary diagnostic step, in patients with suspected Asherman's syndrome, we prefer to use immediate combined laparoscopy with hysteroscopy. By these means the tubal architecture can be evaluated and appropriate therapeutic manoeuvres performed to lyse the adhesions (see later).

Habitual abortion

The outlook for any woman who has had three consecutive pregnancy losses of less than 20 weeks gestation with a fetus less than 500 gms, is less gloomy than Malpas' (1983) original prediction of 75 per cent likelihood of subsequent loss.

Recent work by Poland (1977) has shown that such patients have approximately a 70 per cent likelihood of carrying any subsequent pregnancy to term. These data notwithstanding, these unfortunate patients should be investigated to determine if there is a specific cause for abortion which may be genetic, hormonal, anatomical, immunological, infective or due to chronic systemic disease.

If there is reason to suspect an anatomic uterine lesion, hysterosalpingography and hysteroscopy should be performed early. If no such history exists, investigation of the uterine cavity should be delayed until other more possible causes have been sought and excluded (DeCherney and Polan, 1984). The intriguing subject of the possible immunological component with habitual abortion is beyond the scope of this article. The reader is referred to an excellent review by Scott (1982).

The roles of hysterosalpingography (HSG) and hysteroscopy

In most instances, hysterosalpingography should be the first investigation of the lower genital tract. Earlier, a wide discrepancy between hysterosalpingographic and laparoscopic findings was reported (Taylor and Cumming, 1979). A similar lack of congruence has been observed when the findings of HSG and hysteroscopy are compared. Siegler (1977), Valle (1980) and Labastida et al (1984) have all demonstrated a lack of agreement in about 30 per cent of cases. A dissenting voice was raised by Snowden et al (1984) who evaluated 77 women using both procedures. In 16 (21 per cent), the HSG was positive. In 11 such patients these findings were confirmed hysteroscopically. In 65 in whom no lesion was detected by HSG, hysteroscopically only 1 per cent were shown to harbour an intrauterine lesion. It is possible that this low rate of false negative HSG in Snowden's series reflects most creditably on the accuracy of the hysterosalpingograms performed by these authors.

In most series, the lesions missed by HSG are small and certainly an incidence of 21 per cent of patients with radiologic evidence of such abnormalities is considerably higher than that reported elsewhere (Zondek and Rozin, 1964). Table 16-1 demonstrates our findings in 254 patients. There was a good correlation when the HSG was positive but the radiologic method tended to identify the nature of the filling defects. Hysteroscopy was of particular value in identifying the exact nature of these lesions. The best congruence between HSG and hysteroscopy was noted in the case of uterine malformations.

Hysteroscopic findings

The common hysteroscopic findings are polyps, adhesions, fibroids and septa. Each will be described in detail.

Polyps

Mucous polyps noted within the uterine cavity must be differentiated from dislodged strips of endometrium and myomata. Whereas myomata are fixed, polyps undulate gently with the flow of the distension medium. The final histologic diagnosis of polyps may be difficult to substantiate, reflecting the fact that after removal the typical histological characteristics may be lost. The Hamou MCH, if used at higher magnification, permits *in situ* histological diagnosis. Polyps may also be noted at the tubocornual junction. The significance of these is unclear.

Adhesions

The patient with classic amenorrhea traumaticum of Asherman will present with amenorrhea. Adhesions may occur in patients with no disturbance of menstrual function or with hypomenorrhea. In 69 patients in whom intrauterine adhesions were detected, 23 had normal cyclic menses (Hamou et al, 1983). Etiological agents in their formation include intrauterine manipulative intervention, but most commonly pregnancy. Hamou et al (1983) have alluded to the probable role of vascularisation and fibrosis in placental fragments after delivery or spontaneous abortion. Sugimoto (1978) studied 192 cases of intrauterine adhesions, and concluded that the probable causative event was spontaneous abortion in 72, therapeutic abortion in 59, puerperal curretage in 39, molar abortion in nine, Caesarean section in seven, myomectomy in five and diagnostic curretage in one.

Histologically, these adhesions may be composed of endometrial, myofibrous or connective tissue (Sugimoto, 1978). they may rarely project laterally from the uterine walls but more frequently are noted as central lesions being tethered at both extremeties. A detailed review of intrauterine adhesions has been published by Schenker and Margalioth (1982).

Clearly, the patient with amenorrhea traumaticum is infertile. The significance of less dense adhesions is yet to be demonstrated. They may play a role in habitual abortion and certainly Oelsner et al (1974) have demonstrated an improved live delivery rate in a group of women in whom such lesions were diagnosed by hysterosalpingography and subsequently removed. Sugimoto (1978) evaluated 51 women with a history of habitual abortion in whom intrauterine adhesions had been detected.

Following adhesiolysis, 12 conceived and aborted, and 19 delivered at term while 18 remained infertile. These studies do not permit the conclusion to be drawn that intrauterine adhesions are defined causes of habitual abortion, but they certainly raise a degree of suspicion that such may be the case.

Fibroids

It is probable that submucous myomata are not a cause of infertility (Buttram and Reiter, 1981). It does seem, however, that they predispose to habitual abortion. As many as 41 per cent of women harbouring these lesions may abort. In patients undergoing IVF or GIFT, we routinely perform hysteroscopy if there is any suggestion of the presence of such lesions.

Hysteroscopically their appearances are typical. They bulge into the uterine cavity, the endometrium covering them is thin and they frequently are covered with obvious vessels. They are smooth, firm and may be pedunculated or sessiled.

Uterine malformation

Septa have a typical appearance. The cornua can be seen as dark areas on either side of a central fibrous band. It is probable that anomalies of the reproductive tract do not cause infertility but they have been implicated in the etiology of habitual abortion. Such malformations will occur once in every 700 women (Jones, 1957). The abortion rate was 33.8 per cent in women with a bicornuate uterus, 34.6 per cent in women with a single uterine horn and 22 per cent in women with a septate uterus (Grass and Golbus, 1978).

The prevalence of such findings in an infertile population has been reported in numerous studies. However, whether or not such lesions are causative of infertility still remains moot. Until recently we performed all of our diagnostic hysteroscopies using Dextran 70 as a distension medium. Recently we have had the opportunity to compare the specific hysteroscopic findings in 992 women who were evaluated using Dextran, with 335 women when the hysteroscopy was performed using the Hamou 1 instrument and carbon dioxide as a distension medium (Taylor et al, 1987).

To our surprise, it was noted that in all instances there was a considerably higher apparent detection rate when Dextran was used. We were forced to conclude from their data that many of the findings in our preliminary studies were artifactual, and that while fibroids and septa were detected with roughly the same prevalence, adhesions and polyps were noted much less frequently when carbon dioxide was used. It was interesting to note, however, that the distribution of the lesions remained essentially the same in patients with primary infertility, secondary infertility and those requesting reversal of a previously performed sterilisation (who acted as a potentially fertile control group).

From these data, it was concluded that polyps found hysteroscopically in the infertile patient were probably incidental findings but that adhesions, if present, may play a small but definite role.

Operative hysteroscopy

Hysteroscopy permits accurate diagnosis of intrauterine lesions, and in many instances it permits the performance of therapeutic manoeuvres. The management of polyps, fibroids, adhesions and septa by hysteroscopic means will be discussed and potential therapeutic uses of hysteroscopy will be described.

Polyps

While removal of small intrauterine polyps may not influence the outcome in patients with infertility or habitual abortion, it would seem appropriate that they should be removed at the time of detection. Single polyps can be removed simply with a small hysteroscopic snare or by cauterizing the base. Multiple polyps are best dealt with by removing the hysteroscope, performing curettage and immediately revisualising the uterine cavity. In any residual lesions are noted, they can be removed with the snare or by a second curettage. This approach will ensure much more complete uterine emptying. Englund et al, (1957) has demonstrated that in 164 women previously curetted for abnormal uterine bleeding, hysteroscopy revealed residual lesions in 101. Of these 101 patients, 51 had not obtained relief from their presenting symptom of bleeding. Following hysteroscopic evaluation and repeat curettage controlled by hysteroscopy, only two of these patients returned with the same symptoms within one year.

Adhesions

Filmy adhesions frequently will rupture under the pressure of the distension medium or may be dislodged with the tip of the hysteroscope. If the adhesions are more dense, they can be divided with the use of hysteroscopic scissors. Hamou et al (1983) have introduced the technique of target abrasion. When the Hamou MCH is examined, it will be noted that the distal tip is angled and is somewhat sharp. In the technique of target abrasion the tip of the hysteroscope is brought under direct visual control against one pole of the adhesion and the attachment of the adhesion to the uterine wall progressively abraded with the sharp tip of the hysteroscope. This procedure is repeated at the opposite pole of the adhesion. This technique was successful in 59 of 69 patients as an office procedure.

The remaining ten patients required general anaesthesia because the procedure was too painful or the adhesions were remarkably dense. It has been our practice to remove the adhesions under general anaesthesia because laparoscopic monitoring can be performed. Undoubtedly patients with adhesions have a much more friable uterus and are more prone to uterine perforation (Seigler and Kemmann, 1975). March et al (1978) have recommended a similar approach.

Once the adhesions have been removed in all but the most minor cases, particularly if there has been any diminution in menstrual flow, an intrauterine device (IUD) should be placed within the uterine cavity and the patient should take Premarin 2.5mg daily for 60 days, during the last ten days of which she also takes Provera 5mg twice daily. Once these medications are discontinued, and withdrawal bleeding occurs, the intrauterine device should be removed. An alternative approach to this regimen, made necessary by the virtual disappearances of IUDs from North America, is to administer Premarin and Provera only, and to perform a second look hysteroscopy six weeks after the initial procedure. This second look can be performed as an outpatient procedure using the Hamou MCH. Any residual adhesions can be removed.

It must be remembered that the removal of intrauterine adhesions predispose the patient to a number of potential difficulties in any ensuing pregnancy. In a series of 192 patients in whom adhesions were treated by hysteroscopic lysis, 79 (41.25 per cent) became pregnant and of these 29 (36.75 per cent) aborted spontaneously, two had premature deliveries and 45 experienced at least one term delivery (Sugimoto, 1978). Eight of the patients delivering required manual removal of the placenta or postpartum curettage. There is a distinct risk of placenta accreta following lysis of intrauterine adhesions. In three such cases, two required treatment by Caesarean hysterectomy (Georgakopoulos, 1974).

Fibroids

The management of small submucous fibroids can be achieved by hysteroscopic excision using a modified resectoscope (Neuwirth and Amin, 1976). Pedunculated tumours are easily dealt with by dividing the pedicle. Small sessile lesions can be shaved until flush with the surrounding endometrium. It is probable that this procedure is best carried out under laparoscopic control. When hysteroscopic excision of fibroids is performed, Dextran should be the distension medium.

Postoperatively, bleeding can be controlled by the insertion of a Foley catheter. During the time of its insertion, the patient should receive systemic antibiotics.

In the patient with more extensive tumours, who will have to undergo formal abdominal myomectomy, pre-operative hysteroscopy greatly aids in the identification of any intracavitary lesions, and allows accurate planning of the uterine incisions. If no intrauterine lesion is noted, opening into the uterine cavity can be avoided.

It may well be that in the future such lesions will be effectively dealt with by the use of long acting gonadotrophin releasing hormone analogues. Coddington et al (1986) used such an analogue for six months in six patients. Demonstrable shrinkage in uterine size was noted in all by ultrasonographic means and there was no increase in uterine size for follow up periods as long as seven months following discontinuation of therapy.

Septa

When the presence of a uterine septum is detected by hysterosalpingography, particularly in patients with habitual abortion, the next step should be to perform combined laparoscopy and hysteroscopy. It is only by these means that the exact configuration of the uterus can be determined. No septum with a base greater than 1cm should be resected hysteroscopically nor is hysteroscopy of any value in the surgical management of a patient with a bicornuate uterine deformity.

If the lesion is a septum with a base of less than 1cm thickness, it can be dealt with very effectively by hysteroscopic means. Once the lesion has been visualised it can be divided with hysteroscopic scissors. This is a remarkably bloodless procedure. While both the Argon and Yag laser have been employed in the division of uterine septa, the use of scissors or the resectoscope (DeCherney et al, 1986), is simpler, quicker and requires less expensive equipment.

DeCherney et al (1986) have treated 103 patients by this method. All were treated during the proliferative phase of the menstrual cycle. Dextran 70 was used as the distension medium and all cases were monitored laparoscopically. Incision of the septum was made with a 30 watt per second cutting current. The operating time varied between 20 and 40 minutes. In 103 patients resection was carried out successfully in 72. Thirty-one were considered inoperable. Only one uterine perforation occurred. Following 72 successful hysteroscopic procedures there were 58 successful deliveries. The hysteroscopic procedure clearly is simpler than the Tomkins or Jones metroplasty and can be performed on an outpatient basis.

Potential therapeutic uses

Recently, the management of infertility, particularly unexplained infertility, that due to oligozoospermia, and that due to poor sperm cervical mucus penetration, has been managed by some form of gamete manipulation. Intrauterine insemination, in vitro fertilisation (IVF), and gamete intra-fallopian transfer (GIFT) are finding wider roles. Of these, GIFT may be of particular value in unexplained infertility and in cases of hostile cervical mucus. It does require laparoscopy.

The key underlying all forms of gamete manipulation has been the juxtaposition of sperm with oocyte, initially in the laboratory in cases of IVF and more recently in the ampulla of the fallopian tube with GIFT.

We have demonstrated (Brooks et al, 1988) that it is simple to visualise and cannulate the fallopian tube by hysteroscopic means as an office procedure requiring no anaesthesia. In 72 studied cycles, it was possible in all cases to deposit previously capacitated spermatozoa at the tubocornual junction. Our protocol called for synchronisation of ovulation on a predetermined Provera/Clomiphene Citrate regimen. No pregnancy resulted from this approach and subsequent followup studies demonstrated that our stimulation regimen more often than not produced luteinized unruptured follicle syndrome. This approach, which we called SHIFT (synchronized hysteroscopic insemination of the fallopian tube) is technically feasible and, given effective ovarian stimulation, may open an avenue to the future which could, if successful, provide an alternative to GIFT.

Table 16-1
The comparison between hysterosalpingographic and hysteroscopic findings

	Hysterosalpingographic findings				
		Abnormal N = 22			
Hysteroscopic findings	*Normal (N = 232)*	*Filling defect (N = 16)*	*Adhesions (N = 2)*	*Polyps (N = 1)*	*Septa (N = 3)*
Normal	166	3	—	—	—
Adhesions	45	4	2	—	—
Polyps	18	9	—	1	—
Myomata	3	—	—	—	—
Septa	0	—	—	—	3

References

Asherman, J.G. Amenorrhea traumaticum (atretica). *Journal of Obstetrics and Gynaecology of the British Empire,* 1948; 55: 23.

Brooks, J.H., Mortimer, D., Taylor, P.J. Failure of hysteroscopic insemination of the fallopian tube in synchronized cycles. *International Journal of Fertility,* (in press).

Buttram, V.C., Jr, Reiter, R.C. Uterine leiomyomata: Etiology, symptomatology and management. *Fertility and Sterility,* 1981; 36: 433.

Coddington, C.C., Collins, R.L., Shawker, T.H., Anderson, R., Loriaux, D.L., Winkel, C.A. Long-acting gonadotrophin in hormone releasing hormone analogue used to treat uteri. *Fertility and Sterility,* 1986; 45: 624.

DeCherney, A.H., Russell, J.B., Giaebe, R.A., Polden, M.L. Resectoscopic management of Mullerian fusion defects. *Fertility and Sterility,* 1986; 45: 726.

DeCherney, A., Polan, M.L. Evaluation and management of habitual abortion. *British Journal of Hospital Medicine,* 1984; 6: 261.

Englund, G., Ingleman-Sundberg, A., Westin, B. Hysteroscopy in diagnosis and treatment of uterine bleeding. *Gynaecologia,* 1957; 113: 217.

Georgakopoulos, P. Placenta accreta following lysis of uterine synechia (Asherman's Syndrome). *Journal of Obstetrics and Gynaecology of the British Commonwealth,* 1974; 81: 730.

Grass, R.H., Golbus, M.S. Habitual abortion. *Fertility and Sterility,* 1978; 29: 257.

Hamou, J., Taylor, P.J. Panoramic, contact and microcolpohysteroscopy in gynaecologic practice. *Current Problems in Obstetrics and Gynaecology,* 1982; 2: 1.

Hamou, J., Salat-Baroux, J., Siegler, A.M. Diagnosis and treatment of intra-uterine adhesions by microhysteroscopy. *Fertility and Sterility,* 1982; 37: 593.

Jones, W.S. Obstetric significance of female genital anomalies. *Obstetrics and Gynecology,* 1957; 10: 1039.

Labastida, R., Dexeus, S., Arias, A. Infertility and Hysteroscopy. In Siegler, A.M., Lindemann, H.J. (Eds), *Hysteroscopy Principles and Practice,* J.B. Lippincott, Philadelphia, 1984, 175.

Malpas, P. A study of abortion sequences. *Journal of Obstetrics and Gynaecology of the British Empire,* 1938; 45: 932.

March, C.M., Israel, R., March, A.D. Hysteroscopic management of intra-uterine adhesions. *American Journal of Obstetrics and Gynecology*, 1978; 130: 653.

Neuwirth, R.S., Amin, H.K. Excision of submucus fibroids with hysteroscopic control. *American Journal of Obstetrics and Gynecology*, 1976; 126: 95.

Oelsner, G., Amnon, D., Insler, V., Ferr, D.M. Outcome of pregnancy after treatment of intra-uterine adhesions. *Obstetrics and Gynecology*, 1974; 44: 341.

Poland, B.J., Miller, J.R., Jones, D.C., Trimble, B.K. Reproductive counselling in patients who have had a spontaneous abortion. *American Journal of Obstetrics and Gynecology*, 1977; 127: 685.

Schenker, J., Margalioth, E.J. Intra-uterine adhesions: An updated appraisal. *Fertility and Sterility*, 1982; 37: 593.

Scott, J.R. Immunologic aspects of recurrent spontaneous abortion. *Fertility and Sterility*, 1982; 38: 301.

Siegler, A.M. Hysterography and hysteroscopy in the infertile patient. *Journal of Reproductive Medicine*, 1977; 18: 143.

Siegler, A.M., Kemmann, E. Hysteroscopy. *Obstetrical and Gynaecological Survey*, 1975; 30: 567.

Snowden, E.U., Jarret, J.C., Dawood, Y.M. Comparison of diagnostic accuracy of laparoscopy, hysteroscopy and hysterosalpingography in evaluation of female infertility. *Fertility and Sterility*, 1984; 41.

Sugimoto, O. Diagnostic and therapeutic hysteroscopy for traumatic intra-uterine adhesions. *American Journal of Obstetrics and Gynecology*, 1978; 131: 539.

Taylor, P.J., Gomel, V. Endoscopy in the infertile patient. In Gomel V., Taylor P.J., Yuzpe A.A., Rioux J.E. (eds), *Laparascopy and Hysteroscopy in Gynaecologic Practice*, Year Book Medical Publishers, Chicago, 1986, 75.

Taylor, P.J., Cumming, D.C. Laparascopy in the infertile female. *Current Problems in Obstetrics and Gynecology*, 1979; 2: 3.

Taylor, P.J., Lewinthal, D., Leader, A., Pattison, H.A. A comparison of Dextran 70 with carbon dioxide as the distension medium for hysteroscopy in patients with infertility or requesting reversal of a prior tubal sterilization. *Fertility and Sterility*, 1987; 47: 861.

Valle, R.F. Hysteroscopy in the evaluation of female infertility. *American Journal of Obstetrics and Gynecology*, 1980; 137: 425.

Valle, R.F., Sciarra, J.J. Current status of hysteroscopy in gynaecologic practice. *Fertility and Sterility*, 1979; 32: 619.

Zondek, B.M., Rozin, S. Filling defects in the hysterogram simulating intra-uterine synechia which disappear after denudation. *American Journal of Obstetrics and Gynecology*, 1964; 88: 123.

17
Lasers in female infertility surgery

C. Sutton

Introduction

In the first chapter of Genesis God said "Let there be light" and there was light. However, the physical basis for laser light had to wait until 1917 when Albert Einstein published "The quantum theory of radiation". Even then, the reality of laser light had to wait until 1960, when the first practical laser, a ruby laser was produced by Maiman. For some time it was an invention awaiting an application but it eventually became the first surgical laser and was subsequently used to photocoagulate retinal lesions without an external incision. It was replaced in opthalmology in the mid-1960s by the argon laser because of its more useful absorption properties. The neodymium: yttrium aluminium garnet (Nd:YAG) laser developed in 1961 produces energy in the near-infrared portion of the spectrum and is used for the coagulation of tumours and down flexible endoscopes for the control of bleeding. The carbon dioxide laser, probably the most useful laser in gynaecology, was developed in 1964 by Patel and colleagues at the Bell Laboratories for use in the communications industry. Both these lasers are invisible and require a helium-neon laser to be incorporated into the system as an aiming beam.

The spread of the human papilloma virus and the subsequent development of cervical intra-epithelial neoplasia in young women, which has reached almost epidemic proportions in recent years, led to the search for a method of treatment that would eradicate the disease effectively but avoid the morbidity associated with a cone biopsy performed with a surgical scalpel. The carbon dioxide laser has the unique advantage of being able to precisely vaporise abnormal tissue with minimal damage to surrounding normal tissue. Very little debris remains since the vaporised tissue has been carried away in the smoke plume and healing occurs with hardly any fibrosis or scar tissue so that the end result is healing without anatomical distortion or physiological disturbance. Six weeks later, even when viewed with the magnification afforded by a colposcope, a crater 10mm deep and 10mm in diameter has healed so perfectly that it is often difficult to define the limits of the area that has been vaporised.

Not only is the absence of scar tissue striking but also the regenerated glands produce excellent mucous with no impairment of fertility potential and the cervix performs competently in maintaining a pregnancy and dilating normally in labour. This is in contradistinction to the healing following a conventional cold knife cone biopsy or radical thermocautery with the well known sequelae of dysmuccorrhea, cervical stenosis, incompetence and dystocia (Jones et al, 1979). It is the excellent healing associated with laser vaporisation that has led to its increasing use in female infertility surgery but makes it of no value for sterilisation procedures since the tube heals so well that if often recanalises.

Lasers suitable for infertility surgery

There are many lasers in current use and each one is named after the active medium (be it gas, element, crystal or even free electron) which is used to generate laser light. They have varying wavelengths from near infrared to far ultraviolet and all the colours in between, each one with different physical characteristics and effects on biological tissues. These are tabulated in Table 17-1 with regard to the four lasers most commonly used in gynaecology — Carbon dioxide, Argon, Neodymium-YAG and Potassium-titanyl-phosphate (KTP/532), the latter being a frequency doubled YAG laser.

The carbon dioxide laser, the one most commonly available in gynaecological departments, has the disadvantage that it can only be passed down rigid fibres and is strongly absorbed by water and blood, thus rendering it unsuitable for hysteroscopic applications. Nevertheless, its ability to precisely vaporise tissue with very little scattering of the beam makes it the most suitable for infertility surgery and since this is performed via laparoscopes and operating microscopes the lack of flexible fibre transmission is not of great practical significance.

The carbon dioxide laser

The carbon dioxide laser is a gas laser with a wavelength in the near infrared portion of the spectrum (10,600nm) and the light is therefore invisible and requires a Helium-Neon aiming beam which produces red light, allowing the operator to focus on the target. Laser light exhibits the properties of coherence (the waves are exactly in phase both temporally and spatially), collimation (the light rays are parallel to each other) and a unique wavelength or colour, if visible, so they are monochromatic. Mirrors placed at either end of an optical resonator chamber allow the coherent waves to reflect back and forth many times at 186,000 miles a second between the two ends. Thus, although stimulated emission of radiation is started by high voltage direct current passing through the laser medium, the intensification of laser energy takes place in the resonator and allows the laser light to "leak-out" through a partially transmissive mirror at one end of the chamber. Due to the coherence of laser light the energy can be increased to a very high power density when a lens focuses the beam to a small spot 0.2 to 0.8mm in diameter. This achieves great precision and the fact that the beam is collimated means there is no lateral damage to adjacent tissue on impact. These two properties make the carbon dioxide laser ideal for surgery.

Action of the carbon dioxide laser on tissues

The laser destroys tissue by vaporisation of cellular water at a temperature of 100 degrees Centigrade at the point of impact. The boiling of intracellular and extracellular fluid forms steam, which expands explosively thereby disrupting the tissue and carrying cell debris out of the wound. Some of the debris is charged as it passes through the beam and some actually ignites and burns, producing smoke. The crater thus formed inevitably contains charcoal and it is interesting that subsequent examination of the vaporised area after healing has occurred shows no residual charcoal on the cervix whereas a similar wound on the pelvic side wall shows residual carbon underneath the peritoneum. Presumely this reflects different activity of the leucocytes in removing the charcoal at the different sites but it is of practical importance because the unwary could interpret the black deposits as recurrent endometriosis, since the appearance is not dissimilar.

For the reasons described above, the carbon dioxide laser is able to vaporise tissue with great precision, causing very little damage to the surrounding structures. Histological examination of sections from laser wounds has shown that some cellular damage occurs up to 500μm from the laser impact but that the depth of thermal necrosis is usually less than 100μm. There is therefore minimal fibrosis or scar tissue formation, and laser incisions heal with virtually no contracture or adhesion formation. Since the cell contents are converted to smoke and water vapour, very little tissue debris remains and regeneration of epithelium during the healing phase proceeds rapidly and the adjacent tissue is virtually unaltered (Allen and Stein, 1983).

Bellina et al (1984) compared the tissue damage and healing patterns in peritoneal wounds inflicted by the carbon dioxide laser with those inflicted by the electrodiathermy in the New Zealand white rabbit, and they concluded that the laser wounds resulted in much less trauma to the tissues. It appears, therefore, that if the carbon dioxide laser can be delivered safely either via the laparoscope or the operating microscope, it may offer considerable theoretical and practical advantages over conventional diathermy and the surgical scalpel for infertility surgery.

Lasers in open infertility surgery

The only study that has compared the results of microsurgery using the carbon dioxide laser and electrosurgery has been Mage and Bruhat (1983) who treated 30 cases of terminal salpingostomy with electrocautery with a 17 per cent pregnancy rate and then followed that with 38 cases with the carbon dioxide laser. The laser group had a 24 per cent term pregnancy rate and appeared to get pregnant in a shorter time. This was also the finding of Tulandi (1984) who, in a prospective randomised study, compared the carbon dioxide laser with microdiathermy needle salpingostomy. The pregnancy rates at 10 months were similar (27 per cent to 25 per cent) but the pregnancy procedure interval was less in the laser group, probably reflecting more rapid healing of the tube. Bellina (1983) has produced some excellent results with a 37 per cent rate for correction of bilateral tubal disease and a 32 per cent pregnancy rate for repeat procedures. This was in 230 patients followed for two years.

Chong and Baggish (decribed in Sutton, 1986) have used carbon dioxide laser at laparotomy in the treatment of endometriosis in 23 patients. Their six month pregnancy rate of 61 per cent included 85 per cent with Stage II disease on the revised AFS scale and 38 per cent for Stage III disease, which is impressive, although this may not be due to laser surgery alone, since 78 per cent of their patients were treated with danazol postoperatively. There was no pregnancy in the two patients with Stage IV disease and this is in contrast with the laser laparoscopy results of other authors (*Vide infra*). There would appear to be no great advantage over laparoscopic surgery and the pain, increased cost and increased length of hospital stay are considerable disadvantages.

Delivery systems and technique

At laparotomy, the carbon dioxide laser can either be used with a handpiece attached to an articulated arm to the laser generator or to an operating microscope with a micromanipulator attached to direct the laser onto the tissue. The hand-held probes are fitted with sterilisable linear gauges to indicate the focal length of the lens, which can vary from 125 to 50mm. Magnification can be provided by optical loupes, as the system allows easy control of the spot size but lacks the fine control of the beam that is possible when the beam is directed through an operating microscope.

Delivery of the laser via the laparoscope also offers two choices of equipment. Initially we used an angled laparoscope that allowed the laser beam to be aimed by a micromanipulator down the operating channel of the laparoscope (the single puncture technique). Although equipment for single puncture operative laser laparoscopy is still available, we abandoned this technique because of optical fogging and the difficulty of preventing the beam from reflecting off the side walls of the relatively narrow operating channel. In addition, it was considered hazardous for dividing adhesions, since the long focal length allowed the laser beam to damage structures distal to the adhesions. We used this system for six months before changing to the double puncture technique, which is now in general use and is safer because of the superior visualisation provided by a conventional laparoscope.

In Guildford, we use an 11mm Wolf laparoscope coupled to a Sony Trinitron video camera by a beam splitter although newer and smaller sterilisable cameras are now available that attach directly onto the eyepiece of the laparoscope. Laser energy is transmitted via a lens and mirror through a second puncture probe inserted in such a position that the laser beam is as near as possible to a 90 degree angle of incidence to the target tissue. A third puncture probe is usually inserted in the midline above the symphysis pubis for an assistant to provide traction on the tissue and for irrigation with heparinised Ringer's lactate or Hartmann's solution to remove carbon deposits and to reduce the possibility of thermal damage if laser vaporisation has been prolonged.

Accumulation of smoke and water vapour reduces the power of the laser and seriously interferes with the visibility through the laparoscope. The smoke is extracted through the outer channel of the second puncture probe and in practice we keep the toggles on the gas insufflator on "fast flow" by securing them in that position with adhesive plaster and vent out the smoke by keeping the taps on the second and third puncture probes open all the time we are lasering. Even this is sometimes not sufficient to clear the smoke and it is then necessary to completely evacuate the smoke filled peritoneal cavity and refill it with fresh carbon dioxide. Although this can be very tedious, especially during long procedures, it is nevertheless vital to ensure that the laser is never fired when visibility is obscured by smoke. All our procedures are recorded on a Sony U-matic video recorder on ¾-inch video tape and all operations are viewed simultaneously on a television monitor to enable assistants to provide effective help for the retraction and irrigation of tissues via the third portal probe (Sutton, 1986).

To be able to perform this kind of surgery with skill and confidence requires adaptation to a completely new "no-touch" form of operating technique. The tissue effect of the laser for incising, vaporising and coagulating tissue is entirely a hands-off technique which makes it especially suitable to use via endoscopes. The operator merely controls the exposure time and the power density of the impact of the laser on the tissue. It goes without saying that before embarking on this kind of surgery the gynaecologist must have considerable experience with advanced operative laparoscopy and with the action of lasers on different tissues.

Laser laparoscopy

During the past two decades, laparoscopy has become firmly established as a diagnostic procedure in gynaecological practice to the extent it is now one of the most commonly performed operations in this specialty. With the development of operative laparoscopy, it is now possible to treat many conditions at the same time as the diagnosis is made, thus obviating the need for further operative surgery or medical therapy. Many of these techniques were developed by Semm (1984) and certain operations such as laparoscopic appendicectomy stretch credibility and dexterity to the extreme. Special laparoscopic scissors have been designed for use through a second portal puncture but in practice, they are difficult to use and often cause troublesome bleeding, which can be difficult to control and can result in further adhesion formation. Unipolar or bipolar diathermy can be used for haemostasis or the destruction of endometriotic implants, but the effect is imprecise and high temperatures can be generated (up to 600 degrees Centigrade) which can damage adjacent tissues and can cause serious injury if the bowel is inadvertently touched by the hot instrument (Chamberlain, 1982). For the reasons outlined above, the carbon dioxide laser has none of these disadvantages and is the logical surgical tool for operative laparoscopy.

The first reports of laser laparoscopy came from Clermont Ferrand, France, from the department of Professor Bruhat (Bruhat et al, 1979). Tadhir et al (1984) was responsible for much of the original instrumentation and the technique has been popularised by Daniell and Feste (1985) in the United States, and Sutton and Scorer in Europe (1988).

The most common indications are endometriosis, pelvic or intra-abdominal adhesions, hydrosalpinges and polycystic ovaries (Kelly and Roberts, 1983;

Daniell, 1984; Daniell and Herbert, 1984; Daniell 1987) and advanced techniques have been described for laparoscopic oophorectomy and the conservative treatment for ectopic pregnancy.

Endometriosis

Endometriosis is usually a multifocal disease with ectopic deposits of endometrial tissue on the pelvic peritoneal or ovarian surface with deeper deposits containing haemosiderin and old blood in the uterosacral ligaments and deep within the stroma of the ovary (endometriomas or chocolate cysts). Laparoscopy is considered essential for the diagnosis and the disease should be staged at the same time using the revised classification of the American Infertility Society (1985).

Deposits of haemosiderin can often represent "burnt out" disease and the laparoscopist should be aware of non-pigmented lesions which have been shown to be endometriosis on biopsy and have been well described recently by Jansen and Russell (1986). The laparoscopic staging of the disease often correlates poorly with the severity of the patient's symptoms, sometimes those with a few active deposits appear to have agonising pelvic pain and dyspareunia whilst others with severe disease are often discovered at laparotomy for some other condition and are apparently symptom free.

Similarly, there are those who consider minimal and mild endometriosis to have a casual rather than a casual relationship to infertility, although there seems little doubt that the gross distortion of anatomy caused by severe disease must interfere with tubal function and ovum pickup. It is against this background that the effects of different medical and surgical techniques are difficult to analyse, but laser laparoscopy offers the advantage of being able to treat the patient at the same time that the diagnosis is made and in many cases to avoid prolonged drug therapy, with a plethora of side effects, and to allow the infertile patient a chance to try to conceive before the disease has a chance to recur.

Power densities of between 2,500 and 6,000 watts/cm^2 are effective and safe for vaporising endometriotic implants although with practice one can use higher power and limit tissue exposure by moving the beam rapidly. The laser is used on continuous mode unless the deposits overly the ureter, bladder, fallopian tube or bowel in which case it is safer to use intermittent pulses of 0.05 or 0.10 seconds duration. This intermittent exposure decreases the chance of damage to these vital structures from thermal buildup and it is suggested that the novice steers well clear of these areas and confines himself to the pelvic side wall and the uterosacral ligaments where there is a greater margin of safety until considerable experience has been achieved.

Once the old blood has been vaporised, the area blanches as the stroma is destroyed. The surrounding peritoneal surface tends to dry and some contracture occurs and adequate depth of vaporisation has taken place when the retroperitoneal fat starts to bubble. The high water content of this fat absorbs the laser energy and protects the deeper structures from damage but care should be exercised on the pelvic side wall near the ureters, not only to avoid that important structure but to be careful not to open up thin walled veins, which can cause troublesome bleeding which can be difficult to stop. Once the endometriotic implant is completely vaporised, the area destroyed is irrigated with a jet of heparinized Ringer's lactate or Hartmann's solution to get rid of as much charcoal as possible.

Ovarian endometriomas, which are often notoriously resistent to drug therapy, can be "de-roofed" by a circular laser incision at a relatively high power density. The thick chocolate material is aspirated and the bed of the endometrioma is vaporised at a lower power density to char it and seal off any bleeding vessels. The amount of ovary treated is often quite large and we usually insert a Sterivac drain through the third portal trochar on completion of the procedure to prevent the formation of haematomas from post-operative oozing. Some authors advocate the instillation of 200ml of Dextran-70 but we have not done this.

When patients are complaining of dysmenorrhea or deep dyspareunia in association with endometriosis, we usually vaporise the uterosacral ligaments close to their insertion into the posterior aspect of the cervix. An area one to 2cm long and 1 cm deep is vaporised, usually with the formation of a large amount of smoke. The rationale behind this procedure is to attempt to deprive the lower segment of sensory nerve fibres carried through the ligaments from the sacral nerve plexus. The division of these ligaments is not, interestingly enough, associated with the development of prolapse. Care must be taken to avoid the plexus of thin walled veins lateral to the ligaments and, in practice, it can sometimes be difficult to know if vaporisation is deep enough and, in a surprising number of patients, one or other ligament is very poorly developed and it is then difficult to be certain that one is lasering the correct place. Several authors have reported dramatic pain relief with this simple technique, and in our series of 18 patients with spasmodic dysmenorrhea unrelieved by medical therapy, 13 (83 per cent) patients followed over a year reported an improvement in their symptoms.

Results of laser laparoscopy of endometriosis

We have been using the laser laparoscope at St. Luke's Hospital, Guildford, Surrey, U.K. since October 1982, and have recently reviewed our results of the treatment of endometriosis over a five year period. We have treated a total of 228 patients with either pain or infertility, or both, thought to be caused by endometriosis. A hundred and fifty-three patients complaining of pelvic pain or dyspareunia have been followed up for at least six months and often longer. A hundred and twenty (78 per cent) said they were better after the laser treatment, 33 were no better. Two showed moderate improvement only, whilst six were initially better but subsequently relapsed, supporting the concept that in a number of patients endometriosis is a progressive disease. This was supported by the 33 patients who had a second look procedure between six months and three years after the original laser laparoscopy. Fifteen of these had no evidence of endometriosis on the peritoneal surface but a further 18 still had endometriosis. When compared with the original video recording, the endometriosis was at different sites. No patient had reformed endometriotic implants at sites previously lasered.

Fifty-nine of our patients had endometriosis in association with infertility. Unfortunately, nine were lost to followup and nine had other uncorrectable factors such as oligo/azoospermia. Of the 41 patients who had endometriosis as the sole cause of infertility 27 (68 per cent) became pregnant (four of them twice) resulting, so far, in 31 live births, one neonatal death at 28 weeks and eight abortions.

Daniell (1985) has reported a 72 per cent pregnancy rate following laser laparoscopy in 58 patients without other infertility factors. This is probably the best result reported but they are all more or less the same, the differences being due to the numbers with severe endometriosis. Although the numbers are small, Daniell achieved two pregnancies in three patients with severe disease and Donnez (1987) achieved three pregnancies in seven patients with severe disease.

Although the results for mild and moderate disease may not be significantly better than that achieved by hormone therapy, the figures for severe and extensive disease are impressive when one considers the gross distortion of pelvic anatomy associated with more advanced stages of endometriosis. In addition, the technique offers the considerable advantage that the patient can start immediately to try for a pregnancy rather than delay for six to nine months whilst taking drugs that are expensive and are often associated with miserable side effects.

Laser laparoscopic adhesiolysis

The other area where the precise bloodless destruction of tissue that can be achieved with the laser is an advantage is in the vaporisation of adhesions.

Sometimes these are associated with endometriosis and at other times they can be a reaction to previous infection of surgery. In Guildford we have treated 39 patients with post-operative adhesions involving bowel with the carbon dioxide laser and 78 per cent have remained pain free over a two year followup period. Seven of the patients who failed to show any improvement subsequently had a second look procedure and there was complete lysis of the adhesions in all but two where the adhesions were less pronounced, and these two were both among the first patients we operated on with the laser when we were at an early stage on the "learning curve".

Although adhesions can be divided effectively with the single puncture operating laparoscope, there is always the risk that once the adhesion has been divided the beam can damage structures distal to the target tissue. This could be particularly hazardous in the proximity of the large veins or ureter on the pelvic side walls and also when working among loops of bowel. Some surgeons have manipulated the adhesion in such a way that irrigating fluid or a non-reflective probe is placed behind the adhesion but, in practice, the safest way to deal with adhesions is to use a special adhesiolysis probe made by Laser Industries, Tel Aviv, Israel or Rocket of London.

This has a special non-reflective backstop and I prefer a short 180mm probe with a fixed focus lens for ease of use. For adhesiolysis procedures, the laser should be set at about 35watts with a small spot size to produce the highest possible power density. Traction is applied to the adhesions by atraumatic grasping forceps to assist in vaporisation but care must be taken not to damage the tube itself with the grasping forceps and also not to tear the adhesions with excessive traction since this results in bleeding and defeats the whole purpose of laser vaporisation. To vaporise adhesions between the ovary and the back of the broad ligament (often due to endometriosis), the grasping forceps are applied to the ovarian ligament to rotate it, as the posterior surface is vaporised by a special probe incorporating a reflective surface set at 45 degrees to allow the laser beam to be transmitted at right angles to the normal axis.

Copious irrigation is performed with Hartmann's solution or heparinised Ringer's lactate to remove carbon deposits and debris. This is done at the end of the procedure and any residual fluid is sucked out, but it must also be performed periodically during a long laser adhesiolysis procedure, especially if the adhesions are adjacent to bowel or involve omentum which, with its high water content in the fat, can absorb a great deal of laser energy, which is converted to heat, and requires intermittent cooling to avoid damage to the bowel.

Donnez (1987) has recently reported a group of 54 patients with pelvic adhesions without endometriosis treated by carbon dioxide laser laparoscopy. Those with filmy avacular peritubal and periovarian adhesions had a viable pregnancy rate of 62 per cent whilst those with dense and vascular adhesions had a slightly lower pregnancy rate of 50 per cent (overall total of 31) pregnancies in 54 patients). He had no complication and in eight patients who had a second look procedure three months afterwards, none of the adhesions had reformed. In a smaller series, we have had six viable pregnancies in nine patients (66 per cent) who had adhesions that were distorting pelvic anatomy with no evidence of endometriosis. This is a good indication for laser laparoscopy and even in patients with adhesions and a male factor this technique can be used to prepare the pelvis for GIFT.

Laser laparoscopic salpingostomy

The results of tubal surgery for hydrosalpinges have been notoriously poor and was one of the early reasons to provide alternative assisted conception in the form of in vitro fertilisation (IVF). Daniell (1984) has performed over 100 cases of laser laparoscopic salpingostomy over the past six years. His ongoing pregnancy rate with two years' followup was 28 per cent with about a 15 per cent tubal pregnancy rate, much the same figures as he had achieved with open laparotomy, but with considerably less morbidity and a much shortened hospital stay. On this basis, it would appear reasonable to offer an attempt at this procedure during the assessment laparoscopy for IVF, although it must be realised that the procedure is extremely difficult and time consuming and should only be attempted by experienced laser operative laparoscopists.

Most of this procedures require an initial adhesiolysis, as described above, and this is often best achieved by a combination of carbon dioxide and fibre lasers; the one that we use being the Neodymium YAG laser with an artificial sapphire scalpel which can be used to incise periovarian or peritubal adhesions with minimal bleeding. Methylene blue dye is instilled through the cervical canal to distend the tube and the hydrosalpinx is manipulated with Craft's GIFT forceps in such a way the dimple indicating the site of the original ampullary ostium is positioned as near as possible to a right angle to the laser beam. Using the highest power density possible (maximum wattage and smallest spot size), a linear incision is made, with the dimple at the midpoint, and tissue is vaporised until the dye is released. Two further incisions are formed outwards from the first with the dimple at the midpoint of the cross.

This is one of the few laparoscopic procedures where the single puncture operating laparoscope can be used with advantage and the second and third portals used for grasping forceps to provide appropriate traction on the tissues. As soon as the cruciate incision has been formed, the power on the laser generator is reduced to five to 10 watts and the end of the probe drawn back about 5cm from the normal focal point to defocus the laser so that it can be "sprayed" on the peritoneal surface of the fallopian tube a few millimetres from the end. This causes the peritoneum to constrict and everts the end of the newly formed "fimbria", causing it to open like a flower. This technique is probably better than the earlier attempts to use the laser to "spot weld" the surfaces together since this can cause excessive tissue damage. It would, of course, be possible to use an endosuture on a spring loaded needle holder to secure the everted "fimbria" in position. The neosalpingostomy is irrigated with heparinised Ringer's solution and any excessive fluid removed from the cul-de-sac until it is clear. To avoid any post-operative haematoma formation, we always insert a sterivac drain into the pelvic cavity to evacuate any post-operative collection of sero-sanguinous fluid. The drain is removed after four to 12 hours, depending on the amount of drainage, and the patients usually go home the following day.

Laser laparoscopic vaporisation of polycystic ovaries

Wedge resection of the ovaries has been used as a last resort in those patients with polycystic ovaries who have failed to respond to increasing doses of clomiphene citrate alone or with added human chrionic gonadotrophin. Unfortunately, such surgery, even when employing microsurgical techniques, can result in continuing infertility due to mechanical pelvic factors due to peri-ovarian and peri-tubal adhesions (Weinstein and Polishuk, 1975; Taoff et al, 1976; Daniell and Pittawy, 1983). To avoid major surgery, laparoscopic ovarian biopsy and electrocautery have been suggested as successful therapy for this condition (Campoet et al, 1983; Gjonnaess, 1984), but the former technique is not without risk (Sutton, 1974) and can cause troublesome bleeding and haematoma formation and the hazards of electrocautery have been alluded to above.

For laser laparoscopic vaporisation of polycystic ovaries, a three puncture technique is recommended with atraumatic grasping forceps introduced suprapubically to fix the ovary by holding it by the ovarian ligament. The laser is set at 15 watts and, with the direct laser probe held about 20cm from the ovarian surface, the laser is fired on continuous mode to vaporise all the visible subcapsular follicles on each ovary. This results in about 10–20 laser drill holes about two to 4mm deep on each ovary. The ovaries are irrigated with heparinised Ringer's lactate (5,000 units per litre) to remove charcoal deposits and to allow the ovaries to be inspected for any persistent bleeding. Unipolar cautery should be available and used if significant bleeding persists.

Alternatively the whole procedure can be performed with a neodymium-YAG laser with an artificial sapphire coagulating probe which will seal any bleeding vessels. Two hundred cubic centimetres of 32 per cent Dextran-70 (Hyscon) can be left in the abdomen for its possible post-operative anti-adhesive effects, but we prefer to remove all the irrigant and released follicular fluid from the pelvic cavity and leave a sterivac drain in place for four hours if the patient is treated on a day case basis, or overnight if the patient is to be discharged the following day.

This technique is at present undergoing evaluation but Daniell (1988) has reported some encouraging initial results. He selected a small goup of ten women with anovulatory infertility who were unresponsive to clomiphene with and/or without HCG. Ovulation occurred post operatively within six weeks in eight of the patients and seven (70 per cent) established regular menstrual cycles with biphasic basal body temperature charts and luteal phase plasma progesterones suggestive of ovulatory cycles. All ten patients desired pregnancy and 50 per cent conceived within six months of laser treatment. He had no complication with these procedures and in those who had second look laparoscopies there was no evidence of adhesion formation around the ovaries.

Although this is small series of patients, the results are encouraging, particularly since this technique could easily be combined with the diagnostic laparoscopy which is becoming an integral part of the infertility workup in all patients who are having difficulty trying to conceive. We have started a small pilot study in Guildford in a similar group of patients with polycystic ovarian disease comparing the result of vaporisation of one ovary with the carbon dioxide laser and photocoagulation of the contralateral ovary with the neodymium-YAG laser and assessing the result after six months with a second look laparoscopy if the patient fails to conceive.

Laser treatment of unruptured ectopic pregnancy

The availability of high resolution ultrasound and beta-hCG have enabled the management of ectopic pregnancy to alter from the rather radical laparotomy and salpingectomy to more conservative methods of treatment involving operative laparoscopy and even medical therapy with folic acid antagonists.

Patients presenting with signs and symptoms of ectopic pregnancy (or those who have had previous tubal surgery and are known to be at high risk) have serial beta-hCG measurements performed until the level exceeds 6500 mIU/mL. When this occurs, ultrasound is performed to look for an intra-uterine fetal sac and hopefully to confirm a viable intrauterine pregnancy by the presence of a fetal heart. If no sac is identified, diagnostic laparoscopy is performed to exclude an ectopic pregnancy. Laparoscopy should also be performed if serial hCGs below 6500 mIU/mL failed to double every three days or actually fell without evidence of a miscarriage occurring.

If an ampullary tubal gestation is confirmed, chromotubation should be performed to see if the ectopic can be flushed out of the tube and then sucked out of the pelvic cavity. If this is not possible, Pitressin, diluted 1 in 30 with saline, is injected with a spinal needle transabdominally just beneath the cornu of the uterus and along the mesosalpinx just beneath the ectopic. The segment containing the tubal pregnancy is steadied with grasping forceps and a linear incision is made with either a carbon dioxide laser with the smallest possible spot size and high wattage or a Neodymium-YAG laser with a fine cutting artificial sapphire tip. The advantage of the latter technique is that it seals blood vessels and there is little haemorrhage whereas with the carbon dioxide laser haemorrhage can be quite brisk and point coagulation or pressure from the grasping forceps may be required to stop it.

The area should be copiously irrigated with Hartmann's solution and the ectopic gestation sucked out or flushed out through the linear salpingostomy by chromotubation. No attempt is made to close the salpingostomy. Hyscon can be instilled in the pelvis as described above and we tend to insert a sterivac drain which is left in overnight to avoid haematoma formation and to give warning of any ongoing bleeding. Patients are often given prophylactic antibiotics and are followed by serial beta-hCG determinations until the level falls beneath the limits of detection to ensure that there is no retention of occult trophoblastic tissue.

Pouly et al (1986) has reported on the conservative treatment of 321 ectopic pregnancies using the carbon dioxide laser via the laparoscope. Daniell (1984) in his first two years experience with this technique had no cases of tubal occlusion using fibre optic lasers laparoscopically and had a 40 per cent intra-uterine pregnancy rate and only a 5 per cent repeat ectopic rate. DeCherney and Diamond (1987) have collected the results from several centres where conservative treatment for ectopic pregnancy has been performed by laparotomy and laparoscopy using needle cautery, scissors, carbon dioxide and argon lasers. Although there is no convincing difference between the end results, laparoscopy has to be advantageous with its decreased morbidity, pain and cost and one of the fibre lasers (argon, KTP or Nd:YAG) would seem the logical choice for ease of use.

Argon, KTP and Nd:YAG lasers in infertility surgery

These lasers have the advantage that they can be passed down flexible fibres, can be used in fluid (at hysteroscopy), are absorbed by red pigment, and so are suited to the photocoagulation of endometriosis and in areas that are haemorrhagic.

Keye has pioneered the use of the argon laser and has used it especially in the treatment of endometriosis because of the selective absorption of argon laser energy by the haemosiderin in the endometriotic implants. The uncorrected pregnancy rate was 34 per cent (19 of 56), with 64 per cent of the pregnancies occurring within six months of treatment. Even more impressive, 92 per cent of the patients reported a marked reduction in pain. The argon laser was delivered through a 0.6mm flexible quartz fibre passed down the operating channel of an operating laparoscope. Power settings ranged from five to 12 W with a spot size of 2mm and a two- to five-second delivery time. There was no operative complication and all patients were treated as outpatients.

The Neodymium-YAG laser has been used laparoscopically by Lomano (1988) to photocoagulate endometriosis. Using the bare fibre, the Nd:YAG laser has a considerable depth of destruction beneath the surface (three to 4mm) and also lateral beam scatter, so care must be taken when using this laser near vital structures. To avoid this problem, one of the manufacturers (Surgical Laser Technologies, Malvern, Pennsylvania, USA) has devised an artificial sapphire scalpel and coagulating probe which focusses the energy and allows it to be used in the contact mode rather like a traditional surgical scalpel restoring "the feel" to laser surgery. We have been using for the past year in Guildford and have been impressed by the way in which laparoscopic adhesiolysis can be performed simply and bloodlessly and with much less smoke formation than with the carbon dioxide laser. The disadvantage is the very high initial cost of equipment and the fact that the scalpels have a very short working life. The fibres are also disposable, giving rise to high running costs. There is also a very real risk to the surgeon because of backscatter from YAG laser energy, which could cause retinal damage and resulting blindness. It must never be activated unless a special filter is placed over the laparoscope or hysteroscope and, if used for open surgery, all personnel must wear green protective goggles.

Safety

Intra-abdominal laser surgery should only be performed by experienced surgeons who are also familiar with the biophysics of lasers and are fully aware of the effects of different lasers on different tissues at varying power densities. The surgeon must ensure that all operating room personnel are aware of the hazards, and safety precautions required when a laser is activated, and that warning signs are clearly visible on the outside of the doors leading to the designated laser area. All personnel should wear protective goggles to prevent eye damage from direct or reflected laser light. In the case of the carbon dioxide laser, these can be of clear plastic and spectacle wearers can use their normal glasses. With the neodymium-YAG laser, there is a very real danger of retinal damage from back scatter of YAG radiation, which could theoretically lead to permanent blindness. This risk is also present with the argon and KTP lasers, but to a lesser extent since they are visible and the eye can be protected by the blink reflex. With the YAG laser energy being invisible, however, no such protection exists and all personnel should wear protective green goggles, and the operating department doors should be locked to prevent unprotected personnel straying inadvertently into the laser controlled area.

Other hazards include explosions from inadvertently firing the laser near flammable solutions or anaesthetic agents, but these can be avoided by due care and attention. The smoke plume also constitutes a hazard to the lungs if breathed in and some worry has been expressed by some workers who have found live virus particles in laser smoke (Walker, 1988). Most of these accidents can be avoided by using non-reflective surfaces for laser instruments, moist drapes and sponges, non-flammable sterilising solutions and a properly designed smoke evacuation system.

The carbon dioxide laser has been used intra-abdominally for 15 years and has an impressive safety record, but this is partially due to the understandable care used by those surgeons pioneering a new technique. As laser surgery becomes more popular, there will inevitably be an increase in accidents unless these high standards of safety are meticulously adhered to.

Conclusion

The use of lasers, either delivered by endoscopes or at laparotomy, appears to be a safe and useful technique. Although initial results are encouraging, there is a need for prospective and controlled studies with a longer followup period before their role can be fully established.

It must be stressed, however, that lasers are potentially hazardous, and endoscopic surgery of this nature should be contemplated only by surgeons with considerable experience and skill who are also familiar with the use of lasers and their effects on biological tissue.

Acknowledgements

Finally, I should like to record my gratitude to Sister Annie Parker and her team of nurses and to Dougie Bathie, our Operating Department Assistant and Laser Technician, for all their hard work and enthusiasm over the past five years whilst we have been running our laser service in Guildford.

Table 17-1
Physical properties of different lasers

	CO_2	Nd:YAG	Argon	KTP/532
Wavelength	10.6μm	1.06μm	0.5μm	0.532μm
Tissue effect	Vaporisation	Coagulation	Coagulation	Coagulation
Colour dependent	No	Yes	Yes	Yes
Beams scatter	None	Mod	Slight	Slight
Water absorption	Strong	Slight	None	None
Fibre transmission	No	Yes	Yes	Yes
Penetration depth	0.1mm	4mm	0.5–2mm	0.5–2mm
Visibility	No	No	Yes	Yes
Spectrum	Mid infrared	Near infrared	Green	Green

References

Allen, J.M., Stein, D.S. and Singleton, H.M. Regeneration of cervical epithelium after laser vaporisation. *Obstetrics and Gynecology*, 1983; 62: 700.

Bellina, J.H., Hemmings, R., Voros, I.J. and Ross, L.F. Carbon dioxide laser and electrosurgical wound study in an animal model. *American Journal of Obstetrics and Gynecology*, 1984; 148: 327.

Bellina, J.H. Microsurgery of the fallopian tube with the carbon dioxide laser: Analysis of 230 cases with a two-year follow-up. *Lasers in Surgery and Medicine*, 1983; 3: 255.

Bruhat, M., Mage, C. and Manhes, M. Use of carbon dioxide laser via laparoscopy. In Kaplan I (Ed), *Laser Surgery III — Proceedings of the Third Congress of the International Society for Laser Surgery*, International Society for Laser Surgery, Tel Aviv, 1979; 275.

Campo, S., Garcea, N., Caruso, A. and Siccardi, P. Effect of celioscopic ovarian resection in patients with polycystic ovaries. *Gynecology and Obstetrics Investigation*, 1983; 15: 213.

Chamberlain, G.V.P. Gynaecological laparoscopy. The report of the working party of the confidential enquiry into gynaecological laparoscopy. *London Royal College of Obstetricians and Gynaecologists*, 1982.

Daniell, J.F. and Feste, J.R. Laser laparoscopy. In Keye, W.R. (Ed), *Laser Surgery in Gynaecology and Obstetrics*, G.K. Hall, Boston, 1985, 147.

Daniell, J.F. The role of lasers in infertility surgery. *Fertility and Sterility*, 1984; 42.

Daniell, J.F. and Herbert, C.M. Laparoscopic salpingostomy utilizing the carbon dioxide laser. *Fertility and Sterility*, 1984; 41: 4.

Daniell, J.F. Advanced operative laparoscopic laser techniques. *Laser Medicine and Surgery News*, 1987; 5:3.

Daniell, J.F. Operative laparoscopy for endometriosis. *Seminars in Reproductive Endocrinology*, 1985; 3:4.

Daniell, J.F. and Pittawy, D.E. Short interval second look laparoscopy after infertility surgery: a preliminary report. *Journal of Reproductive Medicine*, 1983; 28: 281.

Daniell, J.F. Treatment of polycystic ovaries by laparoscopic laser vaporisation. Personal communication.

DeCherny, A.H. and Diamond, M.P. Laparoscopic salpingostomy for ectopic pregancy. *Obstetrics and Gynecology*, 1987; 70.

Donnez, J. Carbon dioxide laser laparoscopy in infertile women with endometriosis and women with adnexal adhesions. *Fertility and Sterility*, 1987; 48.

Gjonnaess, H. Polycystic ovarian syndrome treated by electrocautery through the laparoscope. *Fertility and Sterility*, 1984; 20: 41.

Jansen, R.P.S. and Russell, P. Nonpigmented endometriosis: Clinicalogy laparoscopic, and pathologic definition. *American Journal of Obstetrics and Gynecology*, 1986; 155: 1154.

Jones, J.M., Sweetnam, P. and Hibbard, B.M. The outcome of pregnancy after cone biopsy of the cervix — a case controlled study. *British Journal of Obstetrics and Gynaecology*, 1979; 86: 913.

Kelly, R.W. and Roberts, D.K. Carbon dioxide laser laparoscopy: A potential alternative to danazol in the treatment of Stage I and II endometriosis. *Journal of Reproductive Medicine*, 1983; 28: 638.

Lomano, J.M. Photocoagulation of early pelvic endometriosis by the Nd:YAG laser through the laparoscope. *Journal of Reproductive Medicine*, 1988; (in press).

Mage, G. and Bruhat, M. Pregnancy following salpingostomy: comparison between $C0_2$ laser and electrosurgical procedures. *Fertility and Sterility*, 1983; 40: 472.

Pouly, J.L., Mahnes, H. and Mage, G. et al. Conservative laparoscopic treatment of 321 ectopic pregnancies. *Fertility and Sterility*, 1986; 46: 1093.

Semm, K. *Endoscopic intra-abdominal surgery*. F.K. Schattauer, Stuttgart, 1984.

Sutton, C. The limitations of laparoscopic ovarian biopsy. *Journal of Obstetrics and Gynaecology of British Commonwealth*, 1974; 81: 317.

Sutton, C. Initial experience with laser laparoscopy. *Lasers in Medical Science*, 1986; 1: 25.

Sutton, C. and Scorer, H. Four years experience with $C0_2$ laser laparoscopy in the treatment of endometriosis. 1988; (in press).

Tadhir, Y., Kaplan, I., Zuckerman, Z., Edelstein, T. and Ovadia, J. New instrumentation and technique for laparoscopic carbon dioxide laser operations: a preliminary report. *Obstetrics and Gynecology*, 1984; 63: 582.

Taoff, R., Taoff, M.E. and Peyser, M.R. Infertility following wedge resection of the ovaries. *American Journal of Obstetrics and Gynecology*, 1976; 124: 92.

The American Fertility Society. Revised classification of Endometriosis. *Fertility and Sterility*, 1985; 43: 351.

Tulandi, T. Hydrosalpinx: comparison of electrosurgery and laser surgery. *Fertility and Sterility*, 1984; 41: 732.

Weinstein, D. and Polishuk, W.S. The role of wedge resection of the ovary as a cause for mechanical sterility. *Surgery, Gynecology and Obstetrics*, 1975; 141: 417.

Index